OPEN FAMILY AND MARRIAGE a guide to personal growth

OPEN FAMILY AND MARRIAGE a guide to personal growth

Thomas C. McGinnis, Ed.D.

Director, The Counseling and Psychotherapy Center, P.A., and Director, Human Services Center for Education and Research, Fair Lawn, New Jersey; Vice-Chairman, New Jersey State Board of Marriage Counselor Examiners; Board of Directors, International Union of Family Organizations, Paris, France; formerly Associate Professor of Education, New York University, New York, New York; formerly Instructor in Marriage and Family, Fairleigh Dickinson University, Teaneck, New Jersey; Past President, American Association of Marriage and Family Counselors, and Past Vice-President, American Association of Sex Educators and Counselors

Dana G. Finnegan, Ph.D.

Educational Consultant, Oakland, New Jersey; formerly Counselor and Co-Director of the Human Services Center for Education and Research, Counseling and Psychotherapy Center, Fair Lawn, New Jersey

THE C. V. MOSBY COMPANY

Saint Louis 1976

Printed in the United States of America

Distributed in Great Britain by Henry Kimpton, London

Library of Congress Cataloging in Publication Data

McGinnis, Thomas C 1925-
Open family and marriage.

Includes bibliographical references and index.
1. Marriage. 2. Family. 3. Interpersonal relations.
I. Finnegan, Dana G., 1932- joint author.
II. Title. [DNLM: 1. Family. 2. Marriage.
3. Personality development. HQ728 M1450]
HQ734.M18488 301.42 75-31997
ISBN 0-8016-3282-X

VH/VH/VH 9 8 7 6 5 4 3 2 1

To

my wife and children,
who contributed to and brought
alive the principles of this book
and, by living them, enabled our family
to become even more loving and open.

TOM

To

my parents,
who have helped me
become who I am, and to
Nancy, Doug, Susan, Kate, Carol,
Dave, Tim, Steve, Matt, and Karen,
whose change and growth
I joyfully take part in.

DANA

PREFACE

Our society (and the world) is in the throes of a vast and sometimes frightening upheaval. Our two most personal institutions —marriage and the family—seem outmoded and unworkable to many people; to others the very roots of marriage and the family seem threatened by erosion or by an arrant disregard for the values of these institutions.[1,2] And the individual members of our society often seem to feel as if they have been cut adrift in a sea of change and newness without the benefit of old, familiar rules and beliefs by which to chart their life course.[3,4]

To deal more effectively with these distressing and sometimes destructive circumstances, people need to gain some perspective on what is happening around them and to understand the meaning and significance of the events that have changed their way of life. People need to find ways to evaluate the traditional institutions of marriage and the family to determine what about them is worth keeping, what should be changed, and what alternatives are possible.[5-8] People need to understand how marriage and the family work and to learn techniques and skills that will enable them to make these institutions serve rather than limit them.

The subjects of societal change, the institutions of marriage and the family, and the individual's place in society and its institutions are not new, and there are many articles and books that present the *what* and often the *why* of these subjects.[9,10] But these kinds of presentations too often are limited by an emphasis on intellectual understanding. Thus they tend not to focus on preparing people to use what they learn to change and grow as individuals and to develop and maintain qualitative relationships with others.

How then should these subjects be handled? We believe that to teach people how to work constructively with them, a book must definitely provide useful information; in addition, it must help people relate their intellectual knowledge to their own (and others') emotions and behavior. Furthermore, it must teach them to understand how their intellect, emotions, and behavior are interrelated and how to translate this understanding into a healthier style of living.

Open Family and Marriage: A Guide to Personal Growth attempts to provide the means by which you can change and grow and, at the same time, develop healthier, more open relationships. We hope that you will experience this approach as a unique way of exploring and learning about yourself, others, and relationships, especially those of marriage and family life.

The key to our approach is *interaction*—within self and with others. The *interactional approach* assumes that the real heart of any relationship is what is going on inside of each person and what is going on between them.[11] To be aware of, understand, and be able to manage what is going on requires knowledge of self and others, an understanding of intrapersonal and interpersonal dynamics, skillful and effective communication, constructive patterns of interaction, and some knowledge of how all these factors interrelate with and influence one another. The interactional approach draws freely on and shares common views and methods with many other approaches.[12,13] For example, like the *sociological/anthropological approaches,* our interactional approach examines and explains the structure and nature of marriage and the family and the specific environment that influences and helps shape them. Like the *psychoanalytical approach,* it takes into account and works with unconscious material. Like *Gestalt psychology,* it recognizes the importance of working with moment-to-moment experiences in the here and now. Like *behavior modification,* it teaches the alteration of behavior as a way of bringing about changes in personality and in personal relations. The primary theoretical influence, however, is Harry Stack Sullivan's concepts regarding interpersonal interaction.[14,15]

Our version of the interactional approach was developed originally by Dr. McGinnis in his clinical practice of counseling and psychotherapy. Over a period of many years, he formulated a unified theory and approach to help people become free from the restrictive, suppressive patterns of living that prevent them from realizing their potentials as individuals, marital partners, and family members. In terms of this book, he was helping them to become less *closed* and more *open.** Later he translated these principles of clinical practice into teaching educational courses at New York University. These principles proved easy to teach and were easily learned by students (or anyone) interested in and willing to work toward greater personal and interpersonal growth.

Dr. Finnegan, an experienced college English professor, learned the principles of Dr. McGinnis' clinical and teaching style and applied them to her own teaching, student counseling, and personal life. Because she was greatly impressed by the results of this kind of teaching and learning, she accepted Dr. McGinnis' invitation to join him in writing this book. The outcome of this collaboration is a conceptualized, systematized, practical approach to teaching and learning how to change and grow, how to become more open and autonomous, and how to develop and maintain qualitative relationships with self and others.

We have named this approach the *Interactional Therapeutic System (ITS).* We have so named it for three reasons: (1) it is interactional because it focuses on intrapersonal and interpersonal dynamics as the key to individual functioning and relationships, especially those of marriage and family; (2) it is therapeutic in that it teaches ways to become more open and to develop more meaningful relationships; and (3) it is systematized because it presents the dynamics and how-to of interaction in a systematic, step-by-step fashion.

What specifically are you justified in expecting from The System and this book? Here are some expectations you might have and that we hope, at least partially, to fulfill:

1. That you will have available much helpful and practical information about how individuals, marriages, and families function and that you will discover new resources and guidelines for further study
2. That your skill in communicating effectively will increase
3. That you will become increasingly aware of the large variety of alternative ways of thinking, feeling, seeing, tasting, smelling, hearing, touching, and acting
4. That you will become more aware of your strengths, weaknesses, skills, and uniqueness
5. That you will become more observant and respectful of other people's uniqueness—their attitudes, values, feelings, and behavior
6. That you will become both more objective and more subjective about

*Dr. McGinnis coined the term *open family living* in his book, *Open Family Living: A New Approach for Enriching Your Life Together,* Garden City, N.Y., 1976, Doubleday & Co., Inc., written with John U. Ayres. This book is designed to be used separately or along with the material presented in this textbook.

sensing, understanding, and appreciating your own self-system and lifestyle and those of others

7. That you will realize that as your personal freedom increases, so too does your responsibility as a human being and that you will therefore become both a more responsive and responsible person
8. That as you put all of this together you will find that the blend promotes openness, honesty, and spontaneity within yourself and with others and that you will find that experiencing and using this blend can have the effect of helping you build in feelings of adequacy, competence, satisfaction, and joy
9. That you will learn much about the dynamics of relationships, especially those of marriage and the family, and how to apply this knowledge to your own life
10. That you will learn to use The System in all your relationships so that they become more qualitative
11. That you will change and grow and become more open within yourself and with others.

You may have other expectations to add to this list, but for the most part these are the ones we think this book can help you fulfill to one degree or another. The extent to which you do, however, depends in large part on you. How hard are you willing or able to work? How aware or unaware are you at the start of all this? How strong are your attitudes about and your rules against dealing with anything other than the surface? The success you have in fulfilling these expectations thus depends greatly on you and what you bring to this approach. We do believe, however, that almost everyone can benefit to some degree.

We have included a number of *interaction experiences (IE)* in each chapter. They are designed to help you achieve a balanced blend of thinking, feeling, and acting in your learning process.[16-20] Specifically these experiences offer you the following opportunities:

1. They can help you come more alive through expressing yourself—by analyzing, thinking out loud, verbalizing and feeling your feelings, and acting out your thoughts and feelings.
2. They will give you a chance to receive feedback from yourself and from others.
3. They can help you find out more about yourself.
4. They will give you the chance to experience a wider range of alternative ways of thinking, feeling, and acting.
5. They will give you practice in new ways of communicating and interacting. And you (and everyone else) need to practice over and over, since the skills of communicating and interacting are not skills you can learn or build in after one reading or one run-through.
6. Along with the content of the book and your work in and out of the classroom, they can help you put things together to achieve a more balanced blend that maximizes the learning and growing process.

The central goals of our approach are growth and fulfillment, and we offer guidelines and suggestions for achieving these goals. The freedom to work toward achieving these goals is yours. However, the responsibility for achieving them and for applying and using them is yours too. Ultimately you—and only you—are or can be responsible for yourself. Thus we have not written a book that is prescriptive: we have no interest in telling you what you should or should not do. We advance no particular standards of right or wrong, since realizing and acting on one's essential humanness do not fall into strict categories of right and wrong. Whatever moral standards you apply to yourself or to others are those which you formulate. We *are* interested, however, in giving you the information, the guidance, and the help to enable you to make clear and appropriate decisions about your own and others' actions and lives.

• • •

We are very grateful to the staff of The Counseling and Psychotherapy Center, Fair

Lawn, New Jersey, and to our patients and their families and students and friends for the teaching and learning that occurs among us. Many of these people also made important suggestions after reading parts of the manuscript. We would like to express our appreciation specifically to the following people: Dr. McGinnis' colleagues at New York University, particularly Dr. Marian Hamburg, for the opportunity to gain many years of invaluable experience in teaching human sexuality, marriage, and family life with an open approach; Valerie Hurst and Connie Buckley for their editorial advice and assistance, which aided us in giving shape and direction to the earlier drafts of the manuscript; Emily McNally for her interest, support, and invaluable help in revising and integrating the final version; and Joan Cottrell, whose practical help of typing and whose concern, support, and loyalty aided us during the book's creation.

To our families, we are deeply grateful: without their cooperation, their help, and their loving support, this book would not have been possible. Our special thanks go to Kitty and George Finnegan for their editorial assistance, their ongoing concern, and their consistent encouragement; to Tom McGinnis, Jr., for his research, his organizational assistance, and his enthusiasm; and to Mary Yorke McGinnis who has been close to us throughout. In addition to spending hundreds of hours typing and helping to prepare the manuscript, Yorke consistently gave of her energy, strength, and understanding at much personal sacrifice.

To all these people who believed in and supported us and The System, we are truly grateful.

Thomas C. McGinnis, Ed.D.
Dana G. Finnegan, Ph.D.

REFERENCES

1. Hart, Harold, editor: Marriage: for and against, New York, 1972, Hart Publishing Co.
2. Woodward, Kenneth L.: Parent gap, Newsweek, Sept. 22, 1975.
3. Goode, William J.: World revolution and family patterns, New York, 1963, The Free Press.
4. Cox, Frank: American marriage: a changing scene? Dubuque, Iowa, 1971, William C. Brown Co., Publishers.
5. Davids, Leo: North American marriage: 1990, The Futurist **5**:190-194, Oct., 1971.
6. Goode, William J., editor: The contemporary American family, Chicago, 1971, Quadrangle Books.
7. Mead, Margaret: The future of the family, Barnard Alumnae Magazine **60**:6-8, Winter, 1971.
8. Snow, John H.: On pilgrimage: marriage in the 70's, New York, 1971, The Seabury Press, Inc.
9. Leslie, Gerald R.: The family in social context, Fair Lawn, N.J., 1967, Oxford University Press.
10. Broderick, Carlfred B., editor: A decade of family research and action, Minneapolis, Minn., 1972, National Council on Family Relations.
11. Schvaneveldt, Jay C.: The interactional framework for studying the family. In Nye, F. Ivan, and Berardo, Felix M., editors: Emerging conceptual frameworks in family analysis, New York, 1966, The Macmillan Co., pp. 97-129.
12. Burgess, Ernest W.: The family as a unity of interacting personalities, The Family **7**:3-9, March, 1926.
13. Nye, Ivan F., and Berardo, Felix M., editors: Emerging conceptual frameworks in family analysis, New York, 1966, The Macmillan Co.
14. Mullahy, Patrick: Psychoanalysis and interpersonal psychiatry: the contributions of Harry Stack Sullivan, New York, 1970, Science House, Inc.
15. Perry, Helen Swick, and Gawel, Mary Ladd, editors: The collected works of Harry Stack Sullivan, M.D., 2 vols., New York, 1953, W. W. Norton & Co., Inc.
16. Back, Kurt W.: Beyond words: the story of sensitivity training and the encounter movement, New York, 1972, Russell Sage Foundation.
17. Howard, Jane: Please touch: a guided tour of the human potential movement, New York, 1970, McGraw-Hill Book Co.
18. McGinnis, Thomas C.: Sensitivity training in a partly dehumanized environment, Marriage Guidance **12**:515-527, 1970.
19. Lewis, Howard R., and Streitfeld, Harold S.: Growth games: how to tune in yourself, your family, your friends, New York, 1970, Harcourt Brace Jovanovich, Inc., pp. 3-11.
20. Malamud, Daniel I., and Machover, Solomon: Toward self-understanding: group techniques in self-confrontation, Springfield, Ill., 1965, Charles C Thomas, Publisher.

CONTENTS

OPEN FAMILY AND MARRIAGE a guide to personal growth

INTRODUCTION: TOWARD A MORE OPEN SOCIETY

ALL OUR YESTERDAYS

The changes that have occurred in the United States since 1900 alone are phenomenal. In less than a hundred years there have probably been more changes in almost all areas of life than there were in the preceding 350 years. During his lifetime a person who is now in his eighties has seen the horse and buggy yield to the automobile, the airplane, and rockets to the moon.[1] He has seen styles and morality shift from the demand for total coverage of a woman's limbs to the acceptance of almost total uncoverage of a woman's back, legs, arms, and breasts. He has seen changes from gunpowder to the hydrogen bomb; from crude medical techniques to open-heart surgery and human transplants; from home remedies to miracle drugs; from taboos against even mentioning sex in mixed company to open discussions on television of homosexuality, venereal disease, premarital sex, extramarital affairs, and husband/wife swapping; from communication by letter, telegraph, and newspapers to telephone, radio, and television; from the woman in the home and the Negro in his place to the demands and victories of women's liberation and black power. His world and his society have undergone shattering revolutionary and evolutionary changes, and those changes have had an almost incalculable impact on the morals, manners, and mores of American life.[2,3]

What do all these changes mean? What is their significance? Are they essentially the same kinds of changes the world has always experienced in its evolutionary creep through time? Do they perhaps only feel different to us because they happen with greater rapidity and in greater numbers than they used to in other periods of time?[4,5]

Or are we living in a special and different time, a time in which events and changes have taken on additional, new, and more far-reaching meanings than ever before?[6,7] During this century, has the process of evolutionary change turned into one of radical transformation? The noted social historian Plumb[8] seems to believe so because he states:

> We are at the end of ten thousand years of history. We are in the middle of a revolution more profound than any man has experienced, and thus we are affected more deeply than we realize. . . . age-old social institutions are breaking down. . . . Women's liberation, the revolt of adolescence, and the decay of the patriarch are not signs of the sudden fever that has gripped this generation; rather they are the product of a social revolution, of a need for radical readjustment, one such as man has had to make only once before in his history.*

What is this social revolution of which Plumb speaks? Essentially it consists of the move away from a closed society and way of life toward a more open society and way of life. At the beginning of this century American society consisted basically of a structured, authoritarian, patriarchal system. This was a **closed society,** a society

---

*From Plumb, J. H.: An epoch that started ten thousand years ago is ending. . . , Horizon **14:** 4-9, Summer, 1972.

that maintains its stability and the stability of its members by means of a restrictive system of accepted beliefs, expectations, rules, and values. This kind of system supports and is supported by major societal institutions—government, religion, education, the community, marriage, and the family.[9-12] These institutions promulgate and enforce the beliefs, expectations, rules, and values of the closed society; in effect, they tell the individual how to live his life so that he and his society can maintain the *status quo*.

A closed society is by definition one that limits and restricts its individual members by requiring that they conform to group standards. In such a situation the individual tends to have only three alternatives —to accept the standards, to reject them, or to try to modify them. However, in a tightly structured, authoritarian society the price of individual deviation can be high. Some individuals (as is true of all times) are willing to pay the price of nonconformity, but most people accept and actively follow the standards of their society.

Although such conformity is restricting, it carries with it certain important benefits. Clear-cut authoritarian standards and instructions about how one ought to live one's life can provide a great deal of stability. Just because these standards and instructions are clear cut and basically rigid, they enable a person who lives according to them to define himself rather clearly. For example, he can say, "I am a good citizen because I believe in my country, I obey its laws, and I will fight and die for my country if necessary." Or he can say, "I am a good husband and a good father because I act as my society and my religion tell me a good husband and a good father ought to act." Although these examples are rather simplistic, nevertheless, they point out the essential defining function of the closed society.

Although such conformity is limiting in that the individual's identity is defined in terms of externals (institutions, standards, social and occupational roles), this very limitation reduces a certain amount of anxiety. Many of his decisions are already made for him; he does not have to keep carving out an identity for himself. Instead he can accept his place in society. Thus a closed society with authoritarian institutions that teach and enforce definite clear-cut rules tends to provide the individual with a strong and stabilizing "sense of place," a sense of identity. He holds a certain place in his family, in his school, in his community, in his job, in his religion, in his civic duties, in his marriage—in his society. As he determines, accepts, and takes his place, he is relieved of numerous decisions and can gain a strong sense of identity in terms of externals, that is, his society's institutions.

AMERICA'S IDENTITY CRISIS

In the past seventy-five years, however, vast and far-reaching events and changes have swept across the United States and irrevocably altered our way of life. Even a simple list of the basic events and changes is mind-boggling: the shift from a rural to an urban society, the rapid development of technology, increased prosperity, the proliferation of the media and the consequent impact on communication, the secularization of society, the ascendancy of science, the steady inroads made by psychology, and the successes of major protest movements (labor, civil rights, the counterculture, women's liberation).[13,14] In addition to and influencing these changes are significant events that have helped alter the character of our society and our lives—World War I, Prohibition, the Depression, World War II, the bomb, the cold war, the war in Korea, the McCarthy hearings, the discovery of drugs by the young, assassinations, the war in Vietnam, the ecological crisis, and the Watergate scandal.

These and other events and changes have forced American society to change and move away from the closed nature that characterized it in the early 1900s. But in what ways has our society become more open? What does this openness mean?

The realities of the events and changes and their impact on the earlier closed nature of our society cannot be denied. We *have* changed; we *have* become somewhat more open. For instance, it is a fact that denying a person access to any seat on a bus is no longer a socially condoned act. There are laws now against such unconstitutional acts, and many people give intellectual assent to the laws forbidding actions that are unconstitutional. And there seems to be much more intellectual assent to and acceptance of many kinds of situations and actions that were once unthinkable in a more closed society. For example, divorce, premarital sex, teenage freedom, and women's liberation were well-nigh unthinkable in the early 1900s. Now, however, many people at least reluctantly go along with or do not overtly fight against these developments. Either they give grudging intellectual assent or shrug their shoulders in indifferent or bewildered submission.

Much of our behavior also has changed. Because of the impact of events and changes, it is no longer possible to lynch a black man or totally control people's actions by social pressure or ostracism. People are no longer considered social outcasts if they choose not to go to church. If women drink, smoke, or talk about sex in public, they are no longer necessarily viewed as fast, loose, or immoral. The teenager who goes against his parents' commands or wishes is no longer viewed as a freak of nature.

Thus it seems fair to say that in many important ways ours has become a more **open society,** a society that is based on a nonauthoritarian system and that is flexible and tolerant enough to allow for the existence and encouragement of alternative ways of thinking, feeling, and acting. Furthermore, an open society maintains its stability and the stability of its members by means of guidelines rather than strict rules and by means of negotiation rather than authoritarian pressure.

Although this openness has brought many benefits, it has also created three major problems for all of us.

1. Many of the events and changes have occurred so rapidly and with such sharpness that we frequently have had too little time or opportunity to assess, evaluate, assimilate, understand, or accept their meanings and consequences. For example, few people were prepared for the enormous number of technological developments that came out of World War II. The atomic bomb gave mankind the power to destroy itself, but most people were still unable to think in terms of a world community and the responsibilities of power with regard to all of mankind. American society was forced to open itself up to being a world power without knowing how to react to, or deal with, this opening up.

2. Confusion and anxiety have resulted from a breakdown or erosion of old values and old ways. With the challenges to and changes in the old authoritarian systems that governed society have come uncertainty and insecurity. When people are required to perceive their institutions in new ways and in different terms, they then face the problems created by no longer having solid, clear-cut (often rigid) rules by which to measure themselves, others, or life. The external bearings by which they charted their course may become less clear or disappear or seem less valid; then people often begin to feel alienated, unsure, and anxious, since the rules and values that helped them develop their identity no longer offer sufficient direction or else teach ways of living that frequently conflict with the demands of the changed reality in which they find themselves.[15,16]

3. Perhaps the most confusing and anxiety-producing problem of all, since it springs from a huge gulf between what *seems* to be true and what actually *is* true, is that our society seems to be much more open than it really is. The trouble results from the fact that although our society is more open in terms of intellectual assent

and some behavior, it has not really become much more open in terms of basic attitudes, beliefs, values, and especially feelings.

The problem is, then, that although the holding power of our institutions (e.g., marriage and family) and of our old ways (e.g., inherent respect for authority) has lessened considerably, these institutions and ways still remain as our basic frames of reference. And, most certainly, they still exert a strong emotional hold on many, if not most, Americans.[17] Although it is often possible for people to acknowledge change with their intellects, it is frequently difficult for them to accept the change in their hearts. Even if a person truly welcomes a change, he often finds that it is not always so easy to make his behavior fit the new situation or condition because either he does not know *what* new behavior is called for or he does not know *how* to alter his behavior. And even many of those who manage to alter their behavior find that their actions do not necessarily bring the satisfaction they anticipated.

In more specific terms, the problem we all face in dealing with the new and different *now* is that we are still tied, to one degree or another, to the attitudes, values, and feelings of the past. The values promulgated and inculcated by an earlier and far more closed society are still being passed along by many members of each succeeding generation, and a large number of these societal values still pack enormous emotional clout even if they no longer inhibit our behavior. For example, divorce is a fairly common occurrence in our society; yet a frequent concern of the person contemplating divorce is "What will people think?" And although many young people are not regular churchgoers and do not have strong religious beliefs, when they decide to marry, they often are married by a clergyman rather than a government official.

Essentially the problem is that we are caught in huge and powerful **double binds**—situations in which there seem to be only two diametrically opposed alternatives, each of which has great emotional force.[18,19] Thus choosing either alternative means exposure to enormous, often unresolvable conflict about the opposing one, since the choice of either one is unacceptable in the light of the opposing alternative. The person is "damned if he does, and damned if he doesn't." For example, if an individual chooses openness, people who are rather closed tend to criticize him sharply. If an individual chooses closedness, then those who are more open tend to criticize him for that.

More specific examples of a double bind in our society follow. Society (and the family) teaches that to be a good wife and mother, a woman must stay home, take care of the children, and love her role. But she may feel bored, angry, and unfulfilled in this role and want very much to have a career, do something more with her life, and be her own person. Whichever alternative she chooses, she is faced with great conflict. That is a double bind. So, too, is the fact that current circumstances pressure us to experience openness, although the rules and values of the more closed past urge us to see such openness as wrong or unacceptable. For example, people who are currently grandparents are often exposed to the much greater openness of speech, dress, and behavior of their grandchildren. These young people may express anger or disagreement, may wear what are to the grandparents revealing clothes, and may interact with the grandparents in ways that seem disrespectful. If the grandparents wish to maintain a relationship with their grandchildren, they have to struggle with the rules and values of their more closed past. If they want the grandchildren to want to be with them, the grandparents must at least act somewhat accepting. Yet they must also deal with their own rules and values, which teach that their grandchildren's speech, dress, and behavior are really not acceptable.

The dynamic interrelationship among the current and past rules and values of society, family, marriage, and the individual places incredible strains and stresses on all of us.[20,21] Reality has forced society to open up; there has been significant erosion in the authority and credibility of marriage and the family, and the individual has been asked to respond with flexibility and openness to all the changes and new alternatives they present. But at the same time, individuals have been schooled and socialized by society, marriage, and the family according to the old, traditional values of a closed society. It is this interrelationship that has created the double binds in which most of us find ourselves.

These problems have created and lie at the heart of the identity crisis in the United States. Who are we now? How did we get where we are now? How will we deal with these double binds? Where are we going?

It is to these questions and to the needs underlying them that this book addresses itself. Basically it is aimed at helping people to become more aware of, to understand, and to learn to deal constructively with the double binds created by the conflicts between the traditional teachings of a closed society and the individual's own moves toward making himself, his relationships, marriage, and the family more open and meaningful.

APPROACH AND STRUCTURE

The approach and structure of the book are built on the premise that dealing constructively with our identity involves knowledge, awareness, and understanding of the past, present, and future and their interrelationship. Furthermore, change and growth away from closedness toward fuller openness and autonomy require learning about and learning to use certain basic skills and tools of communication and interaction.

Part I: Society

Part I examines and analyzes dating, marriage, family life, and society as they were in the closed past; the impact of changes in these institutions on the individual; effects that the teachings of these institutions have on us in the present; and what characteristics and issues are inherent in marriage and family life and must be consciously dealt with if we are to break into the double bind of closedness versus openness and become more open. The primary focus of this investigation therefore is on how we as a society, as members of marriages and families, and as individuals have arrived at where we are now; what things from the past still affect us in the present; and what conditions in marriage and family life we need to be aware of and work with to become more truly open. Only in this way is it possible to gain an awareness and understanding of *what* problems and conditions we face, an awareness that is the first step in the process of changing, growing, and becoming more open.

Part II: The individual

Part II is devoted to helping people develop an awareness and an understanding of the individual and his dynamics (how he functions and why) because it is the individual who is and who holds the key to whatever changes will take place in dating, marriage, the family, and society.[22] Since the individual is the essential building block of all relationships, whatever changes and moves toward real openness occur in society, marriage, and the family are the result of the changes he makes in himself and in his attitudes toward and use of his institutions.[23]

Part II then is designed to teach how and why the individual functions as he does and how he can bring about changes in his functioning. The approach in Part II is first to explain how a person gets to be who he is now. This consists of looking at how society, parents and other significant persons, and the person himself influenced and contributed to his development. The second step is to show a person how to get in touch with his functioning in the present. This involves teaching him how to use the processes of communication and interaction and apply them to himself and his life. In effect he is being taught to understand and use the Interactional Therapeutic System. Thus this part provides concrete information, knowledge, and practical skills and techniques that can enable a person to work toward becoming more open and autonomous.

In essence, Part II provides the means by which the individual can learn to develop his own guidelines in a shaky society, make appropriate evaluations, change and grow, and develop healthier, more qualitative relationships. It serves both as a helpful guide to individual functioning and as a basic preparation for considering the dynamics of marriage and the family. And it teaches the individual how to change and grow so that he can bring about change and growth in society, in marriage, and in the family.

Part III: Marriage and the family

Part III draws on all the previous material concerning marriage and the family and individual dynamics and looks at what can happen when two or more individuals get together in a relationship and thereby "combine" their dynamics. The purpose of Part III then is to provide an understanding of, an appreciation of, and methods for dealing constructively with the dynamics of human relationships, especially as they occur within the context of the two major personal institutions of marriage and the family. This is done against the backdrop of society, past and present. Carrying out this purpose involves analyzing the effects that each individual's past and present functioning have on marital and family relationships. It means investigating how the match-up between individuals and their dynamics works to create the dynamics of a relationship. And it means considering ways of establishing healthier, more qualitative marital and family relationships.

The overall aim of Part III is to teach how and why marital and family relationships operate as they do and to provide ways—by means of the Interactional Therapeutic System—of making them more open. In effect, this part offers help in vitalizing or revitalizing the beleaguered institutions of marriage and the family.[24-26] It also suggests possible alternatives to the traditional forms of these institutions[27,28] and teaches methods by which people can establish their own guidelines for living.[29]

ALL OUR TOMORROWS

If we are not to be overwhelmed by the loss of stability offered by the past, by the changes and insecurities of the present, or by the inevitable newness and difference inherent in the future, then we have huge and all-important responsibilities to meet. We must learn from the past and work constructively with the present so that our present and our future worlds are healthy, life-giving, and life-enhancing.

If we are to shape our society, our personal institutions of marriage and the family, and our individual lives to our human needs, then we must gain knowledge, understanding, awareness, and practical expertise in the dynamics of human interaction. Most particularly we need to understand and work constructively with the dynamics of the individual and of marriage and the family. If the individual and his personal institutions can change and grow more open, then there is hope that we can establish a present and a future in which society and its institutions serve individuals and help them interact and live meaningful and constructive lives.[30]

We believe that this book and the *Interactional Therapeutic System* it presents offer people viable and usable ways of acquiring and implementing the knowledge, skills, and techniques necessary to becoming more open, more autonomous, and therefore more in control of their lives and their destiny.

REFERENCES

1. Cottrell, Fred: Technology, man and progress, New York, 1972, Charles E. Merrill Publishing Co.
2. Bredmeier, Harry C., and Jackson, Toby: Social problems in America, New York, 1972, John Wiley & Sons, Inc.
3. Etzioni, Amitai: Social profile: U.S.A. today, New York, 1972, Van Nostrand Reinhold Co.
4. Fuller, R. Buckminster: Utopia or oblivion: the prospects for humanity, New York, 1969, Bantam Books, Inc.
5. McHale, John: The future of the future, New York, 1969, George Braziller, Inc.
6. Demott, Benjamin: Surviving the 70's, New York, 1972, Penguin Books Inc.
7. Kahn, Herman, and Bruce-Briggs, B.: Things to come: thinking about the 70's and 80's, New York, 1972, The Macmillan Co.
8. Plumb, J. H.: An epoch that started ten thousand years ago is ending. . . , Horizon **14**:4-9, Summer, 1972.
9. Burgess, Ernest W., and Locke, Harvey J.: The family from institution to companionship, ed. 2, New York, 1960, American Book Co., pp. 209-330.
10. Goode, William J., editor: The contemporary American family, Chicago, 1971, Quadrangle Books, Inc.
11. Kirkpatrick, Clifford: The family: as process and institution, ed. 2, New York, 1963, Ronald Press Co., pp. 3-93.
12. Leslie, Gerald R.: The family in social context, Fair Lawn, N.J., 1967, Oxford University Press.
13. Cudlipp, Edythe: Understanding women's liberation, New York, 1971, Paperback library, Division of Coronet Communications, Inc.
14. Roszak, Theodore: The making of a counter culture, Garden City, N.Y., 1968, Doubleday & Co., Inc.
15. Di Salvo, Charles, with Cox, Claire: Faces people wear: today's identity crisis and how to cope with it, New York, 1968, Hawthorne Books, Inc.
16. Erikson, E. H.: The problem of ego identity, Journal of American Psychoanalytic Association **4**:56-121, 1956.
17. Cox, Frank: American marriage: a changing scene? Dubuque, Iowa, 1971, William C. Brown Co., Publishers.
18. Bateson, Gregory, Jackson, Don D., Haley, Jay, and Weakland, John: Toward a theory of schizophrenia. In Howells, John G.: Theory and practice of family psychiatry, New York, 1971, Brunner/Mazel, Inc., pp. 748-749.
19. Bell, Norman W., and Vogel, Ezra F., editors: A modern introduction to the family, New York, 1968, The Free Press, pp. 571-572.
20. Gordon, Michael, editor: The nuclear family in crisis: the search for an alternative, New York, 1972, Harper & Row, Publishers.
21. Perutz, Katrin: Marriage is hell, New York, 1972, William Morrow & Co., Inc.
22. Fane, Arthur, and Fane, Zenia: Behind every face: a family, New York, 1970, Ginn & Co.
23. Messer, A. A.: The individual in his family: an adaptational study, Springfield, Ill., 1970, Charles C Thomas, Publisher.
24. Davids, Leo: North American marriage: 1990, The Futurist **5**:190-194, Oct., 1971.
25. Schultz, David A.: The changing family: its function and future, Englewood Cliffs, N.J., 1972, Prentice-Hall, Inc.
26. Snow, John H.: On pilgrimage: marriage in the 70's, New York, 1971, Seabury Press, Inc.
27. DeLora, Jo Ann S., and DeLora, Jack R., editors: Intimate life styles: marriage and its alternatives, Pacific Palisades, Calif., 1972, Goodyear Publishing Co., Inc.
28. Rimmer, Robert H.: Proposition 31, New York, 1968, The New American Library, Inc.
29. McGinnis, Thomas C., and Ayres, John U.: Open family living: a new approach for enriching your life together, Garden City, N.Y., 1976, Doubleday & Co., Inc.
30. Toffler, Alvin: Future shock, New York, 1970, Random House, Inc., pp. 485-486.

part one

MARRIAGE, THE FAMILY, AND THE INDIVIDUAL IN A CHANGING SOCIETY

chapter 1

CHANGES IN DATING, MARRIAGE, AND FAMILY LIFE impact on the individual

This chapter examines the sources of the double bind between closedness and openness in which Americans find themselves at the present time. The descriptions of dating, marriage, and family life in the early 1900s provide a clear view of one side of this double bind—the attitudes, rules, and values of a closed society, which still have enormous emotional force even to this day. The descriptions of our current practices regarding dating, marriage, and family life provide a clear view of the other side of the double bind—how our behavior and some of our attitudes, rules, and values have been radically altered in response to events and changes during this century and thus no longer match up with the dictums of an earlier day. In effect, this chapter looks at the reasons why the individual often feels confused and anxious in the presence of society's greater openness.

The center of this conflict is that although society has become somewhat more open and our behavior has become somewhat freer, the individual must struggle with the weight and power of earlier attitudes, rules, and values that are still a strong part of his emotional heritage from the closed society of the past. The struggle is created by the conflict between the present-day force of the old teachings and the greater freedom of behavior available to him. How can he reconcile the old rules against certain kinds of attitudes and behavior with the new "freedom" that says, "Do your own thing," and "Be your own person"? Essentially the struggle centers on the great disparity between what the old teachings say are right and wrong and what an individual's peers and current conditions tell him are right and wrong. He is caught between conflicting directives and values regarding what he *should* think, feel, and do.

Chapter 1 looks closely at the sources of the double binds (the closedness of the past vs. the openness of the present) that confront each individual in society today and examines the impact of these double binds on the individual. Chapters 2 and 3 consider the major characteristics and issues of marriage and the family because these are the phenomena that every person must deal with in some way or another—whether consciously or not.

THE EARLY 1900s

The United States of the early 1900s was a *closed* society, one that maintained its stability and its closedness by a vast network of *accepted* attitudes, expectations, rules, and values. This societal network by and large supported and was in turn supported by all major institutions—religion, government, education, marriage, and the family. The closed society—by means of its institutions—demanded belief in and obedience to authority based on absolutes; there was little, if any, room for relativism or challenge. The underlying assumption was that the *status quo* is good and should be preserved. Thus society required that its individual members fulfill the roles assigned to them and thereby maintain the status quo.[1,2]

Dating in the early 1900s

The expectations, rules and values that governed and controlled dating early in the century were definitely those of a closed society.[3] Although formal chaperonage was no longer practiced (except in certain ethnic groups), the way most dating was set up served essentially the same purpose—control and restraint.

RESTRAINTS ON DATING

Once a boy and girl decided to date, it was expected, if not required, that the boy meet the girl's parents and pass their inspection. Frequently, they already either knew him or knew about him or his family, but whatever the case, most parents required this kind of check on their daughters' dates and expected their own sons to be subjected to the same parental scrutiny.

These arrangements served various purposes. Restricting the ways and places of meeting increased the chances that youngsters would get to know others of their same social class and religion; it also hopefully ensured that young people would date others with similar moral standards. Meeting the boys who dated their daughters was another way of checking on these matters. Furthermore, the boy's meeting the girl's parents no doubt served to impress on him that he was responsible not only *for* her but also *to* them.

Other restraints were also in operation. Most parents set definite curfew hours for their children who dated, and if the young people did not keep to the specified hours, they could expect swift and sometimes harsh discipline. Parents were in evidence, however, not just when their children came home from dates but also as chaperones. Frequently, they or other suitable adults were present during most or all of the date, since much of the dating of young people took place in rather public situations. These included such events as the weekly town dance, gatherings at people's houses, church socials, concerts, church, young people's meetings and outings, picnics, supervised hayrides, and school events. In those situations in which a boy and girl would be alone with each other— or at least not under the watchful eye of a concerned adult—it was expected (and devoutly desired) that their internalized rules and values would prevent them from yielding to their "baser" natures.

What were these major protective (indeed, contraceptive) rules and values? Some of them had to do with roles, and some focused directly on the issues of sexual and moral behavior.[4] As was true in all aspects of living, the male and female roles in dating were sharply defined. The boy was expected to take the initiative. He was also expected to feel and be responsible for the girl's comfort and safety and to protect her not only from any actual danger but also from insult or social embarrassment. Finally, he was, in a sense, to shield her from his own sexual needs—to regard her and treat her as a "lady."

The girl's role was just as stringently circumscribed. She was expected to hold back —to wait to be asked, to be shy, coy, passive. At the same time, however, she was expected to be flirtatious, flattering, and responsive to the male's ego needs. Nevertheless, the ultimate responsibility for holding the sexual lid on the relationship was hers. As her mother had taught her—all men are out for whatever they can get because men are "that way." Her mother had also taught her that women do not really have much (if any) sex drive and, more important, must preserve their virginity at all costs; therefore it was the women's duty to keep the sexual situation under control.

Rules and values like these interlocked with others to form a system that was intended to inhibit or restrain any but a modicum of overt sexual behavior in dating. The major moral position maintained by this system was that premarital chastity was an absolute must for the female. This whole intricate network of assumptions, rules, and values was promulgated and enforced by society, religion, and parents to regulate procreation so that it occurred *only* within the orderly bounds of married life. Added to this network, however, was the double standard. Since men are more quickly and easily aroused, some provision had to be made for their presumably stronger sex drive. Since men do not get pregnant, it was "okay" for them to have premarital sexual relations—as long as it was with women whom they would not consider marrying. Although society and religion branded male premarital sex as a sin, at the same time these institutions acted on a double standard; a young man was expected to "sow his wild oats," sinful though this might be, whereas a young woman was forbidden to do so.

PURPOSES AND FUNCTIONS OF DATING

Every society has some arrangement for selecting mates, whether by parental selection, a matchmaker's services, or pitched battles between males to win the desired female.[5] Perhaps because of the frontier spirit, American society in the ninteenth century began to move away from parental selection or arranged marriages and to develop the institution of dating. By the turn of the century, dating had largely replaced other methods, at least among native-born Americans. However, although the methods changed, the basic purposes did not—until the 1960s. *The primary purpose was to find a person who would be a suitable marriage partner.* Dating served as a kind of social "marketplace": people indicated their availability by showing interest in members of the opposite sex, by presenting themselves in the best light possible, and by being willing to play the social game. The chief functions of dating, were, then, to give young people maximum decent exposure to one another and thus provide a large group from which to choose.

The primary purpose was mate selection, but a secondary one was that *dating was good preparation for marriage.*[6] It gave both boys and girls a good deal of practice in fulfilling their prescribed roles in a nonkinship environment. Boys and girls got a chance to relate to one another on a more serious peer level; they gained experience in listening to, compromising or negotiating with, and making decisions with others from different family backgrounds. In effect, they got a chance to practice some aspects of their later marital roles without the immediate pressure of full commitment to a particular person.

The purposes of serious courtship and engagement were logical extensions of general dating, since each was a successive stage in the process of narrowing down the choices and intensifying the relationships. Engagement was the last stage of the selection process because it meant that the final choice had been made.

The effects and functions of engagement were various. The announcement of a couple's engagement served notice to others that both members of the couple were "reserved," that they were no longer available. It also meant (in most cases) that the parents of each person had agreed to his or her marriage.

For the couple, engagement meant a public and private commitment to one another, an affirmation of preference and choice. But it was an interim commitment; that is, the engagement period was a time (usually a year to a year and a half) during which the couple could be together more, could have a little more privacy, and could thereby have a better chance to test out their compatibility. The engagement period also gave them an opportunity to practice (in primarily nonsexual ways) their future interpersonal roles, now extended to include role relationships with the potential in-laws.

During the engagement period, the couple were also directly preparing in various ways for their marriage. The young man was working hard to save up a nest egg, money to provide some security for the beginnings of the marriage; the young woman, for her part, was busy making and collecting things for her hope chest, such as linens, towels, and dishes. In addition, the engagement period was one in which the man and woman were likely to be preparing emotionally for their future together. It was the time when they could think and talk seriously about their plans: where they might live, how they might wish to live, how many children they might want to have, and what they might want and expect from their life together. Engagement also served one other major function: it allowed a couple to make a commitment but one that was not final. The engagement period was the trial period; if one or both potential partners decided that for some reason the marriage would not work, they still had the freedom to break the commitment. And during a time when divorce was both rare and "disgraceful," this freedom was a practical and necessary safety valve.

Most engaged couples, however, chose not to exercise that freedom but went ahead and took the civil and religious steps necessary to becoming husband and wife. By doing so, they fulfilled the expectations and measured up to the rules and values of their closed society.

Dating, serious courtship, and engagement in the closed society of the early 1900s were hedged around with expectations, roles, rules, and values that sharply defined and limited how people should behave. The restraints imposed by the closed society were primarily designed for two purposes: to restrict and control young people's sexual impulses and to carefully guide the process of selecting a mate to ensure the best possible match-up in terms of such factors as class, religion, background, and education. The focus in dating was not so much on developing the interpersonal quality of the relationships but rather on seeing to it that, within reason, people related to each other according to the approved rules of the closed society's game. The emphasis was on the individual's fitting into the acceptable stereotypes predetermined by the closed society. Hopefully, personal happiness and a rewarding personal relationship would result from the match; however, society's primary concern was that people fit the stereotypes.

Marriage in the early 1900s

Marriage was a key part of this closed society. As such, it was a closed institution with fixed purposes and functions, roles, and rules that had changed little over hundreds of years.[7,8]

The basic purpose (and accomplishment) of marriage was to join human sexual (and emotional) needs with the demands of social and economic necessity.[9]

1. The marriage ceremony served as young people's rites of passage into adulthood. By marrying, a young man assumed the social and economic responsibilities of caring for himself, his wife, and whatever children they would have; a young woman assumed the social responsibility of caring for her husband and their children.

2. Because both society and religion sanctioned only that two-person relationship in which the couple committed themselves "till death do us part," marriage helped to ensure that the woman and especially the children would be protected and cared for. In addition, because marriage was a "forever commitment" to one specific person, it tended to foster stability in society and at the same time meet sexual needs.

3. Another function of marriage—procreation—was what made the first two purposes relevant and necessary. The main purpose of procreation was, of course, to perpetuate the human race.

4. Marriage enabled a couple to pool their resources and create an efficient work unit; by uniting, they could divide their skills and labor to best advantage.

5. Marriage provided the partners with companionship and a certain amount of emotional support. It reduced feelings of isolation and alienation, thus tending to strengthen the overall fabric of society.

The structure and nature of marriage were basically predetermined; a closed society does not—indeed, cannot—produce or encourage an open marital system. The closed marriage of the early 1900s was a rigidly structured authoritarian patriarchy. It was structured according to fixed and inflexible expectations, rules, and values, which were expressed in terms of assigned roles.

These roles were sharply defined and set up a complementary relationship between husband and wife in all major areas of marriage. The husband was head of the household, the authority, and the decision-maker. The wife was expected to obey him, to submit to his authority, and to abide by his decisions without questioning them. (Of course, in reality there were many marriages in which the wife was the real power but disguised the fact by outward shows of conformity to the role.) The husband was expected to perform income-producing work and to do whatever heavy physical labor was necessary in the home; the wife's job was to do the housework, care for her husband, bear children, and take the primary role in rearing them. In effect, the husband's responsibilities and interests involved him in the "outer world" of business; the wife's involved her in the "inner world" of the home.

Other expectations were built in to the husband/wife roles. By and large, sexual intercourse was considered to be a man's need and therefore a husband's right. For the wife, it was her duty. Connected to and supported by these role ascriptions was the double standard, which grudgingly conceded that it might be natural if a husband wandered but asserted that it was unnatural if the wife did so. Other role expectations undergirded the whole, closed, authoritarian patriarchy. The male was expected to be rational, logical, independent, and unemotional—a thinker and a doer; the female was assumed to be illogical, dependent, compassionate, warm, and caring—a nurturer and a doer.

How did a couple in a closed marriage like this deal with the inevitable stresses they encountered? How did they try to keep the marriage together and working? Some couples did not, of course, but the majority managed to do so. Since they had made a "forever commitment," most people were strongly motivated to work at making the marriage function adequately, if not smoothly and pleasantly. Their own commitment was strengthened by societal and religious pressures, which can be extremely strong "glue."

Another kind of glue was that the success of marriage did not depend primarily on personalities or emotional abilities (short of extreme psychopathology); as long as the partners fulfilled their roles, the marriage could work—economically, socially, and physically. Emotional compatibility simply was not necessary to do one's work, procreate, rear children, or fulfill one's societal obligations. There were various ways partners could right (or wrong) the emotional balance: most of them were nonverbal, covert, or at least indirect. For example, one or the other partner might use the silent treatment or make an appeal to a relative to intervene. Whatever the tactics or methods, most people managed to maintain their marriages because they were living according to one of the strongest and most effective emotional directives: "You made your marriage bed; now lie in it!"

Family life in the early 1900s

Since marriage is the fulcrum of the family, it follows that if the marriage was a closed one, the resultant family would be closed also. The extended family* was the rule rather than the exception, a structure that concentrated a large amount of authority in one household or place.

The family had various purposes and functions. Two of its primary purposes were to perpetuate the human race and to protect the offspring of the marital union. A third purpose was to add members to the

*The **extended family** is one in which grandparents, aunts, uncles, and cousins live with or near the basic family of parents and children.

work team; in a rural setting there was usually more work than just the couple could handle. Children were also a kind of "life insurance" for parents. If the father died, the mother could carry on with the help of the children (especially the boys). If the mother died, the daughters could run the household. A fourth function of the family was to socialize the children. This involved teaching them (by means of both models and instruction) all the expectations, rules, values, and roles necessary to being an upright, moral, law-abiding citizen. In essence, to socialize was to civilize. In addition, the socialization process involved educating youngsters—teaching them the skills and methods they would need to become productive workers and citizens. The fifth function was to provide children with a stable atmosphere in which to grow up and to furnish parents with a stable atmosphere in which to live. Hopefully, the family provided a refuge from the cares of the outside world and served as a group that provided opportunities for developing meaningful relationships and for receiving love and approval.

The man and woman's family roles remained essentially the same as their marital roles. The male was the patriarch, the authoritarian head of the household. To this role he added those of disciplinarian and primary masculine model. The female, of course, bore the children, and largely oversaw their growing up. To these roles she often added those of intermediary between father and children about disciplinary matters, of emotional nurturer, and of primary feminine model. With the advent of children, the power balance shifted somewhat. Father kept his original position as most powerful, and mother was still expected to obey him, but the children were expected to obey both parents. Basically the children's roles were to honor and obey their parents, to perform whatever work was assigned to them, and to follow in the footsteps of the same-sex parent.

Essentially the family maintained its emotional balance by pressuring (whether overly or covertly) its members into conforming to their specified roles.[10] The pressures came from nonverbal and verbal communication, awe of authority, approval and disapproval, and dependence on the parents.

• • •

These brief descriptions of dating, marriage, and family life in the early 1900s convey some notion of the tightness, the closedness, of these authoritarian, patriarchal institutions. Closed dating and marital and family institutions meant a closed society and vice versa. ►IE-1, p. 29.*

CHANGES IN DATING, MARRIAGE, AND THE FAMILY

Even before the new century began, events and changes were gathering force and making some impact. By the time this century had started on its seventh decade, the impact of the many powerful events and changes that had occurred had permanently and radically altered the course, the nature, and the quality of American life. The closed societal system that governed life in the early part of the century was challenged, shaken, broken into, disrupted, and (in places) altered beyond recognition. Essentially what had been a closed societal system was *forced* to open up.[11,12]

It is not possible, of course, to cover all the effects of twentieth century events and changes on dating, marriage, and the family. Of necessity our approach is a selective one: we discuss some effects because they are too important to ignore, others because they illustrate the synergistic nature of the changes and their impacts. We also focus more attention on the period after World War II because during this period, the effects of the events and changes have most clearly come to fruition.

*Refer to the preface (p. ix) for a description of interaction experiences (IE).

As you read, keep one point in mind: some of the events and changes have even more far-reaching significance than may be indicated. In addition to their specific impact, many of them have had an overall effect of forcing the closed atmosphere open. Basically they have helped create a general atmosphere of freedom to question and experiment.[13,14]

Impact on values supporting dating and marriage

Until the 1960s, dating was the traditional prelude to marriage, and therefore the values that supported dating practices also supported marriage. Thus when the traditional values underlying dating were challenged by changes, so, too, were those underlying marriage. For this reason the challenges to dating and marriage values are treated in the same discussion. Following this, the impact of changes on the marital relationship and on the family are examined.

Probably the first significant challenge to traditional values supporting dating and marriage was one of technology's first gifts to the new century—the car. By the late teens and certainly by the middle of the Roaring Twenties, the car was available to a number of young people. They found it to be the perfect mobile parlor and sometimes the perfect (although uncomfortable) mobile bedroom. It afforded couples a certain privacy and allowed them to put distance between them and the protective and prying eyes of parents and community. Whether they availed themselves of it, the opportunity for sexual intimacy was there.

Not only the car helped the Roaring Twenties to roar. For a small but well-publicized elite (like those whom F. Scott Fitzgerald immortalized), the twenties became a time of rebellion against the victorian social and sexual morals that had held American society in thrall. Partly the rebellion was triggered by a popularized distortion of Freud's concepts about man's sexual nature[15]: if man is essentially libidinous, then why not accept and act on nature? Partly the rebellion was fostered by the unpopular repressiveness of Prohibition; eventually it became fashionable to break this law. So why not break others too—like those governing sexual and marital conduct? Only a miniscule minority did much sexual acting out; more important, the traditional bulwark of the closed society—authority—was being actively challenged.

Later, especially in the forties and fifties, when the major rural-to-urban migrations occurred, another threat to authority arose. Young couples who lived and dated in the cities or suburbs were harder to supervise. Added to this problem were those generated by World War II—greater sophistication about contraception (partially the result of lectures in the service about sex, VD, and the serviceman); a feeling of "let's enjoy life now because death may come all too soon"; the use of penicillin as a cure for VD; and servicemen all over the globe, far from the comforts of home, comforting themselves with nonmarital or extramarital sexual experiences or affairs and surviving their guilt feelings to tell the tale. In these ways, serious cracks were made in the smooth-faced rock of authority.

Other changes were having their impact too. The slow drift toward a more secular society had been occurring over a long period, and as religion lost more and more of its absolutist, authoritarian power (especially during the fifties), the great commandments against premarital sex and adultery lost some of their moral and emotional force.[16] At approximately the same time, the Kinsey report's findings about Americans' sexual behavior were happily being relayed to the public by the communications media.[17,18] This was possible mainly because of the easing of societal restrictions on what was proper for public contemplation. This easing occurred thanks to changes such as the precedents set by the Roaring Twenties, the greater openness encouraged by World War II, the move toward secularism, and the growing notion that science was somehow above moral reproach. Whatever caused the airing of the Kinsey findings, however, the effects of that airing were to make the unthinkable thinkable (and therefore possibly doable).

The fifties was also a time of a rising standard of living, an occurrence that enabled more and more young people to go to college. College meant greater freedom, freedom from parental and community supervision. It also meant that young people spent more time with their peers than with adults and thus were less exposed to authority figures who might reinforce stricter societal values about dating practices. At the same time, the four to five to six years of college training demanded by many occupations meant as many years' delay in entering the job market and earning a living wage, and many young people were either unwilling or financially unable to marry until they could begin working. Therefore the time between physical maturation and marriage was extended considerably. And since marriage was the only relationship in which sexual intercourse was sanctioned by society, young people found themselves in a bind. Three basic alternatives existed: get married, with or without parental support; avoid having intercourse; or have intercourse. Back in "the good old days," most young people would have refrained from the third alternative. But in the fifties many did not refrain because numerous circumstances were present that tended to open the way to the third alternative of premarital sexual freedom.

One of the major circumstances contributing to this relaxation in the sexual atmosphere had started with the generation who reached adulthood during the Depression and World War II and whose children reached college age in the fifties and early sixties. Because of the more permissive views about child-rearing advanced by psychologists and educators and because of the freer life-styles and attitudes resulting from World War II and growing secularism, this generation of parents granted themselves and their children more personal freedom.[19] Thus in a sense these parents turned away from the closedness of their parents' way of life and in so doing adopted more open life-styles for themselves and granted their children the freedom to have more open life-styles, too.

This greater openness in styles of living extended to sexual behavior, but the fact that there was greater freedom and that people were taking advantage of it was kept under cover for a long time. The rise of the counterculture* in the sixties,[20] however, focused Americans' attention on a truth they had been trying to ignore—that sexual experimentation and greater sexual freedom were here to stay and that society's authoritarian hold on its members (especially its younger members) had been seriously weakened, perhaps even broken. In effect, young people, particularly those of the counterculture, *acted out* the attitudes of greater sexual permissiveness that had been slowly evolving.

The breaking of society's authoritarian hold did not mean just greater sexual freedom. It also meant that the demands placed on people by rigid social expectations, roles, rules, and values were considerably eased. One ironic but healthy outcome of all this was that partly *because* people had greater sexual freedom, sex lost some of its "forbidden fruit" allure; thus people often became better able to adopt a more balanced attitude toward sex and its part in the dating process. In effect, people's perspectives widened considerably, creating more room for developing greater quality in their relationships. In addition, once released from some of those rigid social demands, people had more time, energy, and freedom to pay attention to the interpersonal aspects of their relationships. And young people especially began to do just that in their dating. Increasingly they focused much of

*The term "counterculture" was coined by Theodore Roszak to describe a subculture that developed in the 1960s. This subculture (whose members were under 30 years of age) challenged the views and values of the main culture and developed a life-style which ran counter to that of the main culture.

their dating time and energies on seeking and creating more qualitative relationships with one another. Many of them became concerned with achieving better communication, exploring the how's and why's of relating to one another, and focusing on each other's identity. Rejecting the masks, the strict roles, the limiting rules of the traditionally closed dating game, many young people chose to follow the less formal and less formula-ridden paths of open relating rather than closed dating.[21]

By their attitudes and actions, young people raised serious questions that challenged the traditional rationales for both dating and marriage. They asked the following devastating questions: If sex and interpersonal relationships can be possible, meaningful, and qualitative outside marriage, then why get married?[22-24] Why not just live together, since marriage bonds can create such legal and social wrangles should the couple decide to break up? Why not just live together, since contraception makes it possible to avoid having children and abortion can correct any slipups? Besides, if a couple want to have children, why do they have to be *married* to have and rear them?[25] And if a couple should want to rear their children in a family type of atmosphere, why can't they join or form family communes?[26]

Questions like these challenged various traditional notions of the closed society. The most obvious challenge was directed at the whole institution of marriage,[27] but others were directed at dating and the family.[28] Must dating necessarily be a prelude to marriage? Can't it simply be an experience in and of itself? Aren't other kinds of families just as effective as blood families?

In effect, these questions suggested possible alternatives to the traditional ways demanded by the closed society. The particular alternatives were less important than the basic impact of young people's attitudes and actions. What was so important was that young people, especially the members of the counterculture, shined their psychedelic light on the questions and problems that had been bothering society for a long time but that most people had desperately or righteously or religiously tried to ignore. And the light showed that society was opening up.

Just as the counterculture was hitting its stride and asking its difficult and embarrassing questions, the women's liberation movement was forming and formulating its philosophies.[29,30] Now it was not just "irresponsible kids" who were challenging dating and marriage; adults, too, were indicting the authoritarian, patriarchal views of dating and marriage imposed by a closed society.

Impact on marriage

The changes that were occurring not only challenged the traditional values that supported dating and marriage but also placed strains on already existing marital relationships.[31]

STRAINS ON THE MARITAL RELATIONSHIP

The shift from country or small town to city or suburb usually resulted in a couple's living far away from the extended family[32]; this meant that the couple left behind both the support and the immediate moral pressure of family, friends, and community, which often helped cement the marital relationship. This kind of move usually threw the couple together, alone with only each other at first, and most couples were not too well prepared for such a situation. Other factors combined to place great strains on the relationship: often the couple did not know anyone in their new urban setting, so they had to rely almost exclusively on each other. In addition, at this critical time in their marriage they often lost their unifying work-survival needs; instead the husband alone could almost always earn enough to support them, but his job usually meant that he was totally removed from the household and its environs. Thus the wife was left alone all day to cope as best she could in a strange new environment.

At about the same time as the rural-to-urban shift, the benefits of technological advances and a rising standard of living were creating problems for many of these "displaced" couples. Medical expertise had significantly increased life expectancy, and people had more leisure time as a result of the higher standard of living. Without the relentless pressure of working to survive and with more time to think and to enjoy life, many couples began to reassess their marital commitment of "together forever." *Working* together was one thing; relaxing and *being* together was quite another, especially when forever meant forty, maybe fifty years together instead of twenty-five or thirty. For many couples, being married forever to one and the same person was straining a relationship beyond bearing.

One factor that made the strain greater was that the teachings of psychology were beginning to filter into public consciousness and to be accepted as truths.[33] World War II gave the mental health field its great impetus; after the war, mental health concerns and psychological concepts became public property through community mental health centers, college courses, magazines, books, and television. The teachings that interested the public especially were those which focused on the possibilities of achieving individual happiness and on creating and maintaining qualitative interpersonal relationships. In response, people began to want and expect more from marriage.[34] The wonder is that so many marriages survived the stress created by these desires and expectations, since most people had little idea how to *get* what they wanted.

Psychology's emphasis on individual happiness and qualitative relationships served also to somewhat detach marriage from family life; that is, the growing belief was that marriage is a relationship in its own right and should be regarded and treated as such. This was a big change from the traditional view of marriage as subordinate to and less important than the family. The altered perspective on marriage led many couples to take a long, hard look at their own relationship as distinct from their roles as parents, an evaluative process that often led to discontent or disappointment and sometimes to divorce in spite of the children.

Frequently, the years during the fifties were marked by vague but persistent feelings of dissatisfaction, boredom, and sometimes futility, especially on the part of the wife. Mass production plus postwar prosperity had made timesaving and modernized appliances like washers, dryers, dishwashers, garbage disposals, and vacuum cleaners available and affordable. Such appliances, plus convenience foods, plus convenience services (for example, diaper service) considerably lightened her *physical burden*. Unlike her mother or grandmother, no longer was she an exhausted physical slave to housework and child-rearing. But she was frequently a psychological slave to a boring routine and to a dull, unfulfilling role. World War II had given many women a socially acceptable chance to work outside the home; many never went back to full-time housework. Many women who felt trapped in suburbia envied their working sisters their involvement in the great world out there. Many women who felt constrained from working by their marital roles also envied their husbands' daily contact with the outside world, resented their husbands' absences resulting from business travel, and felt stultified by being cooped up in suburbia with only children and other cooped-up mothers for company. Many husbands, on the other hand, resented what they perceived to be the do-nothing lives of their wives: they found it hard to imagine how deadening but time-consuming their wives' daily routines were. Many husbands resented their wives' "easy life" when they had to work so hard.

Thus it was that many middle-class and blue-collar marriages[35] were beset by boredom, misunderstanding, and resentment. This problem was not soothed by the communications media, which talked about and portrayed other more rewarding and intriguing life-styles. Faced with the question, "Is this all there is to marriage and to life?" many a marital partner began to think and feel that, surely, somewhere "out there" there was something better. And because they were partially freed from major restrictions by greater societal openness and by the rise of secularism, many husbands and wives were ripe for or went in search of an extramarital affair.[36-38] Others were turned on by the promise of the human potential movement, which emphasized and trained people for better interpersonal interaction.[39,40] By the mid-sixties, the often subliminal discontent of many suburban housewives was being discharged into the civil rights and antiwar causes. Then the women's liberation movement gave voice to that discontent, explained it, and urged women to break out of their repressive traditional roles. Women's liberation advocates also argued against women's submission to the patriarchal system of marriage. In addition, however, supporters of women's liberation contended that the traditional male/female roles that marriage helped perpetuate hindered *both* men and women from exploring their own humanness, from experiencing their uniqueness, and from using their full human potential. In effect, the women's movement has sought to free both men and women so that they can have marriages (and other relationships) as equals rather than relationships based on the burdens and putdowns of patriarchy.[41]

DIVORCE AS AN ALTERNATIVE

Contributing to greater freedom in the marital relationship is the freedom to get out of it if need be. Divorce has become a viable, fairly acceptable alternative,[42] but this was not always the case. Only as psychology gained strength and the absolutist views of religion lost strength did divorce become thinkable for many people. Psychology's nonmoralistic, nonblaming views of people, marriage, and divorce gradually encouraged people to accept the reality of marital problems. People became freer to admit they had marital difficulties. They were further encouraged to do so by the media, which publicized all kinds of evidence that yes, people did—and do—have problems. Many couples naturally turned to religion for help, but the clergy could not always give adequate help. And so it was that the mental health professions, including marriage counseling, began to come into their own.[43-45] Although marriage counselors cannot always save a marriage, they can urge that a couple getting a divorce try not to blame each other.[46] In addition, because religion's absolutist moral stand against divorce has been softened by increasingly secular, psychological views, as well as by clergy more attuned to the modern world, blaming the other person has become less prevalent. Contributing to this trend, matrimonial lawyers, enlightened and influenced by psychological and sociological considerations, have fought for no-fault divorce laws.[47] Gradually these are being adopted by various states. The women's liberation movement has also helped influence this move away from blame, partly by questioning the harsh and unrealistic alimony settlements frequently accompany divorce. In effect the argument is that alimony should not be "blood" or "guilt" money.

Basically the move toward divorce as a generally acceptable alternative has meant the freedom to get out of a marriage that is irretrievable.[48,49] Marriage has come a long way—from a closed, restricted, and restricting relationship that, if luck was with them, might still be satisfying to a couple but, if luck was not with them, was a prison built of bars of duty, religious sanctions, and strong societal disapproval.

Impact on the family

The vast changes that were so affecting dating and the viability and nature of marriage were also at work on the family, altering its structure, radically limiting or undermining its basic purposes, transforming the roles of its members, and eroding its potentials for providing psychological comfort to members.

CHANGES THAT ALTERED FAMILY STRUCTURE

The rural-to-urban shift streamlined the family's structure from extended to nuclear.* This change deprived the children of consistent contact with the extra and often more objective role models and surrogates of grandparents, aunts, uncles, and cousins. It also took away the supports that these extended family members could provide and gave the children fewer close people to relate to. In an urban setting, babysitters were usually drawn from the ranks of nonfamily members—a fact that deprived children of contacts which had helped to foster a greater sense of family identity. Thus the long slide of children's alienation from close family identification often began with the rural-to-urban shift.

CHANGES THAT LIMITED THE PURPOSES AND FUNCTIONS OF THE FAMILY

Many of the changes occurring in the United States had a limiting effect on the purposes and functions of family life that had constituted its reasons for being.[50,51] Its principle purposes of procreation, perpetuating the human race, and creating a sizable work force were sharply limited by various changes. Medical advances gradually lowered the infant and child mortality rates so that it was not necessary for a woman to bear as many children to offset a high death rate. Better functioning contraceptive devices made this possible. And as the pioneering work of Margaret Sanger and others in promoting family planning made slow headway against societal and religious resistance, family planning became a reality.[52] This reality joined with another change to cut back family size: the move from country to city eliminated the need for large numbers of children to help with the work. In fact, in an urban, one-breadwinner setting, children became burdens or luxuries, since there was often no productive work for them to do, but they still had to be fed and clothed and cared for.

Other changes also worked against the purpose of procreation. As secularism increased, God's command to "Be fruitful, and multiply" exerted less force as a major reason for marriage and family. As this occurred and as psychology encouraged people to focus on achieving individual happiness rather than merely perpetuating the human race and working constantly, better forms of contraception made it more possible to control family size. At the same time, affluence was making it possible for small families to live in higher style. Thus the trend toward limiting family size ultimately weakened the link between marriage and family, and gradually the subordination of marriage to family became less and less advantageous or desirable.

More recent changes have also had their impact on this growing split between marital and family purposes.

1. The counterculture proclaimed that nonmarried persons could care for children just as well as married people could and proceeded, at times, to prove out their contention in unmarried parenthood and communes. The women's liberation movement came along shortly thereafter and directly challenged the traditional beliefs that biology is woman's destiny and that she gains her "natural" fulfillment only in the roles of childbearer and nurturer. To back up its contention that a woman should have full sovereignty over her body and her Self, advocates of woman's liberation have fought hard for the right to legal abortions. Only when a woman has sovereignty, the movement contends, can she make a free

---

*A **nuclear family** normally consists of two married adults who are parents to one or more children (whether created by the spouses or adopted), all of whom ordinarily live together as an interrelated group. A one-parent family may also be a nuclear family.

choice about her destiny. In effect, the woman's liberation movement has battled to gain feasible alternatives to what has traditionally been most women's only available and permissible role—that of family producer and manager. In fighting and partially winning this battle, the women's liberation movement has helped to widen the already existing gap between marital and family relationships.

2. Another change that has helped to undercut the family purpose of procreation has been the growing concerns about ecology. Now, procreation is almost a dirty word in an era that, it is argued, could benefit most from Zero Population Growth.[53] Thus another reason looms for separating marriage from its original purpose of creating a family.

3. The other purpose or function of the family that has been significantly affected is socialization.[54,55] Many rural children went to school for only six or seven months because they were needed to work the land. Learning was the only activity allowed to compete with work, and work often took precedence; thus schools usually did not offer social or athletic activities. With the shift to urban living, however, the whole picture changed. Children had more time for school. Because they were going to have to compete in an industrial job market, they often needed the verbal and mathematical skills that schools were geared to impart. Schools became more important, and children spent more time in them. Also, since there was far less to do around home, children tended to stay where their peers were. Gradually the schools offered more and more activities of a social nature and thus became the center of young people's lives. Increasingly the schools became the chief socializer, since whoever claims the bulk of the child's time tends to have the chief socializing effect. As time went on and secularism increased, children spent less time not only at home but also in church-centered activities. Again, schools moved into the socializing void. That void had become larger because of the loss of the extended family role models; because fathers spent more and more time at their jobs, and because during and after World War II many mothers also joined the job market. As affluence and mass production fertilized each other, another socializer appeared on the scene—television.[56] Many parents happily greeted television's arrival. It distracted the children and thus gave the parents a chance to have some time to and for themselves.

The children, of course, rarely objected—except when the programs were impossibly bad. By and large, family life lost out in competition with school activities and television entertainment. Thus minimal time for generational togetherness meant that the family functioned less and less as a socializer. In effect the family simply no longer had the same purposes that had once held it together in a much tighter unit.

CHANGES THAT ALTERED THE ROLES OF FAMILY MEMBERS

Family roles did not stay the same. With few exceptions, the changes that occurred in each role category meant an undercutting of the authoritarian patriarchal family system. A number of families experienced this erosion during the Depression[57]: frequently, the man could not get a job, whereas the woman could at least get domestic work. Often this had a devastating effect on the father's self-esteem because suddenly the woman—contrary to both his and her expectations—was the family's support. But even if this kind of situation did not occur in a family, the shift from rural to urban living had its own subverting impact on the patriarchy, since most fathers worked away from the home and therefore could not exert as much influence on the governance of the household. Although many such fathers still maintained their authoritarian stance, for many men the outside demands on their time and energy weakened the impact of their authority. The higher on the job ladder a man was, often the higher the rate of attrition—and many more men moved up the ladder when they were able to get the necessary college degree because of the G.I. Bill and later because of increased prosperity. World War II had already broken the continuity of the patriarchal system by pulling many fathers away from families for the duration (or forever). After the war, many companies began to demand a good deal of travel from its executives, again adding to the "absentee-father syndrome."

Since most families had become nuclear families, absentee fathers meant that much of the time mothers had to fill in for fathers. However, because of their female role training, women tended not to rely so directly on flat-out authoritarianism, a tendency that also undermined the authority of the patriarchal system. It was even further undermined when—encouraged first by World War II's allowance of women into the work force, later by timesaving appliances, and even later by the women's liberation movement—many women entered the job market. That, of course, pulled both parents out of the home, a circumstance that cut down on the time and energy either of them might have to devote to running a tight, authoritarian ship.

One other event that has had enormous impact on the attitudes underlying the patriarchal system has been the publicity about and the slowly growing acceptance of women's liberation. One of the key ideas this movement advances is that the traditional rigid role ascriptions for men and women are harmful to both sexes. The woman's traditional role of passive submission to her husband's authority and the man's traditional role of aggressive authoritarianism prevents each of them from realizing his or her individual potential and blocks each from empathizing with the other's *human* position. The better way, advocates of women's liberation contend, is for each partner to act on his or her own humanness and for them to share the joys and responsibilities equally.[58,59]

This drive to humanize the family by humanizing its members' roles has also extended to the children. Psychology urged and frequently persuaded people to recognize that children are people too. Their thoughts and feelings should be respected.[60,61] Some adults nowadays tend to deplore the "Dr. Spock school of permissive thought" as having gone too far and contributing to the ruination of youth. Nevertheless, the impact of Dr. Spock's books and those of others espousing the individuality of infants and children seems to have provided a necessary antidote to the repressive and rigid role training given to children under the traditional authoritarian family system.[62]

No doubt many children were spoiled by permissive parents, and no doubt such permissiveness seriously undermined the authoritarian system of "the good old days."[63] But permissive child-rearing theories were hardly the only contributor. Parents' own needs and feelings have been deeply involved. Many parents who grew up during the Depression and then made money during World War II but did not have much to spend it on could not wait to shower their children with material goodies. This was their way, apparently, of making it up to their own deprived inner child. In a sense, many parents helped scuttle their own authoritarian ship by being overly permissive.

In other and more constructive ways, parents also undercut the authoritarian closed system. Since World War II, the parental generation has been involved in its own slow move toward openness. As these parents tentatively tried out new attitudes, values, and life-styles, they were challenging the old, closed system.[64,65] And as they did this, their methods of parenting were gradually changing. Because they began to value independence, individuality, tolerance, and experimentation for themselves, they were by extension teaching and encouraging their children to value these goals, too. The concomitants to these values were the freedom or permission to go off in search of them and the security to return home if young people wanted to.

As permissiveness was gaining strength, religious authority was losing strength. With it went much of the moral force that upheld the family patriarchal system, since if the churches lost authority, then the commandment to "honor thy father and mother" lost much of its absolute power. And when those governed by an absolutist authoritarian system no longer believe in or assent to these absolutes, then authority begins to lose its dominance, since the real power base of authority rests primarily on the consent and assent of the governed. If enough of them refuse to accept authority, then authority collapses unless it can back its threats with actual physical force. Even that is not always enough.

The counterculture proved this. The actions of counterculture members also sharply outlined the family's difficulty in fulfilling one of its increasingly important and necessary functions—providing a stable and protective atmosphere in which intimacy, trust, interdependence, and growth were possible. At the very time when a smaller family size and a decrease in the survival motive made stability and security more possible and when security was much needed in an insecure world, the family seemed unable to meet those needs. The impact of various changes had had their corrosive effects. The rural-to-urban shift had delivered the children's time and interest to the schools. The combination of affluence and technological advances had helped drive the wedge between parents and children. The teenager's private telephone enabled him to communicate with his peers rather than with his family, and the second car enabled him to leave and stay away from his family for long periods of time. The television served as a babysitter and distraction and blocked anything more than transitory communication. It is little wonder then that substitute peer group families often exerted more influence on young people than did their blood families.

Through the drug and sexual revolutions and the antiwar protests, the young people of the counterculture pulled away from parental values and life-styles and went their own emotional way. But whether a young person actually belonged to the counterculture, he often shared one experience with its members—the generation gap.[66]

Whichever side of the gap any of us stands on, we all feel to some degree a poignant sense of loss regarding the family. Family unity seems rare; communication is often minimal. Parents feel the loss of their authority and influence; children feel alienated from their parents.

THE LEGACY OF A CLOSED SOCIETY

What is so striking about all these changes that have occurred in dating, marriage, and family life is that we are still not free, still not very open. Most of us, to one degree or another, are still affected by the rules and values of an earlier, more closed society, and many of us are still governed by them. One of the strongest societal teachings is that we should evaluate ourselves and others primarily according to externals. Thus we tend to evaluate people and their relationships in terms of the ways we are taught that people, friendships, and social, dating, marital, and family relationships are *supposed* to operate. As a result, we tend to perceive and assess people and relationships according to their outsides, to externals, even as we long for more intimate and more open ways of relating to one another.

Rules and values from the past

It is important to consider what earlier rules and values about dating, marriage, and family life still exist and therefore may have some degree of emotional hold on us. As you read these lists, try checking your own inside reactions closely to see whether any of these rules and values have even a vestige of influence on your emotions, although you may *think* that some of them are ridiculous or obsolete.

DATING RULES AND VALUES

This list is by no means complete, but it will serve to point out the restrictive nature of earlier (and sometimes current) dating conventions, as well as the emphasis that is placed on appearances.

1. In a dating situation the boy should be aggressive (take the lead); the girl should be passive (let him take the lead). Only in rare and specifically designated circumstances should the girl ask the boy out.
2. On a date the girl should listen and pay close attention to the boy. In effect, she should "feed his ego." The boy should try to impress her; he should show her a good time, spend money on her, and look out for her comfort.
3. In a dating situation, the boy pays their way; the girl repays him with emotional or sexual favors or both.
4. A girl and boy who are going steady should not date or be interested in other people.
5. A girl should never let him kiss her on the first date; if she does, he will think she is "fast." (Perhaps the modern version of this is "a girl should never go to bed with a guy on their first date, or he'll think she's an easy mark.")
6. It's all right for a couple who are going steady to engage in heavy petting, but they shouldn't "go all the way."
7. It's all right for a boy to have sex before marriage but not for a girl (the infamous double standard).
8. When dating, both the boy and the girl should be on their best behavior: they should look their best, act nice, be friendly, and be sophisticated or at least appear adequate to the occasion.
9. A person shouldn't share his or her inner thoughts and feelings with his or her date; that might turn or scare the other person off.
10. A person shouldn't ask his or her date personal questions.
11. "You never really know a person till you marry (or live with) him or her."

Although only a partial one, this list gives some idea of the restrictive nature of the rules and values governing dating behavior. This list also makes clear how societal values encourage shallowness, nonintimacy, and outright deception. Masks and psychological games are the norm established by values like these, since they encourage distortion and reliance on externals and work against openness.

MARRIAGE RULES AND VALUES

The high expectations, demanding rules, and values were not confined to dating but governed marriage too.

1. Marriage partners should love only each other.
2. No matter what one spouse does, the other will love him (her) just because they are married.
3. Marriage is forever.
4. Marriage should offer security, status, meaning, and respectability.
5. When two people marry, they "become one."
6. Married couples should be regarded and treated as a unit.
7. Sex within marriage is the only legal, proper, and "right" kind of sex. It is the wife's duty to satisfy her husband's sexual needs and desires, but even if she does not satisfy him, it is wrong for him to masturbate.
8. Mutual masturbation, oral-genital sex, anal sex, and all but the most common and well-known positions of intercourse are perverted. Such perversions are carried out only by and with prostitutes.
9. All married couples should want to have children.
10. The wife's place is in the home; the

husband's place is outside the home, earning money.

11. Married couples should have no secrets from each other.
12. If I love you, you ought to love me. If I'm nice to you, you ought to be nice to me—because we're married.
13. Married couples should present a united front to the rest of society no matter what their private conflicts and problems may be.
14. Through marriage, each partner can and should try to meet all the physical, emotional, intellectual, and social needs of the other partner.

What is so striking about these rules and values is their limiting, restricting, and sometimes crippling nature. To live up to the expectations that are both implicit and explicit and to abide by the rules and values set forth would be an emotional burden of enormous and far-reaching consequences. Yet many people—perhaps most—did indeed try to abide by these rules and values. And many still do.

FAMILY RULES AND VALUES

As it was with marriage, so it was with family life. There were all kinds of rules and values that explicitly and rigidly directed how family members should think, feel, and act.

1. A family must present a united front to the rest of society no matter what the realities within the family structure. The family should keep its problems to itself: no member should open closets and let skeletons fall out.
2. Blood is thicker than water: don't trust outsiders.
3. You can trust and rely on your family.
4. Family interests are more important than those of individual members; family goals take precedence over individual goals.
5. The allegiance of family members belongs first and foremost to their family.
6. The family's rules and ways are right; family members (especially the children) should not question but should obey them.
7. Family members must protect each other from threats originating outside the home.
8. Each member is expected to believe that if I love you, you should love me. If I'm nice to you, you should be nice to me—because we belong to the same family.
9. Parents must (or just naturally do) love their children no matter what. Children must love, respect, and obey their parents no matter what.
10. Parents must present a united front of love and agreement to their children.
11. Family members should just automatically know what other members feel.
12. Sex should never be discussed in the family as a group. Mothers should teach their daughters, and fathers their sons, the facts of life.
13. Each family member should stay within the limits of his prescribed role; e.g., mother should not try to fix the plumbing, father should not do the wash, and children should act their age and respect their elders.
14. Every family is a unit with agreed on expectations, goals, values.
15. The family affords its members love, stability, and security.
16. The family is the best and the only *right* structure within which to raise a child and have a happy and fulfilling life.

This list of family rules and values is just as disconcerting as the list of those for dating and marriage; their nature is just as restricting and limiting. The family rules and values add other twists, however: they present the family as a monolithic structure that is impregnable, unchangeable, unchallengeable. As these teachings would have it, the family structure leaves little room for the individual to be an individual.

Moreover it prevents the family from functioning as a healthy influence on its members. In a sense, these rules and values portray the family as a semitotalitarian mini-state. If people adhere to, believe in, and operate on the basis of these rules and values (no matter how good their intentions), the resulting family structure is likely to resemble a totalitarian society. ►IE-2, p. 29.

Problems created by the legacy

If you look back over these lists, two things stand out. At least some of these rules and values (or variations of them) are still in effect in our society. And many of them work *against* flexibility, personal freedom and responsibility, effective communication, and open interaction. In essence they conflict with and work against openness because they require the individual (if he is to live by them) to accommodate himself to a rigid mold. They encourage the individual to evaluate himself, others, and life on the basis of appearances, externals; and they also encourage him to play roles, mask, distort, be deceptive, and play games. In short, they perpetuate closedness.

Although many people no longer subscribe to them, these rules and values nevertheless still exert enough emotional influence on us so that even if we go against them, we often have to contend with guilt feelings, feelings of disappointment with self, and/or the disapproval of others. Thus even now in our more open society, many people tend to evaluate themselves, others, and relationships on the basis of outsides and to act in accordance with these outsides. Unfortunately, since most of us have little training in looking or going beyond these externals, we tend either to stay on fairly shallow levels of relationships or to plunge into and flounder in the deeper levels. Whatever happens, however, many of us usually are ill prepared and ill equipped to deal with the *insides* (our own and others' inner thoughts and feelings) of relationships. Yet these are what primarily control and direct the course of our experiences with others.

Still emotionally tied to values emphasizing outsides, lacking the training necessary to knowing how to get in touch with their own and others' inner thoughts and feelings, many people tend to back away from the growing openness in society. The openness arouses anxiety because it has eroded the security offered by the rigidity of old rules and values. For example, an old value like "marriage is forever," although it may have been restrictive, was at least definite. Now, if marriage is not forever, how long will it or should it or can it last? If intimacy (both emotional and sexual) is permissible before marriage, how much is permissible? At what age? And, perhaps most threatening of all, how does a person go about achieving intimacy? In effect the old rules and values that carefully taught us to mask, play games, and evaluate one another and our relationships according to appearances and externals now are being challenged, and many are crumbling. Much of our anxiety comes from not knowing what will take the place of the old values.

Interaction experiences

1. Understanding early family life (p. 16)

Obtain the permission of a person over the age of 65 years to interview him about "the good old days." Explain that this is an assignment for a course and that you would like to get his ideas and feelings about dating, marriage, and family life in the early 1900s. Schedule the interview for at least 45 minutes.

Explain to the interviewee that there are no right or wrong answers to your questions but that you mainly want to get a feel for the climate of the times when he was a young person living in a family, perhaps "courting" or considering marriage. Reassure him that confidential information will not be revealed.

Ask what early societal attitudes, rules, values, and expectations about dating, marriage, and family life your interviewee grew up with. Explain what a double bind is and ask if he recalls situations in which there seemed to be strong, diametrically opposed alternatives. Does he feel his own attitudes and values have changed or stayed the same over the years? What does he think of the state of affairs in these areas today? Would he want to go back to the earlier society or remain in the "now world"? Overall, does the interviewee describe early conditions as conveying closed or open dating, marriage, and family life practices?

EVALUATION: Would you say that you got a good picture of and feel for the "good old days"? Was it an enjoyable experience for both you and the interviewee?

FOLLOW-UP: Write a summary of this experience and consider sharing the nonconfidential parts of it in class.

2. Understanding your rules and values about dating, marriage, and the family (p. 28)

Make a list of your own rules and values about dating, marriage, and the family. Compare your lists with those on pp. 26 and 27 of this chapter. Next, make a list of what you think are your parents' rules and values.

EVALUATION: Are your listed rules and values different from and more open than those given in this chapter? Those of your parents? How do these differences (or similarities) affect your life? If you operate on the basis of rules and values that are more open than those of the early 1900s or of your parents, how does this greater openness affect your life? How does it affect your relationship with your parents? With your peers? With society? Do you experience any feelings of being caught in double binds (as defined and described on pp. 4 and 5).

FOLLOW-UP: Share your lists with one or more members of the class. Discuss your feelings about the differences and similarities and their effects on you. Discuss also how you try to deal with the differences and similarities and their effects on you. You might also show your list of what you think are their rules and values to your parents and share your thoughts and feelings with them.

REFERENCES

1. Calhoun, Arthur W.: A social history of the American family: from 1865 to 1919, vol. 3, New York, 1946, Barnes & Noble, Inc., pp. 283-322.
2. Kephart, William M.: The family, society and the individual, ed. 2, Boston, 1966, Houghton Mifflin Co., pp. 120-149.
3. Turner, E. S.: A history of courting, New York, 1955, E. P. Dutton & Co., Inc.
4. Kenkel, William F.: The family in perspective, New York, 1966, Meredith Publishing Co., pp. 178-183.
5. Ibid., pp. 175-176.
6. Ibid., pp. 172-175.
7. Goode, William J.: World revolution and family patterns, New York, 1963, The Free Press.
8. Goosell, Willystine: A history of marriage and the family, New York, 1934, The Macmillan Co., pp. 355-427.
9. Kenkel, op. cit., pp. 176-178.
10. Ogburn, William F.: The changing family, The Family **19**:139-143, July, 1938.
11. Cottrell, Fred: Technology, man and progress, New York, 1972, Charles E. Merrill Publishing Co.
12. Skolnick, Arlene S., and Skolnick, Jerome H.: Family in transition, Boston, 1971, Little, Brown & Co., pp. 7-30.
13. Rimmer, Robert H.: The Harrad experiment, New York, 1966, Bantam Books, Inc.
14. O'Neill, Nena, and O'Neill, George: Shifting gears: finding security in a changing world, New York, 1974, M. Evans & Co., Inc.
15. Freud, Sigmund: A general introduction to psychoanalysis, New York, 1943, Garden City Publishing Co.
16. Hamilton, Eleanor: Sex before marriage, New York, 1970, Bantam Books, Inc.
17. Kinsey, Alfred C., Pomeroy, Wardell B., and Martin, Clyde E.: Sexual behavior in the human male, Philadelphia, 1948, W. B. Saunders Co.
18. Kinsey, Alfred C., Pomeroy, Wardell B., Martin, Clyde E., and Gebhard, Paul H.: Sexual behavior in the human female, Philadelphia, 1953, W. B. Saunders Co.
19. Goldsen, Rose K., and others: What college students think, Princeton, 1960, D. Van Nostrand Co., Inc., pp. 74-80.
20. Roszak, Theodore: The making of a counter culture, Garden City, New York, 1968, Doubleday & Co., Inc.
21. McGinnis, Thomas C.: A girl's guide to dating and going steady, Garden City, N.Y., 1968, Doubleday & Co., Inc.
22. Berger, Miriam E.: Trial marriage: harnessing the trend constructively, Family Coordinator **20**:38-43, Jan., 1971.
23. LeShan, Eda J.: Mates and roommates: new styles in young marriages, Public Affairs Pamphlet, No. 468, 1971.
24. Rogers, Carl: Becoming partners: marriage and its alternatives, New York, 1972, Delacorte Press.
25. Delora, Jo Ann S., and Delora, Jack R., editors: Intimate life style: marriage and its alternatives, Pacific Palisades, Calif., 1972, Goodyear Publishing Co., Inc.
26. Kanter, Rosabeth Moss: Communes, Psychology Today **4**:53-57, July, 1970.
27. Bernard, Jessie: The future of marriage, New York, 1972, World Publishing Co.
28. St. Andre, Lucien: The American matriarchy: a study of married life in 1997, A.D., Madison, N.J., 1970, Florham Park Press, Inc.
29. Friedan, Betty: The feminine mystique, New York, 1964, Dell Publishing Co., Inc.
30. Statement of purpose, National Organization of Women, Washington, D.C., Oct. 29, 1966.
31. Cox, Frank: American marriage; a changing scene? Dubuque, Iowa, 1971, William C. Brown Co., Publishers.
32. Udry, J. R.: The social context of marriage, Philadelphia, 1966, J. B. Lippincott Co., pp. 25-26.
33. Blanck, Rubin, and Blanck, Gertrude: Marriage and personal development, New York, 1968, Columbia University Press, pp. 9-17.
34. Ellis, Albert, and Harper, Robert A.: Creative marriage, New York, 1961, Lyle Stuart, Inc.
35. Komarovsky, Mirra: Blue-collar marriage, New York, 1964, Random House, Inc.
36. Bird, Lois: How to be a happily married mistress, Garden City, N.Y., 1971, Doubleday & Co., Inc.
37. Hunt, Morton: The affair: a portrait of extramarital love in contemporary America, New York, 1969, World Publishing Co.
38. Neubeck, Gerhard, editor: Extramarital relations, Englewood Cliffs, N.J., 1969, Prentice-Hall, Inc.
39. Back, Kurt W.: Beyond words: the story of sensitivity training and the encounter movement, New York, 1972, Russell Sage Foundation.
40. Howard, Jane: Please touch: a guided tour of the human potential movement, New York, 1970, McGraw-Hill Book Co.
41. Altback, Edith Hoshino, editor: From feminism to liberation, Cambridge, Mass., 1971, Schenkman Publishing Co., Inc.
42. Hunt, Morton: World of the formerly married, New York, 1966, McGraw-Hill Book Co.
43. Fisher, Esther O.: Help for today's troubled marriages, New York, 1968, Hawthorne Books, Inc.

44. Rutledge, Aaron L.: Pre-marital counseling, Cambridge, Mass., 1966, Schenkman Publishing Co., Inc.
45. Silverman, Hirsh L.: Marital counseling: psychology, ideology, science, Springfield, Ill., 1967, Charles C Thomas, Publisher.
46. Krantzler, Mel: Creative divorce, New York, 1973, M. Evans & Co., Inc.
47. Donelson, Kenneth, and Donelson, Irene: Married today, single tomorrow: marriage break-up and the law, Garden City, N.Y., 1969, Doubleday & Co., Inc.
48. Bohannon, Paul, editor: Divorce and after, Garden City, N.Y., 1971, Doubleday & Co., Inc.
49. Fisher, Esther: Divorce counseling—the new freedom: a guide to divorcing and divorce counseling, New York, 1974, Harper & Row, Publishers.
50. Ackerman, Nathan W.: The psychodynamics of family life, New York, 1958, Basic Books, Inc., Publishers, p. 19.
51. Skolnick and Skolnick, op. cit., pp. 7-8.
52. Whelpton, Pascal K., Campbell, Arthur A., and Patterson, John E.: Fertility and family planning in the U. S., Princeton, 1966, Princeton University Press.
53. Erskine, H.: More on the population explosion and birth control polls, Public Opinion Quarterly **31**:303-313, 1967.
54. Kaluger, George, and Kaluger, Meriem Fair: Human development: the span of life, St. Louis, 1974, The C. V. Mosby Co.
55. McNeil, Elton B.: Human socialization, Monterey, Calif., 1969, Brooks/Cole Publishing Co.
56. Cooke, Alistair: Is television changing America? U.S. News and World Report, April 15, 1974.
57. Cavan, Ruth Shonle, and Ranck, Katherine Howland: The family and the depression, Chicago, 1938, University of Chicago Press.
58. Brenton, Myron: The American male, New York, 1966, Coward-McCann, Inc.
59. Janeway, Elizabeth: Man's world, woman's place; a study in social mythology, New York, 1971, William Morrow & Co., Inc.
60. Ginott, Haim G.: Between parent and child, New York, 1965, The Macmillan Co.
61. Ginott, Haim G.: Between parent and teenager, New York, 1969, The Macmillan Co.
62. Levey, John, and Munroe, Ruth: The happy family, New York, 1962, Alfred A. Knopf, Inc.
63. Fletcher, Grace Nies: What's right with us parents? New York, 1972, William Morrow & Co., Inc.
64. Gordon, Thomas: Parent effectiveness training, New York, 1970, Peter H. Wyden/Publisher.
65. Mead, Margaret: Culture and committment: a study of the generation gap, Garden City, N.Y., 1970, Doubleday & Co., Inc.
66. Teenagers discuss the generation gap, Office of Child Development, Washington, D.C., 1970, U.S. Government Printing Office.

chapter 2
THE NATURE OF MARRIAGE

Writing about marriage is not as easy in the 1970s as it once was; so many aspects have changed, so many questions have been raised about it, and so much about marriage has been challenged. Is marriage really dead or dying?[1] Or is it alive and well in most of the cities, towns, and hamlets across the country? Is it any longer necessary? Is it workable? Why bother with it? How is it different from other kinds of relationships? Is it better or worse than other relationship arrangements? Who needs it? Who wants it? Is it the only workable way? Or is there another, better way?

Yet even in the face of all these questions, marriage still seems to be far ahead of whatever is in second place. Apparently the majority of people in this country, if necessary, "would rather fight than switch." The facts are that most people in the United States get married at least once, and the great majority of those who get divorced then remarry. Apparently most people want to, and do, try marriage. Thus it would seem that for all the problems that marriage may be heir to, it also offers many satisfactions. Perhaps one of its chief drawing cards is that it does offer a societally and religiously sanctioned relationship with clear ground rules that can provide guidance and direction to those who enter the relationship. The fact that marriage does have ground rules makes it seem more secure and understandable; people risk uncertainty and insecurity when they set out to create their own "game" and their own rules. Another drawing card is that marriage is, or seems to be, *the* most workable way to have and maintain a relationship between man and woman. There may be other ways, but this one is the most familiar and the one that has worked over a long, long period of time.

THE NEED FOR A CLOSE LOOK AT MARRIAGE

Whatever any of us thinks or feels about marriage and whatever our marital status may be, there are three particular reasons it is important that we take a thorough and careful look at the institution of marriage as it has been and, for the most part, still is in our society.

1. **Marriage** is still the predominant form of long-term heterosexual relationship practiced by the majority of people in this country and is still the one relationship of its kind sanctioned by society and religion. Since this is so, it is necessary to examine marriage closely to understand the central relationship of most people in our society.

2. By its very nature, marriage is the prototype of all long-term relationships: its essential characteristics and the issues particular to it are common to all long-term relationships. Thus whatever is said about marriage applies also (and equally) to *nonmarital* heterosexual and homosexual relationships that are built on long-term commitments. The awareness gained by examining the nature of marriage therefore applies to other long-term, two-person relationships in our society and can form the basis for the opening up process for anyone.

3. Another reason for examining the institution of marriage has to do with a basic tenet of the Interactional Therapeutic System: to make appropriate decisions, it is necessary to have information, insight, and

knowledge of alternatives. Consequently for you to make constructive and appropriate decisions about marriage (will you or won't you marry; what kind of marriage do you want—an open or a closed one), it is important that you learn as much about marriage as you can.

Unfortunately, for a variety of reasons, most people do not look closely enough at marriage before they get married. Some people say (and feel), "I don't want to know how complicated marriage is." Others say, "I don't want to know what the issues are. I'll just deal with them as I go along." Or "That takes all the fun out of it." Or "That kills the romance." Although they may not help to heighten romance, knowledge of and in-touchedness with the nature of marriage will more than likely help enrich the quality of the relationship. Certainly such knowledge and in-touchedness can enable you to make decisions and choices that are freedom granting rather than freedom limiting.

In the closed society of the past the individual's freedom with regard to characteristics and issues was severely limited by a lack of awareness of them or by directives about how he should and should not think, feel, and act in relation to them.

The primary purpose of this chapter is to help you become aware of characteristics and issues of marriage so that you will be in a position to deal consciously, deliberately, and openly with them. Thus you will be able to avoid (at least to a significant degree) getting caught by the power of old directives and by the conflict between that power and the greater openness you might desire in your relationships. By working consciously with these characteristics and issues, you will have the opportunity to gain control over how you will handle them and how you will relate to yourself and your partner.

Values of the past

As you think about the societal (and religious) values that govern traditional marriage, note how limiting and rigid, how fostering of closedness they tend to be. Depending on your background, point of view, and perhaps experience, you may see such limits and rigidity as either advantageous or disadvantageous.

Following are three *possible advantages* of traditional marriage:

1. By adhering strictly to the specifications, you could minimize confusion or doubt about your duties, rights, obligations, and roles. For example, suppose you were raised with a value that "sex is forbidden." However, since both religion and society sanction sexual relations between husband and wife, you at least have support in going against that value once you marry.
2. You gain a societal identity, since by agreeing to the terms of traditional marriage, you have publicly assumed a definite position recognized by your society.
3. By conforming to these specifications, you receive the approval and support of society and religion for your actions.[2]

There are, of course, *possible disadvantages* also:

1. You bind yourself "forever" to a relationship that could change radically over a period of time. For example, suppose you married a person who ten years later began to drink heavily, became an alcoholic, and could not or would not try to stop. By the rules of the original contract, you would have bound yourself to a relationship you never anticipated.
2. Because people regard and treat you and your mate as a unit, you both could lose some of your individuality.
3. As a result of the narrow and rigid role prescriptions, the wife is locked into the stereotype of the domestic, inferior female; the husband is locked into the stereotype of the "hunter," the strong man, the breadwinner. The strain can be great and extremely counterproductive for each of them.

It is true that many married couples do not adhere that closely to these specifications. The current divorce rate alone testifies to that fact.[3] In addition, many married couples who stay married make accommodations to and modify these rules and values. For example, some couples choose not to act primarily as a unit: each cherishes his individuality, each lives his own life, and each goes his own way. Numerous couples do not agree with or try to fulfill the rigid role prescriptions: for example, over 50% of the married women in the United States work outside the home.[4] And all of us know of at least one marriage in which the wife, not the husband, is the real head of the household.

MARRIAGE: ITS NATURE

Essentially the qualities that determine the nature of marriage may be divided into two large categories—characteristics and issues. The characteristics of marriage define its nature by description. Issues define the nature of marriage in terms of content and function.

Core characteristics of marriage

The **core characteristics of marriage** are those characteristics which are intrinsic to the nature of the marital relationship. They are constants; they are always present in this relationship, and they exert continuing and significant influences on each other, on the ways each partner interacts with the other, and on the development of their relationship.

The core characteristics of marriage include intellectual balance, religion, race, ethnic background, socioeconomic class, partners' ages, number of marriages, "age" of the present marriage, and number of children. Since there are such a large number of influences and effects, we will describe only some of the possibilities.

INTELLECTUAL BALANCE

Whether covertly or overtly, consciously or unconsciously, a couple strikes some kind of intellectual balance between them. If they are approximately equal in intelligence and common sense, this kind of balance ordinarily tends to make the fewest "waves" between them. If, however, they are equal but one of them has worries concerning masculine/feminine roles, then trouble may arise. For example, if the husband believes that a man should be smarter than his wife, he may waste a lot of time and energy trying to prove to himself, her, and others that he is really smarter than she.

If the wife has had instilled in her the idea that a woman should *never* appear as smart as a man, that a smart woman is not attractive to men, then she may play down or belittle her intelligence and act less intelligent than she really is, especially when they are together in public. She may retreat into her wifely role and become, for example, superhousekeeper and superhomemaker, leaving the intellectual forum to him.

If one is smarter than the other, the smarter one may lord it over the less-smart one or may simply be himself or herself and let things happen as they will. Or the smarter one may acknowledge his or her intellectual superiority but value the other's common sense or emotional perceptiveness.

Whatever intellectual balance exists, however, is less important than the way each (and both) of the partners reacts to and uses the balance. These reactions and uses will depend, of course, on who each partner is.

RELIGION

Whatever the religious background and affiliation, each partner thinks, feels, acts, and interacts in relation to some religious position (even if it is a nonreligious one of atheism) because every human being must in some way deal with certain moral, spiritual, and philosophical questions. For example, if both partners adhere to fairly orthodox religious beliefs, then they are likely to see marriage as a forever commitment, they probably have strong rules against premarital and extramarital sex, and they are more likely to subscribe to the notion of a relationship based on patriarchal authority. Whatever the specific formal religion may be, in effect the partners operate basically in terms of a closed society, which is described in Chapters 1 and 12.

If the partners do not adhere to formal, orthodox beliefs, they are not as likely to consider marriage as a forever commitment and probably feel freer to consider divorce as an alternative to a miserable relationship.

If the marital partners come from different religious backgrounds, then they may well face other problems that affect their relationship. Suppose a Catholic and a Protestant marry. In some way they have to deal with the Catholic church's fiats about interfaith marriages. For example, if the couple is married in a civil ceremony only, then the Catholic church does not consider them married in the eyes of God. Most certainly, that places some emotional burden on the Catholic partner, and it may arouse resentment in the non-Catholic partner. And if there are children, whose faith will they be raised in? If the Protestant partner insists on their being raised as Protestants, then the Catholic partner is penalized by his church. If the Catholic partner insists on a Catholic upbringing, then the Protestant partner may feel left out of the family (as might the Catholic in reversed circumstances) and angry because of feeling pressure to bow to another faith's demands.

Another example of potential interfaith clashes is the marriage between Jew and non-Jew. Again, the pressures exerted by the formal religion(s) and by outside factors (such as family and friends) can place great stresses on the marital relationship. These stresses and influences inevitably affect the kind of life-style that the marriage develops.

RACE

If the partners are of the same race, then the effects of this characteristic on the marital relationship are minimized. This is especially true if the couple are white. If the couple are from a racial minority, then any prejudices, stereotypes, and discrimination that are directed against the particular race obviously place strains on the marital relationship.

If the marriage is an interracial one, then special stresses are placed on the relationship. For example, if a black and a white marry, which race will they mix with socially? Which race will accept their marriage? Where will they live? How will each of them handle whatever latent prejudices he or she may have? Should they inflict their interracial choice on children? Again, questions and situations like these cannot help but have an effect on the ways the partners interact and on the kind and quality of relationship they develop.[5]

ETHNIC BACKGROUND

Ethnic background often has a strong influence on the roles and expectations of the partners. If both come from the same ethnic group and from families that have fairly similar degrees of adherence to that background, then each partner probably holds essentially the same expectations and sees the husband's and wife's roles in basically the same way. For example, if each is from a fairly strict Italian or Polish or Puerto Rican family, then each is probably used to certain stereotyped roles and expectations: the man is head of the household, the woman is subservient to him; masculinity and femininity are rather rigidly defined; the husband holds a job, the wife bears and raises the children; and the family (the extended family) is more important than the individuals in any given marriage.

If the marriage is between two people from different ethnic backgrounds, then problems may arise. For example, suppose an Anglo-Saxon Protestant woman marries a Puerto Rican Catholic man. She may expect to go on working; he may expect her to quit, stay home, and take care of the household and him. She may agree ahead of time to raise the children as Catholics but may be unprepared for the subtle and not-so-subtle pressures from his family for her to convert. She may end up feeling like a stranger in a strange land who is not used to accepting and not willing to accept always being relegated to the women's group while the men are talking and perhaps drinking with one another. He, on the other hand, may feel embarrassed because his wife comes across as too liberal, too outspoken for a woman, and his relatives therefore do not approve of her. Conversely, her friends and family may not approve of him because his sense of machismo is out of keeping with their values. They may, for example, find him arrogant and domineering.

SOCIOECONOMIC CLASS

Although it is probably less important now than it was fifty years ago, socioeconomic status still has an important effect on marital relationships. For example, the so-called blue collar class often has attitudes about such matters as men's and women's roles, money, social activities, sex, religion, and education that are different from, for example, the upper middle class's attitudes. The blue collar class tends to adhere to more traditional beliefs such as husband dominant/wife submissive and "a man's home is his castle." The upper middle class tends to see itself as more liberated about men's and women's roles. Also the more education a person has and the higher his socioeconomic status, the more willing he seems to be to experiment with new and out-of-the-ordinary sexual practices. For example, the Kinsey report showed that the higher up on the educational and socioeconomic scale people are the more likely they are to engage in oral-genital sex.[6]

Even when there is little if any disparity between the wife's and husband's socioeconomic backgrounds, their joint socioeconomic status as wife and husband influences their relationship. Whether they have too little, enough, or more than enough money and social standing, they still have to deal with the joys and problems generated by their socioeconomic status. Whatever the particular circumstances and even though times have changed considerably, socioeconomic status still has a significant influence on marital relationships.

PARTNERS' AGES

Not only do partners' ages exert a powerful influence on the marital relationship, but their ages also have different effects as they change. Not just the partners' ages at the time of marriage but also their ages at later times can have important consequences for the relationship.

The importance of partners' ages is sharply conveyed by the statistics on teenage divorces. The highest divorce rate occurs in marriages taking place between partners who are between the ages of 16 and 21 years.[7] Marriage demands numerous adjustments, and people in the 16 to 21 age bracket often are unwilling or unable (or both) to make the necessary adjustments. The primary reason for such difficulties is that people of these ages have simply not yet had enough time and life experiences to develop sufficient maturity. Many of them expect too much from their partner and the relationship; many are overly idealistic and tend to romanticize what is actually a realistic and demanding relationship based on the complicated interactions of two complex and unique individuals. Other problems that beset people who marry early are that they usually have had little time to enjoy the freedom from major responsibilities and other personal freedoms that ordinarily are a mark of this age period. Thus when they enter into marriage and face having to take on major responsibilities and give up or make significant concessions about personal freedoms, many young people want out. But whether they want out or to stay in, people who marry during these early years must deal with numerous pressures and situations, and that fact obviously has important influences on the life-style that develops for their relationship.

Perhaps the age group and span that can most justifiably be called "average" for marriage is that in which the partners are between the ages of 22 and 32 years and are close to one another in age (within one to three years). In terms of age, this situation is potentially the least conflictual, although some people in this optimum group may feel regret for not having married someone older or younger.

A marital arrangement that carries with it far more chance of conflict is one in which there is a considerable difference between the partners' ages. The less usual of the two possibilities is a younger man marrying an older woman. An age difference of three to five years would not really fit this category (although it could), but if the woman is, for example, ten years older, then the couple will have to deal with some special stresses. And most of these stresses are not pleasant, since, for whatever reasons, many people in our society disapprove of this kind of age difference. For example, one of the first questions (whether verbalized or not) that is likely to arise is "What's he doing—marrying his mother?" Another is "What is he—a gigolo?" Or "How come she's robbing the cradle?" Or "What could they possibly see in each other?" Whether these specific (and harsh) questions come up is less the point, however, than that people find it hard to emotionally accept a serious relationship between a younger man and an older woman. Somehow many people believe that it is just not "natural," "right," or "healthy." In addition to societal pressure, this kind of relationship faces possible stresses resulting from certain realities. For example, suppose the woman is in her early forties and is not willing to take the risks inherent in having children at her age (e.g., her body is less able to deal easily with the strains of childbirth; children born to a woman in this age bracket run a much higher risk of being born defective). But the man wants children. Obviously they are faced with a major decision. Or suppose he *did* marry her partly because of inner needs for an idealized "mothering" type of wife. In the course of the development of the relationship, he is likely to discover that she is a fallible human being who likes to be other things besides the mothering type.

The more usual type of age-difference marriage is one between a younger woman and an older man. For various reasons, society tends to accept this arrangement with much better grace. Although some people may say, "She's looking for a daddy—sugar or otherwise," by and large, the arrangement is generally accepted. Even so, there are likely to be inner stresses that have some impact on the relationship. For example, suppose she wants children but he already has three by an earlier marriage and does not want any more. Or suppose he just feels he is too old to be a good father. On the other hand, suppose he wants to start a family as soon as they get married, but she wants to have a few years of freedom before they have children.

One other age arrangement should be considered. This is the situation in which two older people get married for the first time. (By older, we mean over 35 years of age.) This discussion can also apply to a marriage in which one or both have been married before but have been unmarried for a long period of time. In this situation there may have to be numerous adjustments, since at least one of the partners has had a good deal of freedom to do as he pleased, go where he wanted, and live his life to suit himself. Marriage then can mean companionship, love, and joy, but it can also mean giving up some of the familiar freedom. By and large, it means adjusting to a new and different way and rhythm of life.

The other major effect that age has on marital relationships occurs because perspectives often change over the course of time. Sexual needs and desires change with age. For example, when women are well into the menopause, some of them become more interested in sex and more sexually active because their inhibitions decrease when they no longer are able to have children. A number of men and women also go through a period of reassessment when they reach their middle or late forties. They may decide to change their way of life—a change that may include divorce, separation, an affair, or simply a shake-up in their usual ways of acting.

If you consider all the different possibilities, age is an important influence on the marital relationship. It is important in terms of the "starting ages" of the partners, as well as their changing ages.

NUMBER OF MARRIAGES

The number of times each partner has been married before has a marked effect on the present relationship. For example, if this is the first marriage for both partners, various important factors are at work. Since they are experiencing, experimenting with, and having to adjust in some way to newness and difference, each partner is bound to feel some anxiety. The way each copes with the anxiety naturally influences the course of the relationship. One method they may use is to rely heavily on traditional roles and expectations; in this way they can cut down on the number of decisions they have to make. Other influencing factors may include questioning whether marriage was the right step, wondering if this is the right person, or regretting the gradual fading of the romantic dream. At the same time, each may be enjoying the new status; the approval and support of friends, relatives, and the community; and each other's company.

The marriage in which one partner has never been married before while the other one has been presents a different set of circumstances. For example, there may be a certain number of comparisons made between this marriage and new spouse and the former marriage and spouse. And the remarried spouse may be guarded about particular issues that were trouble spots in the first marriage.

If both partners have been married before, they may be far more serious and concerned about making this one work, and they may know better what they want. If one or both of the partners has children by a previous marriage, that fact makes the adjustment more involved and complex. Added to these complexities may be others such as some kind of continuing relationship—pleasant or otherwise—with the former spouse and perhaps the in-laws too.

Whatever the specific circumstances—whether this is the first or second or third or fifth marriage—obviously the number of marriages each partner has previously participated in has definite effects on the present relationship.

"AGE" OF THE PRESENT MARRIAGE

Although we will not treat the matter here, we do want to point out that the kind, variety, and amount of dating experience each partner has had obviously affect their marital relationship. Even if a couple have been living together for a considerable period of time (more than a year), if they decide to formalize their relationship by getting married, their decision will have a distinct effect on their relationship.

Whatever the dating background, the first year of marriage (both for those who have never been married and for those who have) is crucially important to the developing relationship.* It is especially during this first year that partners encounter and must deal with a lot of newness and differences.[8] During this year many key matters and issues must be worked out (or at least worked on)—such matters as expectations, roles, communication, and decision-making and such issues as money, sex, and relationships with friends and in-laws. Often the work that is done or not done during this time can contribute significantly to the later making or breaking of the relationship.

By the fifth year,† there has been time for many matters of consequence to occur. For example, there has been sufficient time

---

*So important is the first year of marriage that one of us (T.C.M.) devoted a book to the subject, *Your First Year of Marriage*, Garden City, N.Y., 1967, Doubleday & Co., Inc.

†There is nothing magical about the number of years we pick. They simply are handy numbers to indicate significant amounts of time. The first year, however, is an exception to this, since that particular year is important specifically *because* it is the first.

for the couple to have experienced a variety of different situations—perhaps the birth of children, a change in their socioeconomic status, a shift in occupation, or a change of living conditions—the possibilities are endless. There has been time for all the issues of marriage to have arisen and time for crises to have occurred. In effect, the couple has had a chance to see one another in action; to test out their abilities, inclinations, and disinclinations to work together constructively or destructively; and to measure the stuff of which each of them and the relationship are made. There has been sufficient time for each partner's patterns of behavior (both intrapersonal and interpersonal) to have become somewhat evident to each partner because of their repetition. There has been time for boredom to set in as the result of this knowledge, but there has been equal opportunity for comfort and delight to result from such intimate knowledge of another human being. In addition, some assessment of the road already traveled and of the road ahead probably takes place about the fifth year.

The same factors that apply to the fifth year apply as well to the tenth, but by the tenth year the weight of repetition is even greater. By this year there has been ample time for one or both of the partners to have been tempted by at least one extramarital affair, and one or both may have engaged in such an affair. One factor adding to some partners' vulnerability to a liason is that by the tenth year of marriage, boredom may have become an irritating constant in the marriage.

However, if the marriage has survived this far, there probably is a good deal now to tip the balance in favor of the partners' staying together. By this time most couples have a lot invested in the marriage: time, emotions, children, social position, relationships with others (including family ties), money, status, prestige, and security. And by this time, each partner's priorities may have changed somewhat: romance may now be less important than security; red-hot sexual relations may be less important than the joy of sharing intellectually, emotionally, and physically; and spending time with the children may take precedence over an active social life. By their tenth year many couples have in effect built their own marital institution.

By the twentieth year (or thereabouts) many marriages are entering or going through the stage of *marital menopause.* The children are starting to leave the nest, and in a society that is as child-centered as ours, the departure of the children can create a trauma, not only for mother but for father as well. These are the years of marital menopause also because the partners are often entering or are in their forties, a time when a person has lived at least half his life, a fact that startles many into a life crisis. It becomes a time when an individual tends to reassess his life and to ask, "Who am I?," "What have I done with my life so far?," "Where am I going?," and "What has happened to my hopes and dreams?"

A couple often goes through this kind of reassessment too; suddenly there is time and the occasion for asking, "Who are we?," "What kind of life together have we fashioned?," "Are we satisfied with ourselves and our relationship?," and "Do we want to grow old together, or do we want something quite different?" In the process of reevaluation, the couple may discover that they do not love each other now, if they ever did. Depending on their personalities, they may decide to separate or get divorced, or they may go on a second honeymoon to try to give love or affection a chance. The couple may discover after so many years of marriage that they really do not know one another or they have forgotten exactly what the other is like because they have been so busy raising a family, securing a career, and pursuing status and material goodies. Again, depending on what they are like, the couple may decide they do not want to get to know each other; they may stay together, or they may go their separate ways. Or they may decide to take the time to get to know one another.

Other years and other anniversaries are important too, but this survey at least suggests some of the numerous and varied influences that different time lengths can have on a marital relationship.

NUMBER OF CHILDREN

Like all the other core characteristics, the number of children can also have a powerful effect on the development of the marital relationship. For example, a couple may decide not to have children because they want to have one another to themselves. In this way they are likely to act more in their roles as individuals who are married to one another than in the stereotyped roles of wife and husband. Having no children may free them to build a close and long-lasting relationship, or it may enable them to feel less committed to the marriage and therefore freer to end it.

If a couple has only one child (or if there is only one for a long period of time), the couple may concentrate their time and energy on the child to the detriment of their own relationship. Or perhaps the wife gives most of her time and attention to the child, and the husband feels left out and jealous.

With the second child, the partners may be more relaxed because they now have some experience in parenting and feel more secure. They may get more pleasure out of their parental role, and that pleasure, plus the responsibilities of parenthood, may enhance their feelings of *coupleness.* Or with the second child and subsequent children the couple may become less of a couple and more of a parent unit, thereby lessening to some degree their sense of their marital identity. Or as they experience the pressures of parenting, they may become aware of their needs as individuals and marriage partners and "separate" themselves from the children at times. (This move may well include such ploys as "Go watch TV" and the locked bedroom door for the some-sex-on-Sunday-morning syndrome.)

• • •

If you look back over the nine core characteristics, their importance to and impact on marital interaction become evident. No matter when, where, or under what circumstances the interaction is occurring, the influence of these core characteristics is always present, always shaping the nature of the marital relationship. ►IE-1, p. 47.

The issues in marriage

Although this discussion is not a total or complete survey, the investigation of the issues that fall within the following thirteen categories helps illustrate the nature of marriage: (1) commitment and responsibility, (2) quality of the relationship, (3) power and decision-making, (4) roles, (5) time and togetherness, (6) in-laws (or outlaws?), (7) friends, (8) social life, (9) money, (10) housing, (11) major minimatters, (12) family planning, and (13) sex.

Although only a partial list, the number of issues set forth is impressive and gives some notion of the enormous potentials for complexity and richness of experience in this relationship. Furthermore, this survey clearly indicates both the range and type of issues that those who marry must in some way manage. Whether they manage by ignoring these issues, by working with them directly, by talking about them, by arguing about them, or by negotiating about them depends on the couple, the circumstances, and their relationship. But no matter what their intellectual abilities, age, race, religion, social status, education, or economic bracket, no married couple can avoid having to deal in some way with the majority of these issues.

It is important to remember that issues—in and of themselves—do not cause problems, and they do not bring satisfactions. Instead they raise questions that set up a need for communication and decisions of some kind and that somehow must be dealt with. Issues only cause problems or bring satisfactions in the sense that they elicit intellectual, emotional, or behavioral responses. If one (or both) of the partners is closed, then his perceptions, interpretations, and evaluations of the issues, his own responses, and the other partner's responses may be distorted. Consequently the responses will probably be inadequate, inappropriate, and conflictual; then there will be problems. If, however, both partners are in touch with their insides, are relatively open, communicate effectively, and apply the techniques of The System, their responses will likely be adequate, appropriate, and constructive; then there will be satisfactions. Thus it is not the issues themselves that make the difference; it is the people who handle these issues, the ways they handle them, and the ways they handle themselves.

As you read the following list of issues, you will probably notice that we have used a somewhat different writing style. Our reasons for this are twofold. First, by addressing you as "I" or "we" we are in effect asking you as you read to role play, to take the role of husband or wife or member of a married couple, so that you will get more of a feel for the issue and the responses it might elicit. It is one thing to read about people who worry about money or quarrel about their vacation plans; it is another matter to put yourself in the position of, to experience, the worrying and the quarreling. Our second reason for using this different style is that it invites you to experience (at least vicariously) the "I-you" and "I-they" identity positions as they occur in marriage.

ISSUE 1: COMMITMENT AND RESPONSIBILITY

Every person who thinks about marriage or decides to get married is inevitably faced with the issue of commitment to and responsibility toward the relationship and the chosen partner.[9] Some people resist thinking through the extent or meaning of the commitment because it just seems too awesomely final and total. Their feeling seems to be that once they say "I do," once they have chosen their overall course of action (marriage), there are few if any other choices left and little room for changes or adjustments.

Some people apparently just accept the stereotypes about marriage and make a vague, fuzzy commitment to the whole general matter without investigating any further. The philosophy here seems to be, "I'll play it by ear." Some people go further than that: they think seriously about marriage and what it may involve, and they make an *intellectual* commitment to the relationship. In other words, they think they can accept and commit themselves to what they know and understand about marriage, but they have little feeling for what marriage can and may involve, especially in emotional terms.

Some people react in the opposite way: they make an *emotional* commitment to marriage. They feel deeply about loving, comforting, honoring, and cherishing their partners. But they tend not to think a great deal about the everyday, practical, realistic matters that marriage entails.

In our survey of what commitment can involve, we try to give a broad range of content so that the thinking, feeling, and acting components are all represented. Our reasons for doing this are twofold:

1. We wish to emphasize the far-ranging nature of the commitments that a relationship like marriage can entail.

2. By presenting a large number and a good variety of possibilities, we want to suggest that the commitment a person makes to marriage cannot appropriately be a total or final one. Instead, we believe that perhaps the most appropriate and constructive action a person can take is to commit himself to trying as much and as often as possible to give responses based on a balanced blend of thinking, feeling, and acting.

In a sense the marriage ceremony itself says it all; the vows each person is asked to take are vows of deep and far-reaching commitment. Thus the initial and all-encompassing questions are "Are we willing to commit ourselves to each other publicly, legally, and religiously? If so, what does that commitment involve?"

The words of most traditional marriage ceremonies spell out clearly what is involved. Essentially these pledges speak to two major areas of commitment: the ways we should regard and treat each other and the conditions under which we should operate.

1. The key words directing the ways in which we should regard and treat each other are *love, comfort, honor, cherish, keep (maintain)* one another, and *forsake* all others. Do all these words taken together mean that we should try to fulfill all of each other's needs? Are we committing ourselves to a relationship in which no negative feelings are allowed? What happens if I don't always feel love for you, or you for me? What does "to comfort" mean? The essential issue then is what does each of us commit ourselves to when we take this vow? What do these vows mean to each of us?

2. The marriage pledges indicate that our commitment is a total one; that is, we are saying that we agree to love, comfort, honor, cherish, and keep each other *no matter what happens.*

For better or worse. Through good times and bad, through good moods and bad, through times of crisis, boredom, excitement, and depression—through all this will we continue to love, comfort, honor, and cherish each other? Is that possible?

For richer, for poorer. Am I willing to work so that you can finish or go back to school? Are you willing to do the same for me? Are we willing to scrimp and save, do without, or get extra jobs if there is not enough money? Will I look at you, the husband, as inadequate or weak or unmanly if you lose your job or don't get promoted? Will I look at you, the wife, as "stealing" my role or as "masculine" and aggressive if you get a job or if your job brings in more money than mine? Can we tolerate prosperity?

In sickness and in health. Can I, will I, assume responsibility for you if you get sick? Will you for me? How will you or I feel about the other if one of us becomes chronically ill? What if one of us has severe psychological problems? What if you or I become obese? What if I am scarred in an accident? What if one or both of us becomes addicted to drugs or alcohol? What happens then?

ISSUE 2: QUALITY OF THE RELATIONSHIP

The issue of the quality of the relationship resolves itself into several basic questions: What kind of relationship do we want to have? What do we wish to gain from this relationship? Why have we formed this relationship, and what do we seek from this relationship? What is its reason for being?

Essentially the questions center on the purpose of our relationship—what's it all about? Is it to legitimize a child we created by accident? Is it for sexual convenience? Companionship? Security? Love? Affection? Is it to provide a cook and housekeeper on the one side, a bread-winner on the other? Is it to perpetuate a family name? To escape parental domination? To provide an ego trip (I'm really attractive to another person)? To serve as proof of our maturity? Just what is the nature and purpose of the relationship we have entered into?

Depending on the nature of the relationship, how will we act toward one another? Will we act affectionate in public? Will we fight in public? Will we act one way in front of others, another way when we are alone?

How much sharing will we do? Will we share our intellectual interests? Our emotions? Our pasts? Our secrets? Our talents?[10]

ISSUE 3: POWER AND DECISION-MAKING

Naturally the issue of power and decision-making is a crucial one. Perhaps the key question in all this is—will power *be* an issue in our marriage? Will there be power struggles between us? Will just one of us dominate while the other complains or resents but submits? *Who* will hold the power?

How will we make decisions? Will every

decision involve a power play? Or will we make decisions by means of compromise or, most constructively, by means of negotiation?

Obviously the answers to these questions will have enormous impact on the quality, nature, emotional atmosphere, and conduct of our relationship.

ISSUE 4: ROLES

How we approach and deal with the matter of roles will also have tremendous influence on what kind of relationship we will have. Do we both accept the traditional roles ascribed to the man and the woman? If we do, will we then simply live out the stereotypes? Or will we be able to grant ourselves and each other the freedom to be individuals and to cross role lines as we so desire?

For example, if we hold to the traditional role stereotypes, then presumably we believe that the division of labor is clear and definite: the wife runs the household; the husband earns the money. If the wife works she does so *in addition to* all her other household duties. There is also a clear division of household duties: the wife does all the inside housework; she runs the kitchen; she sews; and she does the laundry and irons. She runs the domestic side of the relationship. The husband does the heavy work like mowing the lawn, raking the leaves, washing the windows, and making necessary repairs.

What if we do not accept these traditional role designations and prescriptions? How do we manage things then? Can we grant each other the freedom and the comfort to be who we are and to do what we have the talent to do, regardless of traditional role prescriptions?

Are we able and willing to be flexible about who does what and about how each of us expresses himself or herself? Can I (the woman) accept your tears when you are moved by something beautiful or sorrowful? Can I (the man) accept your taking the lead in our love making? Have we the ability, the motivation, and the flexibility to experiment,[11] to try new ways of thinking, feeling, and acting? Are we willing to try our best to communicate about and share our feelings as we experiment?

ISSUE 5: TIME AND TOGETHERNESS

How we act in regard to the issue of time and togetherness depends in part on what we decide about another issue—the quality and nature of our relationship. The pivotal question here is that of togetherness. How much time will we spend with one another, and how will we spend such time?

Will we spend the majority of our time together? Or will we spend the majority of our free time apart? How we spend our free time depends on what we think it is for. In other words, do we get together only for sex and room and board? Do we get together just to play, to have fun, and to enjoy life? To avoid being lonely? To have a social life? Do we spend lots of time together because that's what we think married couples are supposed to do? Because we enjoy each other's company, affection, and love?

The quality of the time we spend together depends in great part on what we come together for. When we are together, will we truly communicate or merely "talk at" each other? Will we be like two partial strangers who occupy the same house but go their separate and solitary ways?

What about the time we spend apart from each other? Do I (the husband) spend most of my time off bowling, drinking, playing poker, or talking with my male friends? Do I (the wife) so involve myself in community activities that I'm rarely home when you are? Do I (the husband) work so hard that I have almost no time for you? Do I (the wife) spend hours on the phone talking to my friends so that I barely have time to talk to you?

In effect, then, how do we spend our time? Together? Or apart?

ISSUE 6: IN-LAWS (OR OUTLAWS?)

The subject of many jokes (particularly the mother-in-law type), the issue of in-laws is nevertheless an important one and merits more serious consideration than just jokes.

Many times one of the parents will say, "I didn't lose a son, I gained a daughter" or vice versa. For better or worse, each of us gains a new family. What kind of relationship will I establish with your parents, your brothers and sisters? What kind of relationship will you establish with mine? What kind of ties shall we maintain with our various in-laws? What responsibilities do we have toward them? Or they toward us?

How much time will we spend with them? How often will we visit them? How much will we tell them about our relationship?

Will they try to interfere in or to "run" our marriage? How do we deal with that? What if you dislike or don't get along with my in-laws (or vice versa)?

ISSUE 7: FRIENDS

Whose friends will now be our friends (as a couple)? Yours? Mine? Both of ours? How much time will we spend with our friends? How will we resolve conflicts about our friends? What if I can't stand your friends? Or if you can't stand mine?[12]

ISSUE 8: SOCIAL LIFE

What kinds of things will we do? Will we do them separately or together? How often will we go out? Where? With whom? How often will we entertain? What kind of entertaining will we do? Who will be responsible for it?

ISSUE 9: MONEY

Money is an issue that can raise powerful and far-reaching questions. And, as is true of other issues, the important thing is not whether there is too much or too little, but how we deal with the matter and how we relate to each other.

Following are some of the most important questions: Who makes the money? Who controls the spending? Who spends what? For what? On whom? When? Why? How will we handle our money? Will you give me your paycheck at the end of the pay period and I give you an allowance? How will we divide our money? Will we have a budget? If we both work, do we pool our money? Or do you pay for certain things and I for others?

What if we need more money? Do I (the wife) go out and get a job? Do you get an extra job? Do we *need* more money, or do we *want* more money? What if we have to borrow? Who from? In-laws? Friends? Bank? Loan company? How many and what kinds of credit cards and charge accounts will we have?

ISSUE 10: HOUSING

Although this issue might seem somewhat technical, it also touches on feelings and attitudes. What kind of housing will we try to get? An apartment? A house?

Where will we live? Near your job? Near my job? In the city? The country? The suburbs?

How will we decorate our apartment or house? Who will decide these questions?

ISSUE 11: MAJOR MINI-MATTERS (OR, WHO DIDN'T PUT THE CAP BACK ON THE TOOTHPASTE TUBE?)

Not all the issues are so momentous as commitment, power, sex, and money. Some, like the ones we speak of here, are not issues in and of themselves, but put them all together and they constitute an issue. **Major mini-matters** are all the little details of everyday living that are repeated day in and day out. Their irritation value is far out of keeping with their size, but it is not out of keeping with their constant repetition.

Major mini-matters are perhaps best listed in the form of the eternal accusatory questions each person levels at the other. Who turned the heat up (down)? Why are your feet always so cold? Why do you always have to leave the toilet seat up? How come I never have any buttons on my shirts? Why don't you ever put your dirty underwear in the hamper where it belongs? Can't you ever remember the punch line of a joke? Why didn't you remind me that we were invited to dinner? Why do you always have to interrupt me? How come you always remember your mother's (father's) birthday but always manage to forget our anniversary? How come I always have to put the cat out? Who moved the TV guide? Why can't you ever come when I tell you dinner is ready and on the table? Why can't you squeeze the toothpaste tube from the bottom up instead of in the middle? Couldn't you at least call and say you're going to be late? Can't you ever be ready on time? Do you have to throw your wet towel on the bed? The list is endless. But if the irritations that these little problems can elicit are not dealt with, these mini-matters can become the stuff of major battles.

ISSUE 12: FAMILY PLANNING

The issue of family planning can be dealt with very quickly if both of us do not want to have children. Then all that is necessary is to decide on and use the most effective method of contraception available and acceptable to us. If, however, one of us does want children and the other does not, then we have a problem that we somehow must resolve. Can we talk about why you don't want a child? Why I do? Are we able to communicate and negotiate well enough to reach a reasonable solution?

If we both want children, then we must answer certain questions. When do we want to have our first child? How many children will we have? How far apart will we space them?

If one of us is sterile, would we consider artificial insemination? Or adoption? Are we interested in adopting one or more children rather than having all our own?

ISSUE 13: SEX

As you will note, this particular issue is treated in considerable detail. There are a number of reasons for doing so.

1. For many people, sex is an emotionally "loaded" subject. That is, for many it raises questions about their self-concept, their adequacy, their knowledge and know-how, their sexual identity, their roles, their feelings of masculinity or femininity, their desires or lack of them, their abilities, and their spiritual, moral, and ethical values.

Yet, because sex is also a culturally, religiously, and morally "loaded" issue, too often this subject has been hushed up or talked about in only the most narrow terms or has been reserved as a topic fit only for "adult" ears (whoever those adults may be). A more reasonable and valuable alternative seems to be to discuss sex with frankness, openness, and a strong respect for its natural and delightful place in our lives.

2. Sex is usually the first of the really important issues that a couple encounters directly and in detail. After the wedding, the bills do not have to be paid until the end of the month; social life, friends, and in-laws can wait. But whether or not a couple has sexual intercourse on their wedding night, they still must deal in some way with the issue of sex.

3. How each person treats the other in bed can and frequently does have far-reaching implications for and influences on the development of their overall relationship.

4. Our treatment of this issue will give you a fairly complete run-through of the process of asking the questions that are involved in any issue. Also it suggests that no issue is simple and clear cut, that there are always many different sides.

Sex is considered to be one of the key issues in marriage. Perhaps what makes sex seem like *the* key issue is that most of the questions about the sexual relationship demand some kind of *action answer*. Many of the questions and answers are practical ones, which are then frequently translated into immediate action.[13,14]

The range and scope of these questions are vast. *How often* will we have sexual relations? *When* will we have intercourse? *When* will we *not* have intercourse? *Where* will we have intercourse? Under what conditions?[15]

What about contraception? Will we use

a contraceptive? If we do, what kind? Does each of us understand fully how effective (or not effective) each contraceptive method is? Which one of us will be responsible for the contraceptive protection? Or will both of us take that responsibility? What if we slip up and conceive a child? How will we respond?

What kind of love play, if any, will we engage in? Do I know what really turns you on ?

What positions of intercourse will we use? What sexual roles will we take? Do we subscribe to the traditional designation of man, the aggressor; woman, the passive, submissive one? Can we shed our roles and come together as equal yet unique individuals who will try to respond to ourselves and to each other with sensitivity and caring on a moment-to-moment basis?

How will we deal with the problems, big and little, that may arise? What if you (the husband) just roll over and go to sleep as soon as intercourse is over, leaving me still keyed up, lonely, or wanting to share a time of quiet closeness? What if I (the wife) just lie there passively and make little if any response? What if penetration is painful for me? What if you move too fast for me, or I too slow for you? Will we try to time ourselves so that we can reach mutual orgasm? Do we consider mutual orgasm to be a necessity for a "perfect" sexual relationship? Should we expect or "demand" that I (the wife) have an orgasm every time? Should I pretend I have one even if I don't? Can I and will you help me to have multiple orgasms?[16,17]

If other, more serious problems occur, how will we deal with them? What if I am "frigid"? What if I am impotent? What if I ejaculate prematurely? What if one of us has VD? Will we "ignore" or deny these problems? Will we try to be patient and understanding toward one another? Will we read books or send away for remedies advertised in magazines? Will we seek our friends' or parents' advice? Will we seek professional help?[18]

What about the whole question of marital fidelity? Are we even able to discuss the matter? Does the double standard operate—either implicitly or explicitly—in our marriage? That is, is it okay for you (the man) to have extramarital sexual relations but not okay for me (the wife)? What will happen to our marriage if one of us has an extramarital affair and the other of us finds out? [19,20] What is my (the wife's) attitude toward your activities when you are away from me on long business trips? What is your attitude? What and how do we feel about group sex or husband/wife swapping?[21,22]

Perhaps more important than any other single question about technique or problems is the question: what does our sexual relationship mean to us? Is it merely a physical act we perform together? Is it my (the wife's) duty? Is it my (the husband's) right? Do we regard sexual relations as one more arena for continuing battles between us? Do we engage in power plays even in bed? Do you see sex one way and I another? Do we regard our sexual relations as a total kind of experience that encompasses closeness, intimacy, sharing, fun, tenderness, communication, affection, respect, love? Is sex, in other words, a vehicle (and a delightful one at that) for the full expression of who each of us is?[23,24] ▶IE-2, p. 47.

Working with the issues

These are some of the major issues that any married couple must in some way or another manage. Although these are not all the issues and certainly not all the questions raised by these issues, the list is a formidable one. The range and number of questions that arise about these issues are indicative of the enormous number of decisions that these questions either explicitly or implicitly require. The range and number of questions also suggest that, given the motivation and some skill at communicating, couples will have plenty of exciting material to work with. Certainly, if they choose to deal with the issues, life will not be boring and has the chance of becoming more open.

Interaction experiences

1. Experiencing the differences in core characteristics in a relationship (p. 40)

Imagine yourself married to (or in a long-term relationship with) a person who is different from you in terms of a core characteristic (e.g., much younger or older; of a different race, religion, or socioeconomic class). Make a list of some of the specific differences that would exist between you.

EVALUATION: Try to feel the impact of one of these specific differences on your relationship. For example, if you are a devout churchgoer, how would you feel being married to an agnostic? Of if you are a Christian how would you feel being married to a Jew who celebrates the Sabbath from sundown Friday through Saturday? Try to imagine and feel what it would be like to discuss these differences with your partner to reach some kind of emotional agreement between you. How successful do you think you might be?

FOLLOW-UP: Choose a person in the class who will role play your partner and act out a situation. Discuss with this person the thoughts and feelings you have about the differences between you and the way you managed those differences during the role playing.

2. Learning about the ways your parents deal with a marital issue (p. 46)

Pick a specific question about one marital issue and try to determine how your parents deal with this question (e.g., who decides how the money is to be spent). Try to imagine how they decide how they will deal with the question (e.g., do they discuss the question; do they fight for power; does one of them decide and the other one give in?).

EVALUATION: What does this experience tell you about their marital relationship? How do you feel about their relationship? Can you see ways of communicating and interacting that might be better than the ones they use?

FOLLOW-UP: When you get a chance, either observe your parents as they decide a question or ask them to describe how they do so.

REFERENCES

1. Bernard, Jessie: The future of marriage, New York, 1972, World Publishing Co.
2. Blood, Robert O., Jr.: Marriage, ed. 2, New York, 1969, The Free Press, pp. 5-6.
3. Divorces: analysis of changes, U. S. Government Printing Office, 1973, Washington, D.C.
4. Reiss, Ira L.: The family system in America, New York, 1971, Holt, Rinehart & Winston, Inc., p. 237.
5. Smith, Charles E.: Negro-white intermarriage: forbidden sexual union, Journal of Sex Research **2**:169-177, 1966.
6. Kinsey, Alfred C., Pomeroy, Wardell B., and Martin, Clyde E.: Sexual behavior in the human male, Philadelphia, 1948, W. B. Saunders Co., pp. 369-373.
7. Blood, op. cit., pp. 163-164.
8. McGinnis, Thomas C.: Your first year of marriage, Garden City, N.Y., 1967, Doubleday & Co., Inc.
9. Hilsdale, Paul: Marriage as a personal existential commitment, Marriage and Family Living **24**:142, May, 1962.
10. Foote, Nelson N.: Love, Psychiatry **16**:247, Aug., 1953.
11. Chafetz, Janet Saltzman: Masculine/feminine or human? Itasca, Ill., 1974, F. E. Peacock Publishers, Inc.
12. Chambless, William J.: The selection of friends, Social Forces **43**:370-380, 1965.
13. Katchadourian, Herant A., and Lunde, Donald L.: Fundamentals of human sexuality, New York, 1972, Holt, Rinehart & Winston, Inc.
14. Reuben, David: Everything you always wanted to know about sex, New York, 1970, David McKay Co., Inc.
15. Masters, William H., and Johnson, Virginia E.: The pleasure bond: a new look at sexuality and commitment, Boston, 1975, Little, Brown & Co.
16. Belliveau, Fred, and Richter, Lin: Understanding human sexual inadequacy, New York, 1970, Bantam Books, Inc.
17. Masters, William H., and Johnson, Viriginia E.: Human sexual inadequacy, Boston, 1970, Little, Brown & Co.

18. Kaplan, Helen Singer: The new sex therapy, New York, 1974, Brunner/Mazel, Inc.
19. Boylan, B. R.: Infidelity, Englewood Cliffs, N.J., 1971, Prentice-Hall, Inc.
20. Hunt, Morton: The affair, New York, 1969, World Publishing Co.
21. Bartell, Gilbert: Group sex, New York, 1971, Peter H. Wyden/Publisher.
22. Denfeld, Duane, and Gordon, Michael: The sociology of mate-swapping; the family that swings together clings together, Journal of Sex Research 7:85-99, May, 1970.
23. Otto, Herbert A., and Otto, Roberta: Total sex, New York, 1972, Peter H. Wyden/Publisher.
24. Roy, Rustum, and Roy, Della: Honest sex; a revolutionary sex ethic by and for concerned christians, New York, 1968, The New American Library, Inc.

chapter 3

THE STRUCTURE AND NATURE OF THE FAMILY

In many ways, the view of the family from the seventies is a rather dismal one. Prophets of doom cry out that the family is a breeding place of neuroses and psychoses, a perverted institution that teaches hatred to, inflicts pain on, and distorts the vision and emotions of its members. For example, the thesis of Cooper's[1] book *The Death of the Family* is that the family as it exists now destroys emotional health, indeed produces emotional illness, and should therefore be abolished. And Cooper is not alone in holding these views; other books, articles, and television and radio shows have added to the hue and cry concerning the failing family.[2]

Although some doomsters claim that the family is dead or dying (or ought to be), there certainly seems to be no lack of interest about this institution.[3,4] Before any of us decides that the family is going the way of the dinosaur, however, we need to carefully consider what a family is and what it does.

This chapter therefore focuses on the central question—what *is* the nuclear family? To answer this question, it is necessary to ask and answer others: (1) What actual and psychological conditions comprise its structure? (2) What are the purposes, functions, and limitations of the family structure? (3) What characteristics determine the basic nature of family life? and (4) What issues (and potential issues) are common to the conditions of family life?

Only by answering these questions can we begin to evaluate the role, the meaning, and the importance of the family in our society. And only then will we be able to start determining what the future of the family may be—whether in its nuclear form it is still viable or whether it can survive only if it undergoes a metamorphosis.[5]

THE NUCLEAR FAMILY: ITS STRUCTURE

Although much attacked and subjected to a lot of casual and serious abuse, the family is still the single most important personal institution in our society. As Ackerman[6] notes:

> None of us lives his life alone. Those who try are foredoomed; they disintegrate as human beings. . . . Life is . . . a shared and sharing experience. In the early years this sharing occurs almost exclusively with members of our family. The family is the basic unit of growth and experience, fulfillment or failure. It is also the basic unit of illness and health.*

A definition of the family

Just what *is* this "basic unit of growth and experience, fulfillment or failure . . . illness and health"? The **nuclear family** consists of two married adults who are parents to one or more children (whether created by the spouses or adopted), all of whom ordinarily live together as an interrelated group. Possible variations of this core unit that also qualify as nuclear families include a widow or widower with chil-

*From Ackerman, Nathan: The psychodynamics of family life, New York, 1958, Basic Books, Inc., Publishers, p. 15.

dren, a divorced parent with children, or even a relative (e.g., grandparent, aunt, uncle, even an older sibling) plus children.

Conditions basic to the structure of the traditional family

Certain conditions both actual and psychological constitute the essential structure of the family.[7]

1. Family members live together under one roof as a unit distinct from other family units. Family members regard their family as a distinct entity and tend to be related to as such by "outsiders." Each family constitutes a separate economic and labor unit. That is, a given family does not own or share property or money with other families, nor does it divide its work load with other families (e.g., two families do not join forces and then divide the labor so that one adult female does all the cooking and housework while the other adult female takes care of all the children). But family members *do* share property, money, and work loads with one another.

2. The marital relationship of the parents is the focal relationship. The nature, tone, quality, and style of this relationship significantly affect the nature, tone, quality, and style of the family relationships. For example, if the parents' relationship is hostile and aggressive, then the tone of the emotional atmosphere will probably be hostile, aggressive, punitive, nagging, belligerent, sharp-tongued, and nasty.[8] ►IE-1, p. 65.

3. The parents commit themselves to their own relationship (at least insofar as it bears on the family), to the children, and to the family at least until the children grow up and can live independently.

4. All family members are committed to caring for and about one another.

5. The family unit is structured according to definite roles. These roles are ascribed according to sex, family position (e.g., mother, son), age (e.g., oldest child, oldest son or daughter), and sometimes ability (e.g., the mechanically adept son takes care of mechanical tasks). In particular, the sex roles carry with them distinct sexual and behavioral taboos so that psychological stability and clear bloodlines can be established and maintained.

6. Certain expectations, rules, and values govern the behavior of family members toward one another and toward nonfamily members.

7. Family members are responsible for and to one another under both civil and social (unwritten) law. Parents are legally responsible for their children until they come of age, and children must answer for their actions to the parents.

Of course, there are all kinds of possible variations and qualifications of these conditions. But whatever variations there may be, these conditions comprise the essential structure of the traditional nuclear family.

Purposes and functions of the traditional family

Even a brief survey of the purposes and functions of the nuclear family sharply underscores the difficulty, the complexity, and the extreme importance of the functions that the family is asked to perform.[9] Considering the rather awesome nature of these tasks, the wonder is not that the family does not always do them well but that it does them at all.

The nuclear family is expected to fulfill six major purposes and functions. (For an historical perspective on these purposes and functions, see Chapter 1.)

1. The family is the one societally accepted means of perpetuating the human race; it protects and nurtures the children during their physical, intellectual, emotional, and social development until they are able to care for themselves. Obviously without physical protection and nurture, a child would die. Less obvious but just as important is the fact that without some psychological protection and nurture, that is, without some physical and emotional contact with a caring Other Person, a

child's emotional growth will be stunted, and he may sink into a state of **marasmus,** a form of psychological death, and then die physically as a result.

2. The family is the primary socializing force in a child's life.[10,11] The power and significance of this force is clearly indicated by the biblical proverb: "Train up a child in the way he should go; and when he is old, he will not depart from it" (Proverbs 22:6). "To socialize" means to train and guide a person to become a **social being**—a person who has at least some knowledge of and feeling for who he is as a person and for who he is in relation to other people and to society; a person who knows the expectations, rules, values, and roles that his family and society prescribe and who is capable of trying to fulfill them.

To fulfill its purpose of socializing the child, a family performs certain functions:

a. The family provides role models for a child to imitate and learn from. A little girl can model herself on her mother; a little boy, on his father. In this manner the child can learn the ways of thinking, feeling, and acting that are considered (by society, the family, or both) to be appropriate to his particular role. In addition, the parents' roles within their marital and family relationships serve the child as models for heterosexual, husband/wife, and parental relationships.

b. The family teaches the child his native language—how to form sounds, how to use words, how to construct sentences, and how to make sense out of his and others' language.

c. The family teaches the child personal, family, and societal expectations, rules, values, and guidelines, which help him to organize inner and outer stimuli and help him to regulate the ways he thinks, feels, and acts (Chapter 5). As he learns these, he is also learning patterns of communication and interaction, which he uses to cope with reality. And through this process, he is developing his self-concept and ultimately his life-style (Chapter 6).

d. The family instructs the child about his culture, his background, and his heritage, and this helps to give him a sense of his place in life.

3. The family serves all its members as a kind of built-in "center" for in-depth interpersonal relationships. Belonging to a family means having people of different ages and sexes to talk to, to relate to, to fight with, to be with, to belong to, to care about, to receive care from, to love and be loved by, and to share life with. The family is perhaps the one group in an alienating world that is designed to consistently furnish its members with affection, warmth, acceptance, understanding, love, stability, and intimacy.[12]

4. The family provides its members with a psychological "center," a group to belong to, which family members can use as a reference point for establishing and developing their identities. Sometimes the family serves the constructive purpose of being an identifiable, known entity against which to rebel or test oneself.[13] ►IE-2, p. 65.

5. The family creates and maintains an economic and work unit. By dividing the responsibilities and labors that fall to human beings, the family organization arranges for efficient use of available labor and skills.

6. The family structure provides for the care of the parents in their old age.

Another perspective on the nuclear family

The preceding description of the structure of the nuclear family deliberately avoids making any comment about its workability or any of its possible disadvantages; it is intended simply as a straight account of what the nuclear family is meant to be and do. But such an account ends up sounding idealized, since what the family is meant to be and do and what it actually is and does are usually to one degree or another different. The design of the family is based on ideal standards, standards that are often not attainable even under the best conditions. Rather, they are ideals to strive for. It is a rare family that lives up to them fully.

In fairness to the humanness of the individuals who make up families, let us point out some of the more realistic drawbacks of nuclear family life. This is done not to undercut the earlier description but to fill it out so that the whole description does justice to the realities of family life.

LIMITATIONS OF THE TRADITIONAL NUCLEAR FAMILY

Belonging to a family unit is like being a citizen of a small kingdom: as a citizen you have certain rights and prerogatives, but you also have obligations to fulfill. In effect you are submitted to (and submit yourself to) the rules and regulations which govern this particular kingdom. The family unit is the prototype of group living. It is the original commune. As such it makes certain demands and places certain limitations on its members. Some of these demands and limitations are as follows:

1. You share with other members. For example, if your brother needs a winter coat, you have an old one, and if there is not enough money for two coats, he gets a new coat and you make do with your old one. You also may be called on to share your room, your time, your talents, and your money with other members.

2. You have less privacy than if you lived alone.

3. You have certain responsibilities toward the other members.

4. Your freedom is somewhat restricted: your freedom to come and go as and when you please, to make as much noise as you might like, to do exactly as you please, to ignore others, and to be alone.

5. You are asked (often required) to follow rules, and you often must answer to others—to submit to their judgment, their wishes, their desires, their expectations, and their values.

6. Family members make claims on your time, your energies, your respect, and your affections.

7. You have legal ties to your family: if you do something wrong, your family is the first to be notified.

8. Some limitations can be exemplified by a listing of typical comments young people make about their families: "They don't listen to what I have to say"; "They never let me do anything"; "If my parents love me like they say they do, how come they're always bugging me?"; "The only time my parents pay any attention to me is when I get into trouble or get good grades"; "My parents never like any of my friends"; "How come they're always 'right' and I'm always 'wrong'?"; "I didn't ask to be born into this family."

Other limitations are revealed by parents' comments: "Look at all we do for our children, and they don't even appreciate it"; "No matter what we say or do, it doesn't seem to make any difference"; "Where did we go wrong? Why are they so unhappy?"; "Why is it they take everything and everybody so much for granted?"; "You sweat blood over your children, work your heart out for them, and worry about their futures. Then why can't they even be civil to you? They act like parents are handy people to yell at and talk back to and take advantage of."

9. Another limitation is that many families appear to foster jealousy, rivalry, and competition.

10. Perhaps the severest indictment leveled at the family today is that it does not do what it is supposed to do. Too frequently what exists is an enormous credibility gap. For example, families supposedly consist of people who love and care about one another, but too often family atmospheres resemble a state of undeclared war. Another example is that parents supposedly serve as exemplary models for their children but all too frequently preach one thing and practice another. Parents may say, "Don't smoke pot because it's bad for you," but they may drink heavily on weekends, smoke cigarettes, and frequently

reach for the tranquilizers or the diet pills (or both). Another example is that the children may rebel against and reject their parents, but when they get into trouble, they expect their parents to forgive them and pull them out of trouble.

The family is neither as perfect as we would like it to be nor as flawed as some people claim. It is rather a *human* institution created by and for human beings. As such it has both weaknesses and strengths. Whether an institution is workable, valuable, and constructive or unworkable, miserable, and destructive depends therefore on the people who make up the institution. Specifically the success or failure of the family depends on how family members handle themselves as individuals and members, how they interact with one another, how they deal with the core characteristics of family life, and how they manage the issues that confront them as members of a family.

THE NUCLEAR FAMILY: ITS NATURE

Essentially two things, characteristics and issues, define and determine the nature of the family. Core characteristics define it by description; issues define the nature of the family in terms of content and function.

Core characteristics of the family

The **core characteristics of the family** are those which are intrinsic to the nature of family relationships. They are constants, always present in these relationships, and they exert continuing and significant influences on each other, on the ways members interact with one another, and on the development of their relationships.

The core characteristics of the family are intellectual balance (including intellectual heritage), biophysiological heritage, religion, race, ethnic background, socioeconomic background, number of parents' marriages, "age" of the present marriage, family members' ages, number of children, and children's sex and sibling rank.

Of necessity, this analysis deals (wherever relevant) with the effects of family core characteristics on the four interrelated aspects of family relationships: marital-parental, parent-child, sibling-sibling, and whole family interactions. It includes and focuses first on the marital-parental relationship because ordinarily it sets the direction and tone of all other family relationships. Since the subject of family core characteristics is a complex and large one, there is no attempt to provide complete coverage of the topic. Rather, the discussion presents some representative effects and examples that, hopefully, will suggest other possibilities to you.

INTELLECTUAL BALANCE

If the marital partners are about equally balanced intellectually, and if that balance is basically acceptable to each of them, then the playing of intellectual parental games is likely to be minimized. Each partner contributes whatever intellectual skills he has to the task of parenting and does not tend to use the parental role as a battleground for intellectual one-upsmanship.

If, however, the intellectual balance is not basically equal, then problems in the parental (as well as in the marital) relationship may occur, and these problems naturally affect the children. They may compete intellectually with one another; they may copy the smarter or the "dumber" parent; or they may take sides with one or the other parent.

If the balance among the siblings is unequal (e.g., one very bright, one much less intelligent), this imbalance affects their relationship. The smart one may lord it over the "dumb" one, or the less-intelligent one may pick on the smart one for being an impractical egghead. Or if all the siblings are of average intelligence, one may drive himself to shine more than the other siblings to gain the more intelligent parent's approval. In the event that none of them can get this parent's approval, they may all reject the smarter parent and join forces with the average parent.[14]

BIOPHYSIOLOGICAL HERITAGE

If the biophysiological heritage of both parents is basically one of health, strength, and at least ordinary attractiveness, then this characteristic probably does not exert a particularly significant effect on their parental relationship. Suppose, however, that one of them is handicapped or sickly. Although the two may have worked out their marital relationship in terms of this factor, their parental roles may be strongly influenced by it.

This situation could (and probably would) affect the way the children perceive male/female roles. Furthermore, the children may be drawn to the healthy parent because he or she can tolerate their natural liveliness. Or one (or more) of the children may develop the same kind of illness or symptoms and thereby identify with the sick parent and vice versa.

Suppose both parents are strong, healthy, and well coordinated, but one of the children is weak and sickly. They may be protective of him or intolerant. If the sickly child is a boy and he has a strong, healthy sister, both parents may favor her over him. Or the father may reject him, pay far more attention to the daughter, and unconsciously treat her more like a son, and the mother may complete the balance by favoring and protecting the son and ignoring the daughter. On the other hand, both parents may concentrate on protecting the son and thus pay less attention to the daughter. Whatever the particular circumstance, the effect on the son's and daughter's relationship may be destructive. One may be intensely jealous of the other. The strong one may tend to act like a third parent or may reject him out of hand.

If the parents are basically attractive people and one of the children is rather ugly or fat or skinny, this may lead to trouble. One or both parents may subtly or openly harass the aberrant child. They may be deeply disappointed in him and favor the other children. They may bend over backward to accept him. This child may become the family joke—the target of parental sniping and sibling jokes—or he may become the common family problem or concern.

RELIGION

If the marital partners are of the same religious persuasion, then they are likely to agree basically on their parental role with regard to the religious upbringing of the children.

If, however, the partners' religious backgrounds differ, then this is likely to have some effects on their parental relationship. When there are no children involved, each partner is essentially free to go his own religious way, but when there are children, then certain issues inevitably require parental responses.

If the parents are in conflict about which religion is better and about how the children should be reared, they may engage in an ongoing battle about the matter. In this case, one or both parents may try to enlist the children's sympathy or aid in the struggle. Such tactics may encourage the children to make a definite commitment not only to one or the other parent's faith but also to that parent's emotional side. Or the struggle may turn one or more of the children against religion itself or against the particular faith of one or both parents. Another possibility is that one child may side with one parent, while another may side with the other parent—in which case there may be conflict and struggle between the siblings.[15]

RACE

If there is no significant difference between the marital partners' racial heritage, then race generally has little influence on the partners' parental relationship. If, however, the marriage is a racially mixed one, then the influence can be great. For example, a marriage between a black man and a white woman may work out fine for the husband and wife. They may, for example, find a liberal community to live in and be able to come to satisfactory terms with themselves and their environment. But when children are involved, the effect on the couple's marital and parental relationships may be substantial. The discrimination their child may be subjected to may bring home to them—with a force that nothing else could—the difficulties and problems created by racism. As parents, they may have to deal head on with the pain and humiliation of bigotry; they may have to help their children learn to manage nasty situations and to handle feelings of rejection, hostility, fear, and confusion. And all of this may have to be done in the context of an ambiguous emotional atmosphere not only within the environment but also within the marital and parental relationship. Once the couple have children and must face the effects of prejudice on their children, the partners may begin to feel that they have made a mistake. The partner who belongs to the minority race may blame the partner of the majority race for its bigotry, or the "majority partner" may feel that their troubles are the fault of the "minority partner."

If there are significant differences in the skin color or other racial characteristics among the children, these differences probably have some effect on what child identifies with what parent and vice versa. Favoritism may result because of such identification. If one parent is "top dog" in the marital-parental relationship, then a child who resembles him may act like top dog to other siblings if they resemble the "bottom dog" parent. On the other hand, the family—parents and children—may form a close-knit, supportive unit in response to external pressures of discrimination. The siblings may be protective of one another because of discrimination. Or family members may be more tolerant than many people because they know what prejudice is like and because they live with difference and know it is only skin deep.[16]

ETHNIC BACKGROUND

If both marital partners are from the same ethnic background, then the effect is not likely to be conflictual. However, if the partners' ethnic backgrounds are dissimilar, the potential for clashes in the parental relationship exists. For example, the qualities an American husband and a Japanese wife enjoy about one another as marital partners might contribute to conflict between them in their parental roles. The American husband will probably be away at work during the day and may expect his wife to do the major share of the child-rearing. But the very air of pleasant docility and submissiveness—which the husband may find so charming in his wife—may make it very difficult for her to know how to rear children in the more rough-and-tumble American environment.

If the parents' ethnic backgrounds are similar, they may (depending on their own feelings) rear the children to be proud of their heritage or ashamed of it. Or the children may be ashamed of their heritage if, for example, the parents speak broken English or almost no English and they feel pressured by their differentness outside the home (e.g., if they have trouble in school because no allowance is made for their language background). Outside pressures on the children plus their feelings of shame may drive a wedge between the parents and children and create a difficult, hostile, or alienating atmosphere in the family.[17,18]

SOCIOECONOMIC BACKGROUND

The more similar the marital partners' backgrounds—and the more similar their socioeconomic values—the less the likelihood of parental conflict created by this core characteristic. If, however, one partner comes from a lower or higher socioeconomic bracket than the other's, problems may ensue. When it comes to rearing the children they may clash: a blue-collar father may want to shower the children with all the things he never had as a child, whereas an upper middle-class mother may feel that young people should work for and earn what they get. On the other hand, he may be hard-nosed and autocratic about giving the children spending money, and she may go behind his back and slip them money. Or she may act as the go-between, conveying the children's requests to him and pleading their case with him.

If the family's socioeconomic status is middle or upper middle class, the children may have great and perhaps unrealistic expectations of their parents' ability to provide various comforts. Or their parents' affluence may allow them to feel secure and therefore free to rebel and later make their peace (as often happened with members of the counterculture). If the family's socioeconomic status is lower class or close to poverty, the children may be ashamed of their background and strive to go beyond it. In so doing, they may drift away from or become alienated from their parents.[19]

NUMBER OF PARENTS' MARRIAGES

The fact that neither marital partner has been a parent before affects the couple's adjustment to parenthood. With a few exceptions (e.g., if one of them had the primary care of younger siblings), each is basically inexperienced about parenting. As a result, each may be overcautious and controlling with the first child. As other children are born or simply as time goes by, the parents may become more relaxed about their role, but they may also find that they have less time for each other as marriage partners.

Whether one (or both) of the partners has children from a previous marriage influences the parental relationship. If children from a previous marriage live with the present partners, that has its effects also. For example, the parent of these children may feel the need to defend their behavior, especially if their behavior conflicts with the other parent's concepts about child-rearing. Or conflicts may arise if the partner without previous children feels that the other partner favors the children from his previous marriage over the children of the current marriage.

The children's relationships are inevitably affected by this characteristic. For example, the children from one parent's previous marriage may resent and reject their step-parent, and this might cause trouble between the two parents, or they might obey only the blood parent. On the other hand, these children might prefer their new step-parent to their real parent—a situation that could arouse jealousy in the real parent.

If the children from a previous marriage live with the children of the present marriage, problems may arise between the two sets of children. They may compete with one another for the natural parent's affection. They may try to play one parent against the other. Or they may get along well with each other, especially if the parental relationship is more harmonious in the current marriage. Thus the whole family might be split along old/new marriage lines, or it might be more unified than many families.

"AGE" OF THE PRESENT MARRIAGE

If a couple has their first child in their first year of marriage, they may not have had sufficient time to work out their marital relationship. Having children after a few years of marriage may be an advantage because the couple have had some time to establish and enjoy the marital relationship without the inevitable complications brought about by the presence of children. On the other hand, if during those years the marital relationship has deteriorated, then having children may seem like a way to help the marriage. But such measures often bring more problems than solutions, since rearing children takes hard work, parental cooperation, and some sense of unity and caring.

If the couple have been married for a long time (e.g., ten years) before they have children, they may experience difficulty in shifting for marital to parental gear. They have had considerable time to establish and solidify their marital roles, patterns, and relationship; thus the advent of children may feel like a shocking and surprising intrusion on their settled married life. They may therefore have considerable adjusting to do to become even somewhat comfortable as parents.

Whether the age of the present marriage will have a significant effect on the children will depend primarily on how the parents handle their marriage and themselves. If they are able to communicate and interact with reasonable quality, the effects of the present marriage's age are minimized and are not particularly negative. However, in the event that the parents in any of the previously described situations do not manage their new situation, their marriage, and themselves in a reasonably constructive manner, then the children may have a difficult time. If one or both parents resent the responsibilities of children, the children may feel (and be) neglected and emotionally abandoned. If only one parent neglects or rejects them, they may gravitate toward and form overly strong dependency ties with the other parent. If the parents' marriage is rocky, the children may become pawns in a parental power struggle; they may side with one parent, or they may dissociate themselves from either (or both) of the parents. Any of these outcomes, of course, tends to work against family unity and harmony.

FAMILY MEMBERS' AGES

The core characteristic of family members' ages can be divided into three categories, each of which has its own particular effects: the age span between the parents, the age span between the parents and children, and the age span between the siblings.

Age span between the parents. If the marital partners are about the same ages, then ordinarily the influence of age is minimal. There are, however, two possible exceptions.

1. If both partners are teenagers, their age may work against them when they become parents. As marital partners, they may be happy, since even with the additional responsibilities and restrictions of marriage, they still can retain a good deal of freedom. But parenthood adds further responsibilities and cuts down on freedom. Under such restrictions, teenage parents may chafe, become impatient, and wish they were not married, much less saddled with a child. One or both partners may regret the marriage and its consequences and want out, since being parents seems to block any real chances of having fun and staying loose.

2. If two older people (over 35 years old) of about the same age marry and have children, they may have difficulty adjusting to parenthood because children will further restrict their already somewhat restricted freedom.

In the case of a younger woman marrying an older man, the age difference could seriously affect the parental relationship. For example, if he married her to be a companion and a showpiece, he may deeply resent the time she spends on the children. And she may lose much of her earlier glamour when she steps into her parental role. He may even deny his parental role and refuse to accept her in her parental role. He might, for example, dump most of the parental responsibilities on her but demand that she continue to act and look like the carefree socialite he married. Another problem that can result may be a marked difference in tolerance levels for the natural irritations of child-rearing. He may expect and demand peace and quiet at home and become irritated by the noise the children make. It is possible, however, that he might be more tolerant and easygoing because of his life experience, whereas she might have a short fuse because she is not ready to settle down into domestic tranquility.

Age span between parents and children. If the parents are young (e.g., teenage and early twenties) when they have their children, the relative closeness in the parents' and children's ages may foster understanding and a feeling of companionship among them. The parents are probably better able physically to keep up with the children, which may encourage closeness. On the other hand, if the parents mistake closeness in age for actual membership in the younger generation, friction may result.

If one parent is much older than the other, the gap between the older parent and the children exerts an influence on everybody. In the most general terms, the children are bound to have different relationships with the two parents. If, for example, the older parent is intolerant, then the children may turn to and become close to the younger parent. And, of course, the ages of the children have an effect on this situation too. For example, the oldest child may be closest to the older parent because the age gap between them is the smallest.

Age span between the children. If there is a big age span between the oldest child and the others, he may "parent" or spoil the younger ones, or he may boss them around. The younger children may look up to the older one as a kind of "aunt" or "uncle."

If there are minimal differences in their ages, they may form intense rivalries with one another, or they may become emotionally close to one another. Or two children who are close in age may band together against an older or younger sibling.[20]

NUMBER OF CHILDREN

If there is only one child, the parents may be able to "assimilate" the child into their marital relationship by treating him as a little adult. In this way, they may be able to retain a major portion of their marital freedom. However, they may so dote on this one unique being who is *theirs* that they may "forget" their marital relationship in favor of this new triadic relationship.

The only-child situation is an interesting one, since it means that the alliances the child can make *within* the family are with the parents and not with other children. Being the only child also means that he receives undiluted parental attention (whether negative or positive). The only child may be spoiled. He may be lonely and introverted. He may be far more at ease with adults than with his peers.

If there is more than one child, the children who come after the first one may do much to burst the bubble of exclusivity, and the parents may become more casual about parenthood and may regain some of their former marital and individual identities. On the other hand, they may find that the more children they have the less time they have for themselves as individuals and as marital partners.

The oldest child may be jealous of those who come after him, or he may be happy to have family peers. The advent of other children means that the alliances will probably be somewhat different. For example, the children may band together against one or both parents, or one child or one parent may become the object of criticism or abuse from all the other family members. Or the effect of two or more children may be to create a small community—a built-in group for joint activities (e.g., games, projects). And, of course, if there is more than one child, eventually there will be built-in baby-sitters for the younger siblings.[21]

CHILDREN'S SEX AND SIBLING RANK

If a parent is disappointed with the sex of the first child and the second child is of the other sex, then the balance will presumably be righted. But if the second (and any other children) is of the same sex, then this may compound the parent's disappointment. In the event that all the children are of the same sex, the different-sex parent may feel left out and experience difficulty relating to his or her children or to the family as a whole.

When there are two or more children, the connection between sex and sibling rank affects the relationships of parents and children and sibling and sibling. For example, if the oldest is a boy and the next child is a girl, the parents may demand more of their son than of their daughter. If the second child is a boy, they may demand less of him than of the oldest boy. If three or four same-sex children are followed by an opposite-sex child, this child may be spoiled by both parents and siblings. In the event that the older children are all girls, they may "mother," perhaps spoil a baby brother. Or they may be jealous of the attention given him by the parents. The same jealousy may occur in a reversed sex situation.[22]

SOME COMMENTS ABOUT FAMILY CORE CHARACTERISTICS

For the sake of clarity, most of these family core characteristics have been discussed as separate entities. There is really no way for any discussion to truly capture the complexity and delicate interrelationships of these core characteristics; nevertheless, it is vitally important to remember that none of these characteristics operates in isolation, that each of them has a tempering influence on the others. It is on the complex interplay among core characteristics, family issues, and the inner thoughts, feelings, and actions of each family member that the family's emotional balance depends.

It is also important to keep in mind that although some family core characteristics can present practical problems, by and large, it is not the characteristics but the way family members relate to them that creates problems or brings satisfactions. ►IE-3, p. 65.

Issues raised by and about the family

Although this survey of family issues covers a lot of ground, it is not (and is not meant to be) exhaustive. It is nevertheless an impressive one and indicates the complexities and the vast potentials for rich experiences in family relationships.

Our reason for presenting this survey is to make you aware of the range and type of issues and questions that confront members of a family and that they must in some way manage.

Perhaps the essential and encompassing question is—What kind of family does a particular family want to be? Do family members wish to retain or return to the closed, authoritarian kind of family system of the first half of the century (as described in Chapter 1)? Or are family members willing to risk newness and some anxiety and discard at least the limitations of the older system? In effect, does the family wish to establish and maintain an open family system, which involves tolerance and encouragement of individuality, the fostering of independence and autonomy, honest communication, and non-rule-oriented interaction?

The ways that family members deal with issues (and with core characteristics) are what constitute the dynamics of family interaction.

ISSUE 1: RESPONSIBILITIES TO AND FOR ONE ANOTHER

The question of responsibility affects each and every member of a family and pervades every aspect of family life. What is the father's major commitment—his job or his family? Or can he adequately balance the two? What is the mother's major commitment—to her marriage, home, and children, or is she to have a job in addition?

Another area of responsibility concerns parental care of their children. What exactly are the parents' responsibilities to their children? Which child-rearing procedures should they follow—Dr. Spock, Dr. Freud, Dr. Haim Ginott, "Spare the rod and spoil the child"? What are the children's responsibilities to their parents? Should they be held accountable for their actions when those actions reflect on the family?

How does a family handle the responsibilities that arise from specific family situations? For example, should a severely retarded or disturbed child be reared within the family? Is that fair to the other children? What if a parent (or a child) is an alcoholic? A drug addict? How far does the family's responsibility extend?[23]

ISSUE 2: QUALITY OF RELATIONSHIPS

The emotional atmosphere in a home is the outcome of the kind and quality of relationships in the family. This atmosphere depends basically on members' attitudes and feelings toward one another and toward the family as a whole. Do family members like one another? Enjoy each other's company? Are they indifferent to one another? Do they feel locked into a family relationship out of necessity or in deference to tradition?

What kind of family would they like to be? What are the family's relationships with the "outside world"? Is the family clannish, suspicious of strangers and outsiders? Is the atmosphere one of warmth and hospitality? Is the atmosphere open or closed?

The atmosphere is determined by and in turn helps determine the kind and quality of relationships among family members. What kind of marital relationship do the parents have? What kind of parental relationship do they have with each other? Does one leave or push the responsibility of parenting in the other's hands? Do they share this responsibility? Do they agree or disagree about parenting?

What is the quality of the relationships between the parents and children? Does each parent respect and treat each child as an individual? Do the children see the parents as "gods"? As "monsters"? What are the children's relationships with one another? Do they help each other? Do they play one another against each other? Do they like, respect, and treat one another as individuals? In overall terms, what is the quality of the family relationships? Deep? Superficial? Kind? Hostile? Indifferent? Dutiful?

Does any family member feel that the expectations are too high? Too low? Unreasonable? Impossibly rigid? How does each member feel he measures up to the others' expectations? How does each member feel the others measure up?

Similar kinds of questions may be applied to family rules, values, and guidelines. Are they too strict? Too lax? Too rigid? Too dictatorial? Inappropriate? Overly restrictive?

What patterns of communication exist in the family? Do the parents communicate with one another but not with the children? Should they argue only behind closed doors? Should they present a united front to the children? Or should they feel free to voice independent views, feelings, and decisions? Do the parents talk "at" but not with their children? Does one (or both) of the parents always demand (and have) the last word? Do the parents demand that their children "tell all"? Do the parents encourage free communication—communication without fear of reprisal or disapproval? How much do parents tell the children about difficult or delicate matters (for example, the death of a relative or close family friend; an extramarital affair; an emotional disturbance of a family member; alcoholism, drug addiction, promiscuity, stealing, lying, or cheating on the part of a family member; the breadwinner's loss of a job; the "facts of life"; impending separation or divorce)?

What about the children? Do they communicate among themselves but not with the parents? Do they feel free to say what they really think and feel to their parents? Do they feel free to disagree openly? Do they feel "forced" to tell their parents everything?

What patterns of interaction exist in the family? How do family members treat one another? With kindness? With cruelty? With trust? Without trust? With hatred? With love?

ISSUE 3: POWER AND DECISION-MAKING

Another important set of issues are those pertaining to power and decision-making. What, for example, is the power structure in the family? Who "wears the pants"? Who is the central authority figure? Who gives the orders? Is the reality of power played down or ignored by the family? Are there different kinds of power—parent power, child power, family power? How is the power wielded? What kind of decision-making processes are used? Power plays? Yielding or compromise? Negotiation? Does the family avoid discussing and considering important matters? Do family members support or withdraw from one another? Do they just cling to a vague hope that things will somehow "work out"? Or do they deliberately set out to communicate and negotiate about the matter at hand?

What does the family do in a crisis? Does the family unit disintegrate under the pressure? Do members band together and support one another? Do they try to pick up the pieces and go on as best they can? Do they try to negotiate a new equilibrium?

ISSUE 4: ROLES

The question of roles has significant bearing on the life of the family. Is the family set up primarily along role lines; that is, is the emphasis on who takes what roles and what those roles mean, or is the emphasis on who someone is as an individual and how he acts in terms of his individuality and in regard to other members? Who determines the roles in the family? How are they determined and assigned? By expectations? By demand? By compromise? By negotiation?

Are the family roles limiting or liberating? Are they rigid or flexible? What roles apply in the family? Only the traditional ones such as man, woman; girl, boy; wife, husband; parent, child; son, daughter? Or are other kinds present also? What are the specific expectations for each particular role?

Is it permissible for family members to cross traditional role lines? For example, is there allowance for the father who likes to cook or take care of the children? May the mother keep the family books and decide on its investments? May a teenager take the role of family advisor? How much does the family conform to societally ascribed roles? How different from society's roles can the family's roles be?

ISSUE 5: TIME AND TOGETHERNESS

What is the quality and the quantity of the time the family spends together and apart? What priorities exist regarding the use of time? How do family members use their time together? Working on projects? Talking? Playing? Fighting? Does the family watch television together? Stay up late together? Does the family go on vacations together *always*? Or do members feel free to go on their own?

ISSUE 6: SEX

Perhaps one of the least openly discussed yet most influential family issues is sex. However, even if family members never mention sex—which is possible, although not likely—they still must respond to and in some way deal with the questions that derive from this extremely important issue.

What provisions does (or does not) a family make to ensure members' privacy? Do the parents lock their bedroom door before making love? Are the children trained to knock before entering the parents' (or other siblings') bedrooms? Or is there a double standard—children must knock at the parents' bedroom door, but the parents think nothing of barging into their bedrooms without knocking? What is the minimum permissible degree of undress? Is nudity accepted? To what extent?

How much of their sexual relationship do the parents "act out" in front of their children? Where do they draw the line—kissing, touching, hugging, fondling? How much of their sexual relationships with dates or "steadies" do the siblings "act out" in front of the parents? How much information about their sexual experiences (past or present) do the parents share with their children? The children with their parents?

What about sex education? Who teaches the children? Do the parents leave it to the schools? To the church? To the family doctor?[24] Does the mother teach the daughters; the father, the sons?[25]

What kinds of information and how much will be taught? What attitudes do the parents have toward sex?

What kinds of freedoms and limitations apply to dating? How early will the children be allowed to date? What types of dating are allowed at specific age levels? Are the teenagers expected to "tell all" about their dating experiences? Do the parents question them about their experiences? Are conflicts inevitable because of inherent differences between the parents' and teenagers' philosophies about dating? Or because the parents' ethics are traditional, whereas the teenagers' ethics are situational?

What basic attitudes and feelings toward sex does the family have? That it's dirty? Taboo? Unspeakable? That sex is necessary but causes problems? That sex is fun, that it's healthy and a natural part of life?[26]

ISSUE 7: RELATIONSHIPS WITH RELATIVES

How close are the relationships with relatives? Do the grandparents (on one or both sides), the aunts, the uncles, the cousins live nearby or far away? How often does the family visit with other relatives?

How do the parents of the family relate to their own parents? Do the grandparents try to exert influence—perhaps undue influence—on the parents? Do the parents require the children to treat the grandparents with respect and love? What happens if the family likes one set of grandparents or other relatives better than the others?[27]

ISSUE 8: RELATIONSHIPS WITH FRIENDS AND OTHERS

How do the parents expect and require their children to act toward the parents' friends? Do they demand that the children like the friends? That they be courteous to the friends?

How do the children expect the parents to treat and act toward their friends? Are the parents supposed to like the friends? What if the parents disapprove of a child's friend(s)? What if the parents are prejudiced? Do the parents forbid their children to maintain certain friendships? Do the parents bar certain friends from the house? Are the parents courteous to the friends even if they don't like them? What is the family's basic position on relationships with nonfamily members—"Don't trust outsiders"? "Blood is thicker than water"?[28]

ISSUE 9: SOCIAL LIFE

What kinds of arrangements does the family make about social life? Does the whole family socialize with other families? Are the older children included in some of the parents' socializing, whereas the younger ones are left home with a baby sitter? Or are the parents' and the children's social lives separate? How much and what kind of social life are the children allowed to have? Do they have a family room where they can be alone with their friends? Are they encouraged or discouraged from having an active social life?

ISSUE 10: MONEY

Who earns the money? Father? Father and Mother? Mother? Do the children contribute money to the household? Who decides who spends how much, where, on what, and when? Does one parent or do both parents decide? Or does each individual decide how he'll spend his own money? What are the spending priorities? Do the children receive allowances? Who decides the amount and how? Are allowances tied to good behavior or are they given no matter what? Do the parents pay the children for work around the house? What is the family's philosophy about money? Go now, pay later? Save for a rainy day? Money burns a hole in the pocket?[29]

ISSUE 11: PROPERTY AND HOUSING

If choices are available about where to live and the kind and size of dwelling, then who makes the choices? How are they made? To suit only the parents? To please the children? To get the children into a good school system? To raise or to reflect the family's socioeconomic status? To save money so it can be spent on other things?

What about living space? Do some family members share bedrooms? From choice? Or necessity? How does the family decide who will share bedrooms? Does the family own a car? More than one? Who uses the car(s)? When? For what? What about toys? Does each child have his own toys? Are they "safe" from the other children? How does the family decide on choices of television or radio programs? How do members resolve conflicts over the use of shared property?

ISSUE 12: MAJOR MINI-MATTERS

Essentially major mini-matters cause their pinpricks of discomfort because they result in negative emotional responses (e.g., envy, annoyance) or because they have their roots in a certain degree of carelessness, selfishness, and thoughtlessness and therefore evoke negative responses. All kinds of actions fall into the mini-matters category, for example, the family member who monopolizes the bathroom for long periods of time or the family member who uses all the hot water in extra-long, luxurious showers. Other annoying monopolies are those in which one member takes over the telephone for long, leisurely chats or preempts the car or the television. And what about the person who eats the last piece of cake (or pie or chicken or bread) or who eats something another person was saving for himself (e.g., one of the children eats the diet ice cream mother had brought specially for her diet)?

Other kinds of irritating mini-matters caused by not thinking are various. For example, one (or more) of the family's members may bang doors, talk loudly, rattle garbage cans, shout, or turn the television on loudly while one or more family members are trying to sleep. The disappearing newspaper is also frequently a family bone of contention. One member may want to read it and not be able to find it. And then there are all those annoying instances of toilets being flushed or the dishwasher being turned on just when someone is taking a shower, food and drink being spilled in odd places (like the bedroom rug), and sticky dishes and dirty glasses being left in dark corners only to be found days later attracting ants or growing marvelous molds. Other vexations to the spirit include someone's crawling into a clean bed with filthy dirty feet; squeezing the toothpaste tube in the middle and leaving the cap off; leaving the soap in a puddle of water so that it gets mucky and squishy; not putting in a new roll of toilet paper when the old one has run out; putting feet on furniture; and leaving the toilet seat up.

What about all those irritating habits that human beings are prone to? Snapping gum, talking with a mouthful of food, whistling idly and monotonously, picking the nose, picking the teeth, sucking through the teeth, clinking the utensils at the table, mumbling, giggling, shrieking, belching, whining, teasing, interrupting, not listening and then asking, "What?," talking when the water is running, answering the question "Where are you?" with "Here!," shouting a question from one end of the house to the other end, chattering at the breakfast table.

What about the annoyance factor generated by forgetting? Forgetting to refill the ice trays, forgetting to mail other members' letters, forgetting to feed the pet(s), forgetting to put the cat out at night or walk the dog, forgetting where the car keys were put, forgetting to tell someone he has had a telephone call, not remembering what one was sent to get at the store and returning with the wrong thing, not remembering invitations to parties, not remembering to do certain chores.

Borrowing amongst family members can also induce exasperation. The traditional war cry of the injured party is "Who took my—razor, shaving cream, sweater, radio, TV, power drill, scissors, comb, brush?" The companion cry to the first one is "Where is (are) my ________?"

Another source of aggravation is that of conflicting life-styles. One member likes the house toasty warm; another likes it on the cool side. One member is a bright and cheery morning person; another is a night owl. One is always early or on time; another is always late. One likes to drive fast; another likes to drive slowly. One likes dinner early; another likes it late. One likes a sunny house; another likes cool shade. One likes lots of lights on; another prefers candlelight. One likes hot, spicy food; another likes bland food.

ISSUE 13: FAMILY GOALS AND VALUES

What goals and values do family members express? What ones do they truly believe in? Which ones do they follow in everyday life? What does the family want for itself? What are its values with regard to education, morality, happiness, social conduct, success, health, religion, and ethics? What are the family's goals with regard to education, social conduct, social status, success, happiness, health, morality, intellectual and emotional atmosphere, human relations, and the future?

CONCLUSION

This chapter and Chapter 2 have closely examined the core characteristics and issues of marriage and family life. Hopefully the overall effect of this examination has been to help you become more aware of their existence and the numerous choices inherent in them. These choices can be denied or decided according to rigid values and attitudes, which is the closed approach to the characteristics and issues. The open approach is, however, different. It involves being aware of alternatives, dealing with the choices in a conscious and deliberate manner, appreciating the fact that working with characteristics and issues involves not just self but others, sharing thoughts and feelings with others, and working together in a flexible manner to reach conclusions and choices that each person can live with.

An overview

Part I has looked at the changes in this century that have forced our society, its institutions, and individuals to become more open. It has considered how this opening up has created a double bind between the closedness of the past and the greater openness of the present, the double bind created by the conflict between the continuing power of old values and the rise of new ways of thinking, feeling, and acting. As a part of the process of helping to bring about an understanding of this move from closedness to openness, Chapters 2 and 3 have examined the core characteristics and issues of marriage and the family. Hopefully this examination has fostered an awareness and appreciation of the complexities of marriage and family life and the incredible number of choices that exist.

Part I has therefore provided information necessary to making choices about marriage and family life, which are consciously based on an awareness of your own, others', and society's thoughts and feelings, and knowledge of the characteristics and issues. But intellectual understanding is not enough. There must be changes in the individual's thinking, feeling, and acting. He must implement his understanding if he (and his institutions) are to be more open and able to act in the present. Part II therefore is designed to teach you by means of the Interactional Therapeutic System how the individual can change and grow and become more open both personally and interpersonally. Part II then is devoted to teaching such matters as how the individual got to be who he is now and how he functions in the present. More importantly The System teaches the individual the skills of effective communication and more open interaction, skills that enable him to alter or change his functioning so that he gains greater freedom from the past, can change and grow, and thereby can become more open in the present. Part II prepares the individual for understanding and applying the knowledge and skills taught by The System to the dynamics of marriage and family life, which is presented in Part III.

Interaction experiences

1. Examining the impact of your parents' relationship on the family (p. 50)

How would you describe your parents' relationship? What impact do you feel their relationship has on the nature, tone, quality, and style of your family's relationships? For example, how would you characterize the emotional atmosphere of your family, and what contributions do you feel your parents' relationship makes to this atmosphere? For example, if your parents frequently are sarcastic to one another, is the atmosphere tense and anxious?

EVALUATION: Can you think of any changes your parents could make in their relationship that would help the family? What do you think would happen to the family's relationships if one (or both) of your parents suddenly started acting in ways that are opposite to the ways he or she acts now?

FOLLOW-UP: You might try discussing this matter with your parents and seeing what their view of their relationship and its impact on the family is.

2. Discovering the psychological "center" your family provides (p. 51)

What kind of psychological "center" does your family provide? A stable, protective reference point? A group to rebel against? A motivation for striking out on your own? An overpossessive, dependency-creating net? A warm, loving haven?

What kind of center would you *like* your family to provide if you could make it different? Write a classified ad in which you state the attributes you would like your new family to have. (Or if you are satisfied with the way your family is now, write an ad that would sound attractive to a prospective seeker of a new and more satisfying family.)

EVALUATION: How did you feel as you wrote out your ad? Were you pleased? Upset? Surprised? Anxious? Were you able to put your likes into words? Did trying to do so give you a clearer view of and feel for your family?

FOLLOW-UP: Share your ad with other members of the class and see whether there are many points of comparison between your views of your families.

3. Identifying the effects of a core characteristic on your family (p. 59)

Take one of the core characteristics discussed previously and determine its specific manifestations in your family. Try also to determine some of its effects on the relationships in your family. After this, imagine what your family would be like if this same core characteristic had taken a different form. For example, suppose you are an only child. Imagine the effects on your family if you had one or more brothers and sisters.

EVALUATION: Were you able to get a clearer notion of your family through this experience? What did you think and feel as you figured out some of the effects of a core characteristic? Did imagining a difference in the core characteristic help you see your present family more clearly? What thoughts and feelings did you have during this experience? Do you prefer the way your family actually is, or would you rather have your imagined core characteristic be the reality?

FOLLOW-UP: Try this same experience using other core characteristics.

REFERENCES

1. Cooper, David: The death of the family, New York, 1970, Pantheon Books, Inc.
2. Skinner, B. F.: Walden two, New York, 1948, The Macmillan Co.
3. Vincent, Clark E.: Family spongia: the adaptive function, Journal of Marriage and the Family **28**:29-36, Feb., 1967.
4. Otto, Herbert, editor: A family in search of a future, New York, 1970, Appleton-Century-Crofts, pp. 1-9.
5. Ibid., p. 9.
6. Ackerman, Nathan: The psychodynamics of family life, New York, 1958, Basic Books, Inc., Publishers, p. 15.
7. Parsons, Talcott: The social structure of the family. In Anshen, Ruth Nanda, editor: The family: its function and destiny, New York, 1959, Harper & Row, Publishers, pp. 241-274.
8. Blood, Robert O., Jr.: Marriage, ed. 2, New York, 1969, The Free Press, pp. 11-13.
9. Reiss, Ira L.: The family systems in America, New York, 1971, Holt, Rinehart & Winston, Inc., pp. 3-6.
10. Blood, op. cit., pp. 446-462.
11. Ackerman, op. cit., p. 21.
12. Ackerman, op. cit., pp. 23-25.
13. Ackerman, op. cit., p. 21.
14. Zajone, Robert B.: Dumber by the dozen, Psychology Today **8**:37-40, Jan., 1975.
15. Babchuck, Nicholas, Crockett, Harry J., Jr., and Ballweg, John A.: Change in religious affiliation and family stability, Social Forces **45**:551-555, 1967.
16. Heer, David M.: Negro-white marriages in the U.S., Journal of Marriage and the Family **28**:262-274, Aug., 1966.
17. Glazer, Nathan, and Moynihan, Daniel P.: Beyond the melting pot, Cambridge, Mass., 1963, MIT Press.
18. Nye, F. Ivan, and Berardo, Felix M.: The family: its structure and interaction, New York, 1973, The Macmillan Co.
19. Ibid., pp. 54-70.
20. Forer, Lucille K.: Birth order and life roles, New York, 1969, Charles C Thomas, Publisher.
21. Nye, F. Ivan, Carlson, John, and Garrett, Gerald: Family size, interaction, affect and stress, Journal of Marriage and the Family **32**:216-226, May, 1970.
22. Belmont, Lillian, and Marolla, Francis A.: Birth order, family size and intelligence, Science **182**:1096-1101, 1973.
23. Blood, op. cit., pp. 288-292.
24. Kilander, H. Fredrick: Sex education in the schools, New York, 1970, The Macmillan Co., pp. 217-229.
25. McGinnis, Thomas C.: Sex education and the battleground of controversy. In Silverman, Hirsh L., editor: Marital Therapy, Springfield, Ill., 1972, Charles C Thomas, Publisher, pp. 107-122.
26. Luckey, Eleanore B.: Helping children grow up sexually, Children **14**:130-135, July-Aug., 1967 .
27. Duvall, Evelyn Millis: In-laws pro and con, New York, 1966, Association Press.
28. McGinnis, Thomas C.: Your first year of marriage, Garden City, N.Y., 1967, Doubleday & Co., Inc., pp. 143-154.
29. Cobleigh, Ira U.: Building a successful family investment program, New York, 1967, Association Press.

part two

THE INTERACTIONAL THERAPEUTIC SYSTEM AND THE INDIVIDUAL

chapter 4

FOUNDATIONS OF THE INTERACTIONAL THERAPEUTIC SYSTEM

THE INTEGRATION OF THINKING, FEELING, AND ACTING

Traditionally our culture has placed the highest value on intellect—reason, logic, facts, information—usually with the implied devaluation of emotion and spontaneous action. Certainly emotions, or outward shows of them, have long been suspect as difficult to deal with if not downright dangerous. This tendency to overvalue intellect, logic, and tightly-controlled emotion is mirrored in American folklore. From Cool Hand Luke to James Bond to the President of the United States, traditionally it has been the man who plays it cool and "close to the hip" who gets our respect and admiration, whereas contempt is the reaction evoked by the so-called weak sister who lets his emotions get in his way.

There is a whole set of legends about another type of hero—he who shoots first and asks questions later; the strong, silent man of action; the slugger, the mover, the killer. And then there are the heroes with simple and direct instincts—brawling, two-fisted giants of the rivers, the mountains, and the forest—Paul Bunyan or John Henry.

But where in any of our legends or folklore is there a celebration of the balanced, integrated person? Where is the person who is revered because he thinks *and* feels and who acts well on the basis of his thoughts and feelings?

A balanced blend of thinking, feeling, and acting

Far too long our culture has ignored the need for and the desirability of a balanced blend of thinking, feeling, and acting. Only now do we seem to feel the stirrings of a move toward that balance. In a world of cold technology and shrunken frontiers and enforced togetherness, we have begun perhaps to look inward. Our physical and psychological survival now depends not on cold intellect alone, not on emotional response alone, and not on decisive action alone. It depends instead on a balanced blend of all that we have within us and on all the elements of our experience. All human beings think, feel, and act; all human experience incorporates thinking, feeling, and acting. To deal with ourselves and our experiences in ways that are growth producing and life enhancing, we must learn to blend these three components wisely and well. For us to become healthier, more open, and more autonomous, we must seek and achieve this kind of integration. It is this kind of integration that is the ultimate aim of The System.[1]

To help you visualize this integration, draw three equal-sized interlocking circles, two on top and one on the bottom. Label the left top circle "Thinking," the right top circle "Acting," and the bottom circle "Feeling." We urge you to draw these circles whenever you are working with the concept of the balanced blend.

THE BALANCED BLEND AND LIFE-STYLE

If a person's life-style is basically an open, healthy one, then even though one faculty may be stronger or dominant, there is still a fair degree of balance among the parts. But the person who overintellectualizes most situations tends to deny or ignore feelings. Thus he is out of balance; he is in effect operating primarily on one cylinder instead of three. If you were to draw the three circles for the Overintellectualizer, you would make the "Thinking" circle much larger than the "Acting" and "Feeling" circles. The Overemotionalizer has the same general problem: specifically he is barely able to think about the feelings that wash over him and direct his actions. The Acter-Outer, on the other hand, seems to think and feel very little; mostly he acts out whatever seems to strike him at the moment.

Each of these personality types is crippled by the lack of balance in his style or make-up. The Overintellectualizer needs to get in touch with his emotions so that he can feel who he is and so that his actions will be based on more than cold logic. The Overemotionalizer needs a stiff dose of rational understanding and intellectual discipline so that he can sort out his feelings and make appropriate decisions about them and about himself. The Acter-Outer needs to think more before he acts and be more aware of his feelings, which frequently touch off his seemingly "mindless" actions.

In this discussion we have drawn on three extreme styles to underline the need for balance. In this case, teaching balance to people with styles that are distorted properly falls within the realm of psychotherapy. But the principle of balance, of integration, is not confined to therapy. If they are to fulfill their potential, all human beings need to seek this balanced blend of thinking, feeling, and acting. Unfortunately too few people manage to achieve this blend; too often people have an overdose of one style or perhaps they have a mixture of two extremes—for example, the person who acts on his feelings with little thought of what's going on. Thus we find that many people need to be *taught* how to seek and find that balanced blend. ►IE-1, p. 75.

THE BALANCED BLEND AND SENSORY RESPONSES

This whole question of balanced or unbalanced life-styles bears directly on the ways that a person takes in and responds to the world through his senses. All human beings have a large number of sensory faculties and therefore an enormously wide range of responses. Each sense can be stimulated by and can respond to communication. In addition, each person can stimulate and evoke responses in another person through that person's senses. Furthermore, since people's senses are interlinked and sensitively attuned to one another, if one sense is stimulated, others are likely to be also.[2,3]

For example, suppose you are asleep and are awakened by the sound of footsteps in the next room (and you know you are all alone in the house). Your *hearing* sensor is what is initially stimulated. But that sets off a chain of communications to other sensors: you *think*, "A BURGLAR!"; you *feel* terror; you *look* hard at the darkness; you sit upright in the bed, then freeze in that position *(behavioral);* your *heart* pounds; your *guts* churn; your *mouth* gets dry and *tastes* like copper; you break into a cold sweat and your skin creeps *(tactile)*.

People's life-styles strongly affect their sensory responses. If a person has an open, balanced style, then his senses are attuned to incoming communications and respond in appropriate ways. He maintains an appropriately balanced blend of his sensory responses. If a person's style is closed, depending on what his specific style is and *how* closed he is, he tends unconsciously to "damp down" or turn off some of his sensory responses. For example, the severely depressed person tends not to be very sexually or sensuously responsive; he is too wrapped up in his blanket of gloom. The Overintellectualizer's intellectual senses will be all aquiver, but his heart and gut may be "sleeping." He notices and deals intellectually with facts, information, statistics, and details, but he tends to deny or ignore his emotions. The passive individual's physical senses operate somewhat halfheartedly. Usually it takes a major jolt to get him moving and responding.

The person whose life-style is underpinned by many repressive rules about sexual matters may block out most if not all of his sexual responses. In addition, since early sexual curiosity leads a child to touch, to smell, to listen, to look, to taste—in other words, to explore and experiment—his rules, more than likely, not only put the clamp on sexual exploration but also the free use of his five senses. So now he blocks off both overt sexual responses *and* a great many of his sensory responses. At the same time, however, his intellectual senses may be finely tuned. In essence the person with a closed style tends to not use or only partially utilize many of his senses. The balance in his specific life-style determines which senses he does and does not use.

THE BALANCED BLEND AND LEARNING

Our philosophy of teaching is that the best, the fullest, the most meaningful kind of learning (both book learning and "life learning") results from blending and balancing thinking, feeling, and acting (the cognitive, the affective, and the behavioral components). As is true of psychotherapy and of all growth experiences, teaching needs to offer all three kinds of learning so that people can get whatever proportions they may need. This is possible only if the whole range of learning experiences is made available.

Because traditional education has so often been geared only to the intellectual, we tend to reverse direction and begin with the heart and either move down to the feet or up to the head, or we may begin with the feet and move to the heart and then the head, using interaction experiences as the vehicle. The reason for this approach is to try to get people feeling and moving first; this helps them come alive. Too often a straight intellectual approach leaves people untouched, uninvolved with either themselves or the subject.[4]

It is, of course, appropriate at times to start a class by giving or asking for facts and then discussing ideas or to start with facts and then ask how people feel about the matter. But more often, our move is toward emotional and behavioral learning. For example, we may ask people to play (act out) a childhood game. This is a physical, behavioral reliving of a past emotional position and can help people get in touch with earlier, perhaps more spontaneous feelings. Sometimes acting out helps people feel something faster and more sharply, and then they can grasp its content better.

The point of this discussion is not, however, that one should necessarily start with one way and not another. The point is that teaching should tap and facilitate thinking, feeling, and acting in appropriate proportions and that it should consistently offer this broader range of learning experience. At least this broader range gives people a chance to see and feel what they may need and an opportunity to begin filling in whatever gaps exist in their learning and life experience.

BASIC PREMISES OF THE INTERACTIONAL APPROACH

For you to be able to move on to more specific explanations and analyses of The System, you should first be introduced to the premises which form the basis of the interactional approach.

1. This approach is **humanistic** because its primary focus is always on the individual—on how he functions, on how he affects the relationships and groups he belongs to, and on how these relationships and groups affect him.[5,6]

2. The orientation of this approach is **holistic** because it concentrates not just on the individual but also on his interrelated-

ness with others, especially in marriage and family life, and with his society.[7]

3. Every human being is **unique.** Although every person is similar to and different from every other person, the *way* a person combines and lives out these similarities and differences is what makes him unique.[8,9] Similarly, every marriage and every family is unique.

4. Every person's **whole self** is comprised of two interlocking and mutually influencing "parts": his insides and his outsides. A person's **insides** are *intrapersonal* phenomena, that is, his inner thoughts, feelings, and experiences—both conscious and unconscious.[10] A person's insides consist of his thoughts and feelings about himself; the ways he treats himself; his expectations, rules, and values; his thoughts and feelings about the external world; and all those interactions with the external world that he carries on totally within himself (imaginative interaction). A person's insides then are all those thoughts, feelings, and actions that occur solely within him—the territory of his inner world. They are private unless he chooses to reveal them through communication.

A person's **outsides** are *interpersonal* phenomena, that is, his conscious and unconscious external expressions and manifestations of his insides.[11] Outsides are thoughts, feelings, and actions a person transmits either intentionally or unintentionally to others, and they are governed by his insides. Outsides are public in the sense that they can be observed, sensed, interpreted, experienced, and understood by others. They are the external representation of a person's inner world.

Similarly, every marriage and every family has both insides and outsides.

5. A person can be understood. He is what and who he is because of the experiences he has had and the people he has known. A person is not the product of some mysterious and magical process that cannot be understood.[12]

So, too, marriages and families are what they are because of the participants' experiences within themselves, with each other, and with others. Marriages and families can therefore be understood also.

6. Every person has a life-style. All the consistent ways a person manages life by means of characteristic patterns of thinking, feelings, and acting constitute his **life-style.**[13] "*Life-style*" is an operational term; it describes the observable, dynamic manifestation of his personality. If you take the time and trouble to understand what a person's experiences have been and the ways he has learned to manage life, then a person and his life-style will make sense to you. They are not unfathomable; they can be understood, reacted to appropriately, and dealt with constructively.

Marital relationships and families also develop "personalities" and life-styles. For example, a married couple may come across consistently as friendly, outgoing, and warm; another couple may come across as petty, backbiting, and hostile. One family may be open—warm, friendly, kind, accepting of differences in its members, and able to communicate. Another family may be closed—unfriendly, rigid, intolerant of differences in its members, and disapproving of attempts at open communication.

7. Every person, every marriage, and every family has a life-style that, although it may be similar to other life-styles, is at the same time unique.

8. Individual people, marriage partners, and whole families live by innumerable sets of self-made and self-imposed expectations, rules, and values, and these may enhance or interfere with personal and interpersonal growth.[14]

9. In the process of growing up, *everyone* develops both psychological scars and strengths: how disturbed or how healthy a person is is a reflection of the quantity and quality of those scars and strengths.[15]

In like manner, each marital relationship and each family group bears the psychological scars and strengths gained from living and interacting. For example, what family does not have some skeletons in its closets? And what family does not have its own unique blend of dignity and strength (a blend that sometimes becomes evident when one of the skeletons falls out of the closet into public view)?

WHAT HAPPENS NOW?

This book focuses primarily on "fingertip" material, that is, the thoughts, feelings, and notions about behavior that you have at your fingertips but which, too frequently, you do not or cannot quite put your hands on. This is the stuff that is "on the tip of your tongue" but that frequently eludes you. It is the thing you see out of the "corner of your eye" but cannot quite remember. It is the movement you started to make but never carried out—the hand half raised to say goodbye.

The main intent of this book and of this approach is to release that which is almost ready for release: **"fingertip" material**—those ideas, feelings, and actions that are just beneath the surface of awareness, or that you know about but cannot quite get at or have not yet implemented. Understanding, dealing with, and learning to manage this fingertip material is what leads to new and better ways of living—to being in closer touch with yourself and others and to being better able to use your full potential as a thinking, feeling, and acting human being.[16]

The individual: his identity and abilities

Certain key ideas lie at the heart of the interactional approach. These relate to who the individual is, how he acts, and what he can do.[17,18]

A person is what and who he is now as a result of his heredity, his environment, his background, and his responses to these influences and forces.[19] Depending on these factors and innumerable variables that influence them, he may turn out, for example, to be kind and loving or mean and hostile or well adjusted or poorly adjusted. And who he is will help determine the kind, nature, and quality of the relationships he establishes and maintains.[20] Whatever any human being may be like, however, generally he does the best he can with the equipment he has.[21] For example, most parents really do want the best for their children, but things like anxiety, personal problems, and unreal expectations get in the way. Nevertheless, even though our very humanness can block us from serving our own or others' best interests, most of us do try to be decent human beings.

In addition to this view, however, there is another, more optimistic one. Whatever a person may be like now, he *can* change and grow. By acquiring the necessary communicational and interactional skills, he can learn to live more constructively and appropriately. Thus the life-style you have now need not be a straitjacket that keeps you from ever thinking or feeling or acting any differently from the way you do now. Although you *can* remain essentially the same as you are right now (and you may choose to do so), you do not *have* to remain that way. The power and the ability to change and grow lies within you: no one can force you to change and grow, but no one can prevent you.[22,23]

HOW DOES A PERSON GROW?

What follows is a necessarily oversimplified description of the process of growth. The person who engages in the process of change and growth does numerous things. He begins to observe himself in action and to communicate with himself and thereby get more in touch with his inner thoughts and feelings. ►IE-2, p. 75. He becomes more aware of who he is and what he is like—of how he thinks, feels, and acts. In so doing, he gains awareness and appreciation of his own uniqueness and of his life-style. He begins to see and understand how and when and why he responds in consistent, often automatic ways. As he does this, he is acquiring insight about himself and his functioning (the ways he thinks, feels, and acts). He then implements his insights, altering or modifying or changing his automatic responses to make them more appropriate to what is really happening. ►IE-3, p. 76.

In addition to learning from his interactions with self, he is learning from his interactions with others. He becomes more aware and appreciative of their uniqueness and their life-styles by observing and by communicating with them. His communicating means telling it like it is to *himself* as well as to others, getting feedback, sharing, clearing away distorted ideas and feelings, and setting straight the misassumptions that most human beings are prone to make about themselves and others. As he tries these new experiences, he is becoming aware of, learning about, and developing new alternatives to his old ways of thinking, feeling, and acting (both within himself and with others). And as alternatives become possibilities, life begins to open up, to reveal more of its infinite variety. When a person does or experiences any or all of these things, he is changing—maybe just a little, maybe a great deal. But he is changing and growing.[24,25]

The ingredients of change and growth

Change and growth come about as a result of at least partly conscious and deliberate attempts to use the process of interaction* (and its primary vehicle, communication) in constructive ways. What then are some elements involved in this process? The process of interaction encompasses the following questions (and their answers): *Who are you? How well do you communicate with yourself? How "in touch" with yourself are you?* For example, do you think one thing and say another? Do you just smile when you really feel like smashing somebody? Do you think you would like to do something but find that you block yourself from doing it? These questions all have to do with not being fully in touch with yourself; they have to do with a break in communications with yourself. Part (and a vitally important part) of what this book teaches is how to communicate effectively and meaningfully with yourself and how to understand yourself as a whole person—your thoughts, your feelings, and your actions.

Interaction also involves other questions: *Who are you in relation to other people? How do you come across to them? They to you? Do you react to them in set automatic ways, or are your responses flexible and appropriate to them, the situation, and the moment? What kinds of things do you communicate to them and they to you? How well do you communicate with them?* For example, how do your parents see you? As a child? Is that the way you see yourself? Can you communicate your feelings to them? Can you see them as human beings in their own right? Or do you simply put them into that vast and rather depersonalized category of "parent"? Another (and an equally important) part of what this book teaches is how to understand other people, how to see yourself and be aware of your feelings as you interact with others, how to make your responses more flexible and appropriate, and how to really communicate with other people so that both you and they have a clear idea of who you are and who they are. It is by acquiring and learning to use these skills that people can interact with themselves and others with far greater understanding, meaning, and fulfillment.

We believe very strongly that expertise in communication and interaction—in effect, expertise in being human—can be taught, that it can be learned.[26,27] All of us are learning all the time, but too often we learn expertise in inhumanness. We learn all too well the lessons of prejudice, hostility, aggression, aloofness, "privateness," noncommunicativeness, rejection, and rigidity of thinking, feeling, and acting.

---

*__Interaction__ refers to whatever verbal and nonverbal activity (action) transpires within one person or between/among two or more people. The **dynamics of human interaction** refers to the forces (e.g., each person's self-system, life-style, communication) that create and constitute this activity and the interplay among these forces.

If we are so good at learning those things, there seems to be no reason why we cannot be equally good at *un*learning some of our negative lessons and at learning more positive ways of dealing with ourselves and others. There are reasons, of course, why it is difficult to unlearn the negative and to learn the positive. Whatever is new and unfamiliar tends to arouse discomfort or anxiety or both and to elicit defensive reactions in us. But from our own experience we have found that people are capable of learning to communicate and interact more effectively, of changing, and of growing. We have also found that once people get involved in learning about, acquiring, and implementing communicational and interactional skills (i.e., once they begin to learn and practice The System), once they begin consciously and deliberately to change and to grow, they usually find it to be the most exciting experience that being human has to offer.

We hope that your experiences with this book, this course, yourself, and others will be primarily a positive one. Much of what can help to make your experience a positive one is that you are involved with others as you learn. People need people, and people can help each other.

We urge you therefore to draw on other people for support and feedback and to try to share your inner thoughts and feelings with them. Such sharing can help you become aware of how similar your feelings and reactions are to other people's, can help you appreciate your own and others' uniqueness, and can help enhance the tremendous excitement inherent in moving toward greater openness.

Interaction experiences

1. Focusing on less active components of your style (p. 70)

Try to determine what balance exists in you among your thinking, feeling, and acting components. Draw the three circles mentioned on p. 69 in proportion to the balance you think you have. Now, focus on one of the components represented by one of the smaller circles and try to give it more "play" than you ordinarily do. For example, if you are primarily an Acter-Outer, then concentrate on thinking at more length before you carry out a specific act. If you are an Intellectualizer, concentrate on what you are feeling as you think about something, or consider acting on your thoughts rather than just thinking them.

EVALUATION: Is it difficult for you to give more attention to your less dominant component(s)? Did you feel uncomfortable? Were you surprised by your responses to this experience? Were you pleased? Turned off? Turned on?

FOLLOW-UP: Try paying more attention to and encouraging one (or both) of your less active components as you go through your day.

2. Getting in touch with your inner self (p. 73)

Too many of us are not very aware of who we are and what we feel in the *here and now*. To help you get more in touch with yourself in the here and now, try the following experience when you can be uninterrupted for 5 or 10 minutes.

Close your eyes. Make no noise; just try to tune in on the sounds that surround you. Without attempting to identify what they are, really listen to each different sound that you can hear and then to all these sounds together. Try to get in touch with your feelings in relation to these sounds.

Keep your eyes closed. Try to become more sharply aware of your senses of touch and smell. Try to get in touch with how your body, your clothing, and the air feels. Try to become aware of whatever odors are present around you.

Now, with your eyes still closed, move about slowly, trying to be closely in touch with yourself and your surroundings. Touch, listen, smell, taste—really feel and experience yourself and the physical world around you.

EVALUATION: What emotions did you get in touch with during this experience? Was the experience pleasurable? Anxiety-provoking? Disconcerting? Fun? Exciting? New and different? Did you become more aware than you usually are? Are you surprised by the number of sensory stimuli present in your surroundings?

FOLLOW-UP: Ask a friend to lead you around while you keep your eyes closed. Have him give you a guided tour of different sensations in your environment. For example, he might see to it that you touch something cold and something warm, something rough and something smooth, and so forth. After this, reverse roles, and you lead your friend around. In this manner, you both will have a chance to become more aware of yourselves, your environment, and the relationship between you. After you have both led each other around, share your feelings about the experience.

3. Becoming more aware of automatic behavior (p. 74)

Perform some act that you ordinarily carry out automatically or semiautomatically (e.g., brush your teeth, comb your hair, light a cigarette, drink some water, eat something, write your name, put on your shoes, cross or uncross your legs). Then perform the same act again, only this time do it much more slowly and deliberately. As you do so, try to get in touch with what you are thinking and feeling.

EVALUATION: Does what you think and what you feel during this have much (or anything) to do with your behavior? How aware were you of what you were actually doing?

FOLLOW-UP: For an 8- or 12-hour period, try to get and stay more in touch with what you are thinking and feeling as you act.

REFERENCES

1. Sullivan, Harry Stack: The interpersonal theory of psychiatry, New York, 1953, W. W. Norton and Co., Inc., p. 93.
2. Gunther, Bernard: Sense relaxation below your mind, New York, 1968, Collier Books.
3. Schulz, William C.: Joy: expanding human awareness, New York, 1967, Grove Press, Inc., pp. 25-50.
4. Leonard, George B.: Education and ecstacy, New York, 1968, Dell Publishing Co., Inc., pp. 1-21.
5. Burgental, James F. T., editor: Challenges of humanistic psychology, New York, 1967, McGraw-Hill Book Co.
6. Severin, Frank T., editor: Humanistic viewpoints in psychology, New York, 1965, McGraw-Hill Book Co.
7. Lewis, Howard R., and Streitfeld, Harold S.: Growth games: how to tune in yourself, your family, your friends, New York, 1970, Harcourt Brace Jovanovich, Inc., pp. 3-11.
8. Mannes, Marya: Who am I? In Hoopes, Ned E., editor: Who am I?: essays on the alienated, New York, 1972, Dell Publishing Co., Inc., p. 9.
9. Montague, Ashley: The humanization of man, New York, 1962, Grove Press, Inc., p. 16.
10. Rogers, Carl R.: The organization of personality. In Hamachek, Don E., editor: Human dynamics in psychology and education, Boston, 1970, Allyn & Bacon, Inc., p. 615.
11. Mullahy, Patrick: Psychoanalysis and interpersonal psychiatry: the contributions of Harry Stack Sullivan, New York, 1970, Science House, Inc., pp. 245-246.
12. Jourard, Sidney M.: Disclosing man to himself, New York, 1968, D. Van Nostrand Co.
13. Symonds, Percival M.: Origins of personality. In Hamachek, Don E., editor: Human dynamics in psychology and education, Boston, 1970, Allyn & Bacon, Inc., pp. 580.
14. Ibid., pp. 587-590.
15. Symonds, op. cit., pp. 591-592.
16. Maslow, A. H.: Personality problems and personality growth. In Hamachek, Don E., editor: Human dynamics in psychology and education, Boston, 1970, Allyn & Bacon, Inc., p. 649.
17. Erickson, Erik H.: The problem of ego identity, Journal of American Psychoanalytic Association 4:56-121, 1956.
18. Rogers, Carl R.: On becoming a person, Boston, 1963, Houghton Mifflin Co., pp. 107-124.
19. Bruce, Paul: Three forces in psychology and

their ethical and educational implications. In Hamachek, Don E., editor: Human dynamics in psychology and education, Boston, 1970, Allyn & Bacon, Inc., p. 577.

20. Williams, Thomas Rhys: Introduction to socialization: human culture transmitted, St. Louis, 1972, The C. V. Mosby Co.
21. Lair, Jess: I ain't much baby—but I'm all I've got, Garden City, N.Y., 1972, Doubleday & Co., Inc., pp. 11-22.
22. Jersild, Arthur T.: In search of self, New York, 1965, Teachers College Press, pp. 99-100.
23. Otto, Herbert A., editor: Explorations in human potentials, Springfield, Ill., 1966, Charles C Thomas, Publisher.
24. Fagan, Joel, and Shepard, Irma Lee, editors: Gestalt therapy now, New York, 1970, Harper & Row, Publishers.
25. Perls, Fredrick S.: Gestalt therapy verbatim, Lafayette, Calif., 1969, Real People Press, pp. 1-4.
26. Lair, op. cit., pp. 171-184.
27. Leonard, op. cit., pp. 18-19.

chapter 5
PRESCRIPTIONS FOR LIVING

Part I focused on the double binds created by the conflicts between the old values of the closed past and the newer values and behavior of the more open present. Now it is time to examine more closely the sources, functions, meanings, and strength of the values that underlie our past and present behavior and the ways in which those values direct and govern our behavior.

PRESCRIPTIONS FOR LIVING—PFLs

We have named the values, rules, and expectations that govern our lives and tell us how to live "prescriptions for living" (PFLs—pronounced "piffles"). Basically **PFLs** are internalized expectations, rules, and values, both conscious and unconscious, that provide the content, shape, impetus for, and direction of the ways a person operates and manages himself. These PFLs make up the conscious and unconscious code or formula according to which a person lives. Prescriptions for living are the source of signals, messages, influences, forces, regulations, commands, directions, instructions, guidelines, and models that "tell" and "teach" a person *who* he should be; *what* he should be like; *what* he should think about, feel, and do; and *how* he should think, feel, act, and react. In effect PFLs *prescribe* his thoughts, feelings, and actions and reactions in terms of *what, when, where, with whom, how much, how long, how often,* and *why.*[1]

For example, a PFL such as "children should be courteous to their elders" (an expectation) tells a child how he is expected to act. "Believe what I tell you because I have more experience than you do" (a rule) commands that the person think in a certain way. "A nice girl doesn't go to bed with a man before marriage" (a value) places restrictions on a particular kind of behavior and suggests that the girl who does not subscribe to this value is of lesser worth.

Although PFLs can be and often are restrictive and negative, they are not necessarily so. All of us have them, and many PFLs are extremely useful. In fact, we all need some PFLs. For example, a child needs PFLs like "don't cross the street without first looking both ways" and "don't pull the cat's tail; he might get angry and scratch you." An adult profits from having PFLs such as "be sure to read and understand the fine print of a contract before you sign it" or "a person should be willing to listen to another person without interrupting him or censuring him for his ideas and feelings" or "it's good to be in touch with your feelings."

Packets of PFLs

Every person has many, many PFLs about many, many things (e.g., sex, money, education, trust, honesty, marriage, family). But an individual's PFLs are not randomly distributed; rather they tend to cluster together in what we can think of as packets. **Packets** are comprised of a number of individual PFLs that naturally group themselves together because they are closely related to one another according to specific subject matter (e.g., success, intelligence, time), attitudes (e.g., tolerance, honesty), emotions (e.g., anger, love), and/or behaviors (e.g., taking drugs, taking responsibility).

For example, suppose a person has a PFL that warns, "Don't trust strangers." More than likely there are other, closely allied PFLs that cluster together with this warning PFL and support and reinforce it. Other companion PFLs might be "people are just out for what they can get," "you never know what another person may be thinking," "strangers are usually up to no good," "you've got to know a whole lot about someone before you can be very sure of him," and "avoid people you don't know or aren't sure of."

These individual PFLs cluster together to form a packet of PFLs that are closely related to one another in terms of the specific subject of strangers, an attitude of distrust, and the behavior of being suspiciously avoiding.

Composite PFLs

Out of a packet or perhaps two or three packets of interlocking PFLs will arise a **composite PFL**—one dominant PFL that synthesizes the directions given by all the interrelated individual PFLs in a packet into a powerful basic prescription about how the person should think, feel, and act. Thus it is the composite PFL (supported by all the related individual PFLs in the packet) that prescribes how a person should be and live. In the case of the packet of PFLs just described, the composite PFL might be "don't trust strangers," which directs the person to *think* that strangers cannot be trusted, to *feel* suspicious, mistrustful, and uneasy around strangers, and to avoid dealing with strangers whenever possible *(behavior)*.

Patterns

It can (and does) happen that a person will think, feel, and act from time to time on the basis of an individual PFL within a packet. The more frequent occurrence, however, is for a person to think, feel, and act according to the powerful prescriptions set forth by a composite PFL. When a person repeatedly and consistently implements (i.e., thinks, feels, and acts according to) an individual or composite PFL, then we term his implementation a **pattern.**[2] Thus PFLs provide the shape, the impetus for, and the direction of patterns.

The composite PFL, "Don't trust strangers," might be implemented in a *pattern* of suspicion and mistrust of other people. This pattern of suspicion and mistrust is an interpersonal one.

But it is important to note that PFLs, packets of PFLs, and composite PFLs underpin and direct *both* intrapersonal and interpersonal patterns. **Intrapersonal patterns** are the consistent, inside, private ways a person thinks, feels, and acts within and toward himself.[3] **Interpersonal patterns** are the consistent, public, outside ways a person thinks, feels, and acts with and toward others. For example, suppose a person has the following packet of PFLs: "People who praise themselves are egotistical and selfish"; "Pride goeth before a fall"; "Modesty is a virtue"; "The higher you climb, the farther you fall"; and "Look out—just when you're feeling pleased with yourself, something bad will happen to you." The composite PFL for this packet might be "don't feel good or think good thoughts about your achievements—it's dangerous." From this, the person might develop an *intrapersonal pattern* of denial; that is, he would consistently block out or ignore feelings of pride in or appreciation of his personal achievements. On an *interpersonal* level, he might develop a pattern of denial also, but interpersonally his denial might take the form of self-mockery or self-depreciation. Or he might act self-conscious and brush aside any compliments to him.

As this example shows, the intrapersonal and interpersonal patterns that develop from a packet of PFLs and the composite PFL may be similar. However, it is also possible for the two kinds of patterns to differ somewhat. For example, suppose a person had the packet of PFLs: "You are your own best friend," "Always rely on yourself," "Keep your own counsel," "Trust your own judgment," and "Make your own decisions." Suppose the composite PFL is "be self-reliant." From this, the person might develop an intrapersonal pattern of self-trust and self-regard. But he might develop an interpersonal pattern of aloofness and disdain toward other people and their ideas.

Every person has a number of both intrapersonal and interpersonal patterns, all of which are interrelated and mutually influencing; that is, they interlock with, support, and reinforce each other. Thus there is an internal consistency among a person's patterns, and for this reason, most people function in fairly consistent ways. For example, if a person has an interpersonal pattern of deep distrust of others, he probably does not have a contradictory pattern of being warm, friendly, and accepting. Rather, he is likely to have another pattern of backing off from others.[4]

One exception to this should be noted. It is possible for a person to have a number of contradictory PFLs and patterns, yet function in a consistent manner.[5] His consistency results from his alternating between two conflicting PFLs, patterns, or sets of them. For example, a person might have one set that says, "It's no fun to plan ahead. Do things on the spur of the moment; that's what makes life exciting" and "Always act on your first feeling or impulse; trust your hunches." But suppose he has another set that says, "Look before you leap. You can get in a lot of trouble if you don't look ahead and check out the possible consequences" and "Look ahead; plan for the future. You never know what's around the next corner." Depending on many variables, the person who has the conflicting sets may alternate back and forth between them or stick with one set.

In specific terms, there are two major kinds of **conflicting PFL** sets. The first is created by the child's reaction against PFLs he has been taught. He reacts by constructing an opposing set and acting on it most of the time. But he may occasionally fall back into the PFLs he is reacting against. The second kind consists of two sets of directly conflicting PFLs, which demand that the child make a decision between them. If one set is stronger or delivered by a more influential parent, the child may ultimately operate primarily in terms of that set. Or both sets may have equivalent force (double bind PFLs) so that the child's choices are haunted by a "damned if he does, damned if he doesn't" quality. Whatever the particular case, however, the child will experience anxiety as a result of having to choose from and operate on conflicting PFLs.

THE NATURE OF PFLs

The PFLs that are verbally and nonverbally conveyed to the developing child usually take three basic forms: (1) expectations, (2) rules, and (3) values. Although there are others (e.g., wishes), these three forms are the most common and taken together essentially cover the basic concerns of living.

1. **Expectations.** These are most commonly communicated through the word "expect" ("I expect you to . . ."), but they are also frequently delivered as "should" or "ought to." Many societal or cultural expectations are expressed in this way ("children should . . ."; "a married woman should . . ."; "a single man ought to . . ."; "a parent should . . .").

2. **Rules.** These are easy to spot, since they are most commonly communicated through "do"/"don't" ("don't go with . . ."; "do be like . . ."). Rules are also frequently expressed as "must/must not," "can/can't"; and "have to" ("I must . . ."; "you must not . . ."; "I can . . ."; "you can't . . ."; "I have to . . ."; "you have to . . .").[6,7]

3. **Values.** These are sometimes more subtle and therefore more difficult to detect than are rules and expectations, but they are usually communicated in the form of "good" and "bad" ("it's bad to . . ."; "it's

a good idea to . . ."). Values can also be stated as "worth something/worthless," "important/unimportant," and "right/wrong" (". . . has never been important to this family"; "it's always right to . . .").[8]

All of these prescriptions are applied, of course, to all three areas of functioning: thinking, feeling, and acting. An example of this follows. In the time prior to the women's liberation movement, many a father might have expressed (verbally and/or nonverbally) these expectations to his daughter: "Because you are a girl, I expect you to *think* in a slightly illogical manner"; "I expect you to *feel* deeply and intensely and to operate on the basis of your feelings, not your intellect"; "I expect you to *act* nonaggressive, demure, 'feminine.'" If the growing girl accepts this particular package of expectations (as well she may), she will tend to think, feel, and act in accordance with them. And she will be likely to measure herself (and other females) against these criteria.

The PFLs that each partner brings to a marriage can strongly affect how each will think, feel, and act in the relationship and can therefore influence the course and quality of the relationship.[9,10] For example, suppose a husband has a value PFL about the issues of work and money that says, "A wife can't respect her husband if he doesn't carry the full financial responsibility for their marriage." But suppose the wife has her own value PFL that says, "To lead a meaningful life, a person must develop her talents," and she decides to get a job. Because of his PFL, her husband may *think* that she really does not respect him, he may *feel* angry and threatened, and he may *act* resistant to her seeking a job. She may *think* her husband is acting like a stupid, mean-spirited chauvinist, she may *feel* angry and rebellious, and she may *act* by redoubling her efforts to get a job. Obviously, unless these people communicate honestly with each other and constructively negotiate the conflict based on their PFLs, each one's PFL will restrict and distort the way each thinks, feels, and acts and will thereby be harmful to their relationship.

These two fairly simple examples give some taste of the power and influence that PFLs can wield in a person's life. If you recognize that every human being is exposed to an enormous number of PFLs, you can begin to appreciate the importance and complexity of the developmental process that every child experiences.

Prescriptions for living may be conceived of as seeds that are planted in the child's mind and heart. Some will never see the light of day because they will wither from lack of nurturance. But many of them will grow to be like strong and sturdy plants and trees. Some will become flowers, but others will become weeds, ugly and threatening. Some will become misshapen, twisted, gnarled, and perhaps diseased trees, whereas others will grow into magnificent evergreens or giant redwoods.[11]

Sources of PFLs

Where do prescriptions come from? Parents are usually the major transmitters. But other Significant Persons such as siblings, grandparents, other relatives, peers, and teachers can also contribute greatly to the "planting." In addition, many seeds are borne on the winds of culture. For example, look at all the societal prescriptions that are handed down to us:

Expectations: Adults shouldn't act childish; the family should be preserved at almost any cost.

Rules: Don't murder; don't commit adultery; don't commit incest; don't lie, cheat, or steal; respect the law; be kind to animals; do unto others.

Values: Marriage is a blessed and lawful state; patriotism is good; politics is dirty business; premarital sex is wrong; each person has the right to live as he pleases as long as he doesn't hurt anybody else.

In addition, as a result of his own experiences and his perceptions of those experiences, a child will create other PFLs. For example, he may make friends with children of another race and thereby develop his own values about and expectations of members of that race.[12]

How PFLs are communicated

Prescriptions can be communicated both nonverbally and verbally.

NONVERBAL TRANSMISSION OF PFLs

Many of the earliest and most crucial instructions about what and what not to do are conveyed to the child nonverbally long before he can talk or really conceptualize. In response to the feeling tone, the emotional atmosphere of his environment, and the ways significant people treat him, the child "feels in his bones" the impact of many unspoken PFLs.[13] For example, suppose an infant's mother is subject to rapid mood swings: one moment she is patient and tender with the infant; the next moment she is irritable, nervous, and rough with him. Over a period of time, this child may build in a vague sense of anxiety, which, if it were verbalized in PFL form, might be expressed as, "Watch out; you never know what's going to happen next." Although this set of experiences alone might not create a permanent PFL, there may be other, similar experiences with his mother that add to this PFL and perhaps make it permanent. At the very least, early experiences like this create fertile ground for the planting of later, conceptualized PFLs.

Other PFLs can be transmitted almost as subliminally by means of parental patterns of thinking, feeling, and acting.[14] Although the parents may never overtly express certain PFLs, the child sees the PFLs in action, since patterns are the implementations of PFLs. For example, if a child sees his father rather consistently treat his mother and other women with contempt and scorn, he may deduce and build in one or more of the following PFLs: "Women are inferior," "It's alright for men to treat women with contempt and scorn," or "All men are naturally mean to all women." If a child sees his mother rather consistently complain about and belittle his father and other men, he may deduce and build in one or more of the following PFLs: "Men are a pain in the neck," "It's alright or natural for women to put men down," or "All women dislike or think ill of all men." On the other hand, if a child sees his parents frequently help out less fortunate relatives or friends, he may infer a PFL such as "helping others is good" or "those in need deserve to be helped out." If he sees his parents treat each other with concern, consideration, respect, and love, he will probably develop a PFL such as "marriage is a good thing" or "marriage means caring and loving" or "you should always treat your mate well." Thus as these examples illustrate, a child may learn many PFLs without their even having been verbalized.

Another form of nonverbal communication of PFLs is that of omission.[15] Parents may avoid mentioning certain subjects, but their very silence sends special messages about these subjects. For example, if parents say absolutely nothing about sex, their silence may plant a seed in the child's mind that sex is dirty, mysterious, forbidden, dark, or sinful. Since children make up their own PFLs if they have no other frame of reference, silence on a subject as important and as fascinating as sex allows the child to grab PFLs out of the atmosphere and plant them in the rich soil of his imagination. And the prescriptions (or suggestions for them) are there for the taking in magazines, in sex books, in movies, in pornography, in graffiti, in the gutter, and in things the child sees and hears (such as doors closing, his parents' bed squeaking, moans and groans, muffled laughter, and sudden activity as the lights go back on, the water runs, and the toilet is flushed). Thus, although the parents may say nothing at all about sex, their silence communicates just as surely as if they had sat down and talked at length about sex. The child fills in the gaps created by their silence by constructing PFLs to explain what his parents do not explain. To dispel his own confusion and anxiety, the child reacts by creating PFLs, which in some way help him to understand this unmentionable subject.

VERBAL TRANSMISSION OF PFLs

PFLs can be (and frequently are) communicated verbally.[16] For example, a child may take in values by hearing adults in the family discuss with scathing contempt the actions of the girl down the street "who'll sleep with just about anybody." Or he may hear his parents speak of how the "wops" or "niggers" or "spics" or "honkies" are ruining the value of local real estate, or how those "Pope-worshippers" (or "kikes" or "Holy Rollers" or any other religious group) are ruining the country or have taken control of world finance. Even though these comments may not be made directly to him or their content taught to him as outright PFLs, the child may take in their content and meaning as PFLs. Thus he may internalize his parents' epithets about other races and religions into a PFL such as "people of other races and religions are undesirable and should be avoided" or "people of other races are destructive."

Of course, many PFLs are taught directly as PFLs: "Don't get too friendly with people, they might make demands on you," "Don't talk back to your parents," "We expect you to act like a man," and "No respectable girl would make out in public." Often when PFLs are expressed so overtly, they carry a great deal of force, but by the same token they may be the easiest to resist or rebel against. ►IE-1, p. 91.

RESPONSES TO PFLs

When a prescription for living is introduced into a child's life, if it has enough force or weight that it does not just fall by the wayside unnoticed, the child must relate to it in some way. What are the possibilities?

Rejection

One direct way a child can respond to a prescription is to reject it outright.[17] If there is an obvious gap between a PFL and reality, he may realize this and reject the teaching. For example, suppose a mother gives her daughter, this rule: "Don't have anything to do with the neighbors; they don't like us and they laugh at us." But suppose the daughter knows from her own experience that this simply is not so. Then the daughter may reject her mother's prescription. In addition, the daughter may reject or take with a grain of salt many other of her mother's prescriptions; at the least, the daughter will probably check out many of her mother's statements before accepting them. It is probable that the wider the gap between a PFL and reality the easier it is for a child to reject the prescription. Conversely, the narrower the gap and the more subtly the PFL is conveyed the harder it is for a child to discriminate about and resist accepting a PFL.

A child or an adolescent may have another reason to reject PFLs: he may rebel and refuse to accept what he is taught. He may do so because he is angry at the "teacher," because he feels that he knows a better way, or because his peers' prescriptions mean more or make more sense to him.

If a person does reject one or more prescriptions, however, he must then create his own as replacements, since PFLs are absolutely necessary for living. He may construct his own PFLs on the basis of what he learns from other significant persons, what he learns from his own experiences, or a combination of the two, or he may significantly modify an existing PFL.

Building in and elaboration

A second possible way for the child to respond is to follow the prescription almost exactly as it is stated: he behaves, thinks, or feels (or all three) as the PFL directs him to.[18] If the child is told that he must pay attention to what his father says, he pays attention; if he is told that it is not good to cry when he gets his feelings hurt, he tries to build in this value and teach himself not to cry.

Another kind of response is a variation of building in PFLs. A child may take certain

PFLs, interpret them according to the way he sees the world, and elaborate on them—a process that sometimes results in a distortion of the original intent of the PFL.[19] For example, suppose a father impresses on his little daughter that she should never accept candy or rides from strangers, especially strange men. His intent is to protect her from child molesters. Her elaborations of this stated rule might be as follows: (1) "Don't accept candy or rides from strangers"; (2) "Be very careful and wary of strangers"; (3) "Be suspicious if a strange man gives you something because if he does he wants something from you"; (4) "He might touch you and do bad things to you"; (5) "He might try to hurt you"; and (6) "He might kill you." If this elaborated PFL is reinforced by other "suspicion-type" PFLs and perhaps by some experiences, this girl may grow up to be a young woman who believes that men are only out for what they can get and that when men ask her for a date, they do so only to get her sexual favors in return.

It should be noted that only *one* PFL and its elaborations is obviously not the sole cause of a major attitude such as this young woman's mistrust of men's motives. If a PFL is this strong and this significant, others will support it either in terms of subject matter (men, sex, motives) or attitude (suspicion, mistrust, fear) or both. ►IE-2, p. 91.

PFLs AND PATTERNS: THE LARGER CONTEXT

Up to this point, the discussion and explanations have focused on the power and importance of PFLs as the dynamic underpinnings, the determiners, of the patterned ways an individual thinks, feels, and acts. But, most certainly, the individual and his personal PFLs do not develop or exist in a vacuum. Rather, the individual learns his PFLs from other individuals, from his parents, from other family members, and from his society. In effect, what is constantly occurring is a reciprocation of influences between the individual and these other entities. Thus it becomes important to examine the other entities that have and are directed by PFLs and that influence and are influenced by the individual and his PFLs.

Societal PFLs

Society and its institutions (e.g., government, education, religion) is a vast and powerful propagator and enforcer of innumerable **societal PFLs.**[20] The areas that societal PFLs apply to are practically limitless. They cover such disparate yet interrelated areas as social conduct, private conduct, morality, ethics, sexual behavior, religious behavior, male/female roles, social and private roles, folk wisdom, dress, family, and marriage. Some societal PFLs take the form of actual, written laws—"Don't steal"; "Pay your income tax"; "Don't run a red light"; "Don't attack, injure, or kill others"; and "Don't speed." But perhaps the bulk of societal PFLs take the form of unwritten laws, expectations, rules, and values. For example, there are PFLs relating to ideals: "Being a good citizens means being informed and exercising the right (and privilege) to vote"; "Education is the right of every person"; and "America stands for the principles of liberty and justice for all." And there are PFLs about everyday things such as the following: "Men shouldn't cry in public (and rarely in private)"; "Women are the weaker sex and need to be protected"; "Childhood is a time of natural innocence"; "Don't have sex before marriage"; "Women shouldn't be passionate or enjoy sex very much"; "A penny saved is a penny earned"; "The strong should protect the weak"; "Do unto others as you would have them do unto you"; "The family that prays together stays together"; "Boys may be (and should be) adventuresome and self-reliant"; "Girls should be gentle and nurturing"; "Family members should be loyal to one another"; and "You can't truly love more than one person at a time."

The list is long, since there are innumerable societal PFLs. Although many societal PFLs can be restrictive and limiting, they also serve positive purposes. One is to provide a kind of societal "glue" that holds people together in a type of loose confederation of general agreement about various aspects of life. Another is to furnish a structured approach to life, which is derived from people's past experiences and shared beliefs, goals, and instructions. A third is to help determine and define what life means by, for example, establishing what is right and what is wrong. A fourth purpose is to regulate the ways people behave toward one another in the myriad situations, roles, and relationships that make up life in any society. ►IE-3, p. 91.

Family and marital PFLs

One of the primary means for passing on societal PFLs from one generation to the next is the family. In effect the family serves as the local transmitter and administrator of the culture's PFLs. As parents teach their children how to be social beings, they are handing down prescriptions distilled from the wisdom, prejudices, perceptions, fears, and hopes of many prior generations and of a long-term social structure.[21]

In addition to the societal PFLs it hands down, the family develops its own sets of family PFLs, some of which result from the living out of societal PFLs about the family.[22] For example, there are numerous societal PFLs about the ways family members should relate to one another (e.g., family members should love each other); what each kind of role requires (e.g., a father should be a firm disciplinarian; it is a mother's function to toilet train the children); and the family's relations to the rest of society (e.g., parents are responsible for their children's behavior).

Other family PFLs come from the PFLs that each parent brings to the new family from his or her own family background and from a combination of the two parents' individual and family PFLs. Naturally, the forerunner of the process whereby each parent's PFLs are merged with the other's is the merger that occurs between the marital partners' PFLs about life, themselves, marriage, and family life, since it is the marital relationship that forms the core of the family and its relationships. As the marital partners work out their relationship, they gradually form their own easy or uneasy combination of PFLs and patterns regarding the marital issues that confront them.[23] For example, suppose the husband has a PFL that says the man should handle all the finances, whereas the wife has a PFL that says whoever has the most talent or ability for a particular job should do it. Assuming a certain degree of good will and skill at communicating, they work out the potential conflict between them. Perhaps the wife is able to convince her husband that his masculinity does not depend on his filling a particular role and that following some version of her PFL leads to a more mature relationship between them. They both learn to integrate the work and chores of married life according to each one's talents and abilities and thus establish a pattern of respecting, sharing, and negotiating. If this husband and wife are able to deal with most of their differences (and similarities) in these constructive ways, they will develop a basically flexible, open, marital life-style.

However a marital couple works out differences and similarities in their PFLs and patterns, the result will be a marital life-style based on this blend. The PFLs, patterns, and life-style they develop as a marital couple determine in large part what they teach their children and therefore what PFLs, patterns, and life-style the family develops. In the case of the couple just described, the PFLs that their family develops include ones like "the person who has the ability to do a certain thing should be the one to do it" and "respect each person's uniqueness." The patterns that naturally arise include respect, flexibility, and self-confidence. And the family style will be a healthy, open one.

The matter of family and marital PFLs, patterns, and styles is, of course, far more complex than this discussion indicates, but a more thorough and detailed analysis of these subjects occurs in Part III. Before closing this subject of societal, marital, and family PFLs, patterns, and styles, it is important to consider the underlying principles that essentially determine the quality and character of the relationships based on societal, marital, family, and individual PFLs.

Directives and guidelines

Whether relationships (and institutions) are closed or open depends ultimately on the nature of the PFLs on which they are grounded. If a society, its institutions, and the relationships within it are based primarily on directives, then they tend to be closed; if they are based primarily on guidelines, they tend to be open.

The differences between directives and guidelines are as follows: Essentially a **directive** sets up restrictions that try to cover every occurrence of a situation and that imply *always*. A directive allows for few if any exceptions (unless the exceptions are stated as part of the directive). Thus a directive offers its "owner" or "obeyer" little room to choose, since it is not the nature of a directive to admit alternatives. That is, a directive is usually a flat, unequivocal statement ("do this"; don't do that"), which is designed to be applied consistently and without question to all similar or similar-*seeming* situations. The question of the appropriateness of its application does not fall within the scope of a directive's nature. Thus with a flat directive, a person need make only one choice—to follow or not to follow it. If he decides to follow it, he releases himself from the need to make further choices. This fact explains, perhaps, why there is security to be found in following directives. It also explains why the strict directive follower tends to be relatively closed, rigid, and non-autonomous.

The nature and effects of guidelines are different. Far from dictating, a **guideline** suggests various possibilities and alternatives. It allows for exceptions and leaves the choices or decisions about appropriateness up to the person who subscribes to the guideline. For example, a directive would flatly state, "It's wrong to show or express anger," whereas a guideline might say, "Showing and expressing anger can be healthy and appropriate at times. Evaluate the situation and act accordingly." Obviously there is less security in guidelines but far more freedom—freedom that rests on exercising sensitivity, choice, judgment, and responsibility. This may explain why the person who operates primarily according to guidelines tends to be relatively open, flexible, and autonomous.

It should be made clear that some directives are necessary just for staying alive. For example, a very young child simply is not equipped to use a guideline about playing with matches. However, the process of growing toward healthy autonomy involves a gradual increase in guidelines and decrease in directives.

If a society, its institutions, and its members operate primarily according to directives, the result is closedness—an authoritarian atmosphere, restricted choices, and an often severely limited number of alternatives. As described in Chapter 1, American society was essentially closed at the beginning of this century. But because of vast upheavals and changes in both physical circumstances and ideological outlook, the United States has gradually moved toward greater openness based on guidelines rather than directives.

It has been, however, just this move away from directives toward guidelines that has prompted a good deal of anxiety for people in the present. Although many directives of the closed society have fallen away or have lost much of their force, many people have been at a loss about how to establish guidelines to replace the directives. In addition, when people do establish new PFLs and guidelines, they often find that the old directives still have great—and contradictory—force. The resultant double bind frequently engenders much conflict and **anxiety**—generalized, unfocused feelings of uneasiness, apprehension, and discomfort. Basically this anxiety results from an emotional disequilibrium created by newness, difference, and conflict.

The ways that people deal with this state

of disequilibrium are what The System is all about.

DYNAMIC EQUILIBRIUM

Every human being is constantly and continuously engaged in establishing and maintaining his **dynamic equilibrium,**[24] a vital balance by which a person keeps his sense of self and stability intact, while at the same time allowing for and adjusting to newness, to difference, to change, and to the unfamiliar. In effect, each of us is always trying to get and stay comfortable within ourselves, with others, and in relation to circumstances and the situation.

Before birth until death, each person is confronted by a barrage of stimuli to his senses: the sights, sounds, smells, tastes, and touches; the events; the people; and the thoughts, feelings, actions, and reactions that make up life. From moment to moment, these stimuli come at and to a person at an almost overwhelmingly rapid rate. Like the ocean, they swirl about him; he is flooded by stimuli. Unlike the ocean, however, these waves of stimuli do not necessarily come to him in a steady, regulated, organized way—in a way that would enable him to anticipate them.

What is his natural response? It is to seek and, if possible, find and maintain stability in this flux. That is, each person attempts to organize, to control, the innumerable swirling, disorganized moments of life experiences in such a way that he can manage them. How does he go about organizing and controlling them? The two primary means he uses are his prescriptions for living and his patterns.

PFLs as organizing principles

A person looks at the world through the windows of himself and supplies a system of organization to the stimuli "out there." He assesses, evaluates, and categorizes these stimuli according to how they measure up to the criteria established by his PFLs. For example, suppose Alice has a prescription that says, "Most people who smile pleasantly and act in a friendly manner can probably be trusted." Thus Alice tends to categorize people who act this way as probably trustworthy—before she has even met them. Suppose Zack has a PFL that tells him, "All loud and forceful women are aggressive and want to dominate men." Thus Zack will classify all women who act this way as wanting to dominate men (himself included). By classifying and categorizing simuli according to PFLs, a person confers a certain amount of consistency, stability, and manageability on external stimuli.

Another way that prescriptions for living help a person to reach outside himself and organize stimuli is by guiding his **selective processes,**[25] that is, how he selects what he will respond to. He sets up processes of selective awareness: selective attention and inattention, selective sensitivity, selective forgetting and remembering, and selective action and reaction. For example, think about how much you cut out of your consciousness; television or music in the background; light and noise when you are napping; other conversations when you are listening to one person or are talking yourself; the whole rest of the world when you are making love.

Each person is free to do this kind of selecting because of his PFLs. For example, a person may have a prescription telling him that it is dangerous not to listen when someone in authority speaks to him but that it is safe not to pay attention when the little child next door chatters to him. Selectivity makes life less demanding and more manageable because it enables a person to short-circuit a lot of stimuli before they even reach him. He simply blocks them out; he prevents them from bothering him or from making a difference to him. Selectivity therefore allows a person to concentrate more fully on those stimuli he does choose to let through.

PFLs also enable a person to make life more stable and manageable by helping him to deal with that which is new and unfamiliar. Newness, especially a lot of it, tends to arouse anxiety. To lessen anxiety, a person immediately attempts to make the new somehow familiar. He does this by seeking and finding (or creating or imagining) that quality in the new experience which is the same or *seems the same* as something his PFLs and experiences have already made familiar to him.[26] For example, suppose you meet someone for the first time. Rather than relate to him as a totally unknown quality, you quickly "slot" him according to your PFLs. Suppose he does not look you in the eye when he talks to you. Aha! Just as your parents taught you—people who don't look you in the eye are hiding something, so don't trust them. Or maybe he does look you straight in the eye the whole time he is talking to you. Then you are inclined to trust him. It is, of course, impossible here to run through all the ways you might respond to a new person according to your PFLs. Perhaps it is sufficient to point out that any new person will present you with many stimuli and that you will measure him according to not just one PFL but according to a whole network of them. In this way, each of us applies control and order to anxiety-producing newness: we categorize it in such a way as to make it familiar and therefore comfortable.

Prescriptions for living then help every person to cope with the innumerable stimuli that come at and to him. Using his PFLs, he sifts and sorts the stimuli of life: he categorizes them, he selects among them, and he makes the unfamiliar ones familiar by linking them to that which he already knows.

Patterns as organizing techniques

In addition to organizing external stimuli, a person organizes himself by means of patterns of thinking, feeling, and acting so that he is ready and able to respond to categorized stimuli. In effect, he preprograms himself to respond in consistent ways to particular kinds of stimuli.[27] For example, one of Zack's PFLs tells him that all loud and forceful women are agressive and want to dominate men. Another prescription warns him that if you give this kind of woman the slightest encouragement, she will try to get you involved in a relationship with her. Another PFL cautions him that if you get involved with this kind of woman, she will make life hell for you. A composite PFL logically evolves from this network of PFLs: "Don't be nice to this kind of woman" or "Avoid this kind of woman if you don't want to get hurt." Also suppose that Zack has watched his loud and forceful mother aggressively dominate his meek and mild father. What is the outcome? Zack develops an *interpersonal pattern* of avoiding loud, forceful women. (He may by extension develop a pattern of avoiding anyone, male or female, who is loud and forceful.) When Zack meets a woman who acts this way, he avoids her. He is preprogrammed to respond in a particular way to a particular set or category of stimuli.

Not only does a person organize himself to handle external stimuli, he also does so to manage *internal stimuli.* He organizes the ways he thinks, feels, and acts in response to his *inner* thoughts, feelings, and actions. For example, I may react to my feelings of anger by withdrawing into sullenness; you may react to your feelings of anger by lashing out at others. You may feel challenged by thoughts about the future, whereas I may feel threatened. Whatever our differences are, however, we each have patterns of responses to help us cope with our internal stimuli. ►IE-4, p. 92.

PFLs and patterns then are what enable a person to achieve and maintain a sense of control, a sense of order, and a sense of management of himself, his environment, and his reactions to it. Once he categorizes stimuli according to his PFLs and thereby makes them familiar, he can have his patterns of response ready. That reduces the elements of surprise and anxiety; he does not have to fish around to find the right response. In effect, each person *predetermines* how he will let life present itself to him, and he *predetermines* how he will think, feel, and act toward life. Thus he meets, organizes, and manages life on his terms. This process of applying PFLs/patterns is what enables a person to feel comfortable, to maintain his dynamic equilibrium. And as long as he can continue to use this process successfully, it will be a self-reinforcing one.

Usually the ordinary functioning of an individual's personality* is adequate to the task of maintaining dynamic equilibrium in the midst of the flux. However, often something (a thought, a feeling, an issue, an event, another person) comes along and threatens or actually disrupts a person's dynamic equilibrium. Such threats or actual disequilibrium evoke feelings of anxiety.

The closed person

Everyone's dynamic equilibrium is threatened or disrupted from time to time, and everyone uses his psychological defenses when this occurs. But some people use their defenses more often than others and, for the most part, use them in an unconscious manner. The person who tends to employ his personality primarily in a defensive manner is the closed person. The **closed person** is one who has little self-awareness and awareness of others and who is governed largely by unconscious, automatic, and repetitious ways of thinking, feeling, and acting.[28]

What are the characteristics of the closed person?

1. He is essentially not available to new and different experiences; he tends to back away from trying new and different ways of thinking, feeling, and acting. He feels threatened by or anxious about what is not familiar to him: the unknown involves risks that he feels too insecure to take.

2. It is difficult for him to accept individuality. He is far more comfortable around those who conform to the same PFLs and directives as he does. If people are rather (or even somewhat) different from him—either socially, economically, racially, culturally, sexually, religiously, ethnically, politically, morally, physically, emotionally, or intellectually—he has trouble relating to them, or he may reject them outright. He tends to seek out and mix with "his own kind."

3. He is not very flexible. If a person or a situation requires him to bend a little or to think, feel, or act in ways that are different from his usual ones, he has a difficult time doing so (if he even tries). He tends to stick to his tried and true patterns of living, and he tries to get others to change to his ways if possible. If he can control people so that they fit his predetermined criteria, he feels comfortable. But if he is asked to change or to act outside the bounds of his criteria, he becomes anxious and defensive and probably balks.

4. He is not freedom granting. He believes people should act in certain acceptable (to him) ways. He has problems in "allowing" others to be who they are. If he has control over others, he tends to clamp his rules, his values, his expectations, and his ways of doing things on them.

5. He himself is not a free person. By and large, his life-style, which is basically rigid, inflexible, and highly automatic and repetitious, strongly restricts and limits him. He is not likely to try new and different experiences; he sticks with what is familiar; he does not move out to meet, or accept, people who are different from him. He stays "close to home" if possible; if not, he carries that "emotional home" with him wherever he goes. Thus his closed life-style tends to limit his growth, to curb his curiosity, and to inhibit his creativity. It also tends to restrict

*We try to avoid using the term "personality" because the concept it stands for is so large and all-encompassing that it is difficult to relate to it as a single entity. Thus whenever possible, we deal with smaller, more manageable concepts that are parts of the largest concept of personality. Nevertheless, because the term "personality" and the concept it represents are so much a part of our language, our thinking, and our ways of viewing people, it is necessary to provide you with our definition of the term.

Our definition is as follows: **Personality** is the dynamic interaction between and among a person's biophysical and psychological components, the results of which inform and control both his characteristic and unique thoughts, feelings, and actions.

his relationships, since it interferes with his communication and leads him to distort the meaning and intent of his relationships.

The closed person is obviously limited by his closedness; his life-style is **dysfunctional.**[29] Although he does function (he holds a job or goes to school; he may be married and have a family; he interacts), his functioning is limited and/or impaired. It is less qualitative, less healthy, less constructive than it might be.

The open person

No one is perfect: even the open person plays "games" at times.[30] But ordinarily the open person does not play games because he is able to achieve his psychological ends and to establish and maintain his dynamic equilibrium by direct, undistorted, and appropriate ways of thinking, feeling, and acting.

The characteristics of the **open person**[31] are as follows:

1. He is available to new and different experiences; that is, he is able to try out and to experiment appropriately with new and different ways of thinking, feeling, and acting. He is willing and strong enough to take the risks that accompany newness and difference.
2. He is accepting of individuality; he does not demand that others be a certain way before he will accept them. He meets and interacts with people in terms of who they are, not in terms of who he might like them to be or who he thinks they should be.
3. He is flexible. People do not have to act according to what *he* believes in, and circumstances do not necessarily have to go his way. He can and does negotiate with himself and with others about how he wishes to respond. And if necessary and appropriate, he can and will change or adapt his responses to new and different people and situations.
4. He is freedom granting. People do not have to fit a particular mold. His philosophy is—*I am who I am, and others are who they are; I will do my best to communicate and interact with them in appropriate and constructive ways. But I do not believe in prejudging people, in trying to restrict them, or in trying to force them to act in particular ways.*
5. The open person is himself free—free from the limitations and restrictions of a rigid, inflexible, highly automatic and repetitious life-style. Consequently he is more experimental, more excited and exciting, more alert and aware, and more alive. He is open to his own being, to others, to life.

The open person's life-style is **functional.**[32] His functioning (the ways he thinks, feels, and acts) is basically qualitative, healthy, and constructive. He is in touch with his inner thoughts and feelings and his life-style; thus he is not dominated by unconscious forces and does not usually operate on the basis of distorted information or feelings. Although he is perfectly capable of defending himself when necessary and appropriate, his personality is not primarily geared to rigidly defending his dynamic equilibrium.

CONCLUSION

This chapter has focused on the relationship between PFLs/patterns and our past and present behavior, that is, on the ways PFLs and patterns contribute to our closedness or openness. Chapter 6 will examine the process by which the individual learns to be who he is in the present (e.g., how he acquires PFLs and patterns). In effect, the next chapter investigates the process of developing an identity.

Interaction experiences

1. Evaluating parental PFLs (p. 83)

If possible, identify five major prescriptions your father lives by. Identify five major prescriptions your mother lives by. Write them down in full sentence form and identify at the end of each sentence whether the PFL is a verbal or nonverbal one. Compare you mother's set of five with your father's set of five. What does the comparison "say" about each of them? For example, are your mother's PFLs all negative? All positive? Mixed? What about your father's? Is each one's set of PFLs, for example, those of a passive or an aggressive or a relaxed or an authoritarian person?

Select a partner. *Nonverbally* role play (act like) your mother as she would act on one of her PFLs. Do the same for your father. As in charades, let the other person try to guess what PFL it is you are acting out. Negotiate with your partner to determine if he wishes to role play one of his parents' PFLs.

EVALUATION: Discuss with your partner what effects these PFLs had on each parent's behavior and the effects of that behavior on you.

FOLLOW-UP: You might wish to share your lists with your parents and to discuss your experience with them.

2. Experiencing the power of your PFLs (p. 84)

Try to determine what some of your PFLs are and list them. In so doing, remember that we all have PFLs which govern all areas of our lives (e.g., success, intelligence, time; tolerance, honesty; fear, affection; work, taking responsibility, play). Next, try to determine a packet of PFLs that you have about a specific area and then the composite PFL for this packet.

First, act according to one of your individual or composite PFLs. For example, suppose you have a PFL that says, "Never be late for anything." Act on it in the way you usually do; that is, consciously and deliberately be on time to your next time commitment. Try to get in touch with what your thoughts and feeling are as you do this.

Second, act *contrary* to this same PFL. For example, consciously and deliberately *be late* to your next time commitment. Try to get in touch with what you are thinking and feeling as you do this.

EVALUATON: What differences in your thoughts and feelings did you experience as you acted these two different ways? What does the comfort you felt in acting as you usually do and the discomfort you felt in acting contrary to your PFL tell you about the power and the automatic quality of your PFL? Do you feel that your PFL restricts your freedom of choice and action?

FOLLOW-UP: Try this same experience with other of your PFLs. In this way, you can gain greater awareness and understanding of the rules, values, and expectations that govern your life.

3. Experiencing the emotional force of societal PFLs (p. 85)

Probably all of us conform in many conscious and unconcious ways to societal dictates, since we are reared with a vast number of societal PFLs about conformity such as the following: "Don't make waves"; "Do the right thing"; "Don't draw attention to yourself"; "Don't be different"; "Don't violate the unwritten codes of behavior."

Either fantasize doing so or, if appropriate, actually go against a PFL about conformity. For example, speak out in class if you usually do not do so or speak to a stranger.

EVALUATION: What were your thoughts and feelings as you went through this experience? Were you uncomfortable? Anxious? Did you feel silly? Ridiculous? Humiliated? Embarrassed? Defiant? Aggressive? Hostile? Did you feel the strength of this PFL? Of the societal pressure attached to it?

FOLLOW-UP: Try this same experience with other societal PFLs. Also, share your feelings about your experience with others.

4. Working with consistent patterns (p. 88)

Take some time to sit down and think about your consistent patterns. You might think in terms of how you consistently think, feel, and act when you are with particular people or groups of people or in terms of how you consistently think, feel, and act in response to such things as criticism, praise, anger, joy, sarcasm, annoyance, fear, loneliness, and affection.

Do not try to think of all your patterns at one time—just two or three.

When you have determined one or more of your patterns (either intrapersonal or interpersonal), check with another person who knows you well to see if he or she has observed and is aware of the pattern.

After this, try two experiences.

1. With an intrapersonal pattern, ask another person to be you. Instruct him about what to say to you to carry out the pattern. (In effect, he plays one part of you that talks to the other part, which is played by you.) As you experience how he treats you according to your intrapersonal pattern, try to get in touch with what you feel in response to this enactment of your usual treatment of yourself. For example, suppose you discover that you have a pattern of "yelling" at yourself when you make mistakes; that is, you make belittling comments to yourself like "that's really dumb" or "that was ridiculous" or "oh, c'mon you stupid jerk" or "there I go—klutzing around again." In this experience, you will be hearing these things said directly to you by *another* person.

Two other ways to carry out this experience are as follows (and you might try them both):

a. You treat another person the way you treat yourself.

b. Have two other people act out the way you treat yourself.

EVALUATION: Do you like the way you treat yourself? What were your feelings during this experience? Would you treat another person the way you treat yourself? Can you think of different and better ways to treat yourself?

FOLLOW-UP: The next time you catch yourself treating yourself in a particular negative way, you might try to deliberately treat yourself more constructively and pleasantly. Also try having another person act out your pattern and then do it differently (act more pleasant, treat you better).

2. Try this same experience with an interpersonal pattern of yours.

REFERENCES

1. Montague, Ashley: The humanization of man, New York, 1962, Grove Press, Inc., pp. 145-158.
2. Perry, Helen Swick, and Gawel, Mary Ladd, editors: The collected works of Harry Stack Sullivan, M.D., vol. 1, New York, 1953, W. W. Norton & Co., Inc., pp. 103-104.
3. Ackerman, Nathan W.: The psychodynamics of family life, New York, 1958, Basic Books, Inc., Publishers, p. 54.
4. Mullahy, Patrick: A theory of interpersonal relations and the evolution of personality. In Sullivan, Harry Stack: Conceptions of modern psychiatry, Washington, D.C., 1947, William Alanson White Foundation, pp. 122-123.
5. Montague, op. cit., p. 147.
6. Ruesch, Jurgen: Synopsis of the theory of human communication. In Howells, John G., editor: Theory and practice of family psychiatry, New York, 1971, Brunner/Mazel, Inc., pp. 238-239.
7. Symonds, Percival M.: Origins of personality. In Hamachek, Don E., editor: Human dynamics in psychology and education, Boston, 1968, Allyn & Bacon, Inc., p. 592.
8. Ackerman, op. cit., pp. 335 and 337.
9. Dicks, Henry V.: Experiences with marital tensions seen in the psychological clinic. In Howells, John G.: Theory and practice of family psychiatry, New York, 1971, Brunner/Mazel, Inc., pp. 274-279.
10. McGinnis, Thomas C.: Your first year of marriage, Garden City, N.Y., 1967, Doubleday & Co., Inc., pp. 14-16.
11. Mead, George H.: Mind, self and society, Chicago, 1934, University of Chicago Press.
12. Ford, Donald H., and Urban, Hugh B.: Systems of psychotherapy: a comparative study, New York, 1964, John Wiley & Sons, Inc., pp. 549-550.
13. Chess, Stella: Your child is a person, New York, 1965, The Viking Press, Inc.
14. Jersild, Arthur T.: In search of self, New York, 1965, Teachers College Press, p. 3.
15. Symonds, op. cit., p. 587.
16. Mullahy, op. cit., p. 130.
17. Symonds, op. cit., pp. 588-589.
18. Symonds, op. cit., p. 589.
19. Ackerman, op. cit., pp. 197, 333, and 339.
20. Ackerman, op. cit., p. 19.
21. Laing, R. D.: The politics of the family, New York, 1971, Pantheon Books, Inc.
22. Ackerman, op. cit., p. 18.
23. Montague, op. cit., p. 168.
24. Jersild, op. cit., pp. 19-20.
25. Mullahy, op. cit., p. 131.
26. Jersild, op. cit., p. 20.
27. Symonds, op. cit., p. 581.
28. McGinnis, Thomas C., and Ayres, John U.: Open family living, a new approach for enriching your life together, Garden City, N.Y., 1976, Doubleday & Co., Inc., Chapter 3.
29. Satir, Virginia: Conjoint family therapy, Palo Alto, Calif., 1964, Science & Behavior Books, Inc., pp. 9-92.
30. Maslow, A. H.: Personality problems and personality growth. In Hamachek, Don E.: Human dynamics in psychology and education, Boston, 1968, Allyn & Bacon, Inc., pp. 647-649.
31. McGinnis and Ayres, op. cit., Chapter 3.
32. Satir, op. cit., pp. 92-94.

chapter 6
THE PROCESS OF DEVELOPING AN IDENTITY

Chapter 5 focused on PFLs and patterns as determiners and vehicles of the ways we think, feel, and act. As such, they are key components of human identity. This chapter takes a fuller look at identity, especially the process that brings about its development. **Identity** includes who a person is in the here and now, how he got to be the way he is now, and who he may become in the future.[1-3]

The person who knows and appreciates his identity is aware of and understands the following:

Who he is in the here and now. To know and appreciate this part of his identity requires that a person be reasonably in touch with his insides and his outsides. Not only is he fairly aware of what they are, but he also knows a lot about how they function in his life and why.

How he got to be the way he is now. To know and appreciate this part of his identity requires that a person have a basic understanding of how he as a child developed his insides and outsides, who influenced him, how they influenced him and to what degree, and what experiences have left their mark on him.

Who he might become. To know and appreciate this part of his identity requires that a person have a good, working knowledge of the other two parts. By knowing basically who he is now and how he got to be the way he is, he can understand what it is about himself that he may wish to add to, modify, or alter, so that he can change and grow in whatever ways he chooses.

In effect the following discussion concentrates on three factors: how the family in particular influences the child's development of his identity, how this developmental process assures that the individual is likely to build in a large portion of teachings from the past (in the form of PFLs and patterns), and how an individual becomes who he is in the present.

This chapter then explains how the past and present shape identity, what influences are at work, and how a person builds in these influences. If you understand how your identity has been shaped and what you have built in, you are in a position to reshape your identity to your desires, to build *out* whatever elements you wish to, and to build in whatever new and different elements seem appropriate and desirable to you. The remainder of the book is devoted to teaching you how to accomplish these things.

THE JOHNSON FAMILY

Until you get directly involved in and begin to practice with the concepts discussed in the book, they remain essentially abstract and perhaps seem unreal. Therefore to give you something more tangible to work with, we have created a "sample" family, the Johnsons, with whom we want you to become thoroughly familiar. (See Appendix A.) We have several reasons for urging you to understand and to really develop a feel for who they are, how they got to be who they are, and who they might become.

1. Since the Johnsons are presented both as individuals and as a family group, they

will serve as living examples of individual functioning, marital dynamics, and family dynamics.

2. Since they are described and analyzed in considerable detail, they can, for example, illustrate what prescriptions for living, patterns, and life-styles are and how these are communicated and passed on from parents to children.

3. This basic family will be used and referred to throughout the book so that once you come to know them they can serve as touchstones for explaining various other concepts.

4. This family will give you tangible individuals and a tangible family group on which to practice. Hopefully you will then be able to take what you have learned from the Johnsons about individual, marital, and family dynamics and apply your understanding to your own family and to your other relationships.

In other words, the Johnson family gives you a group to work on that allows you to remain somewhat objective as you learn the principles of individual and group dynamics. That objectivity will protect you to some degree from the anxiety that might arise if we asked you to start working directly on your own family group. On the other hand, you may choose to get involved with, work with, and practice on both this mythical family and your own family at the same time. Whatever you choose to do, this family will serve you well as an illustration of the principles and dynamics of individual, marital, and family interaction.

THE DEVELOPING INDIVIDUAL'S WORLD

The development of an individual's identity is an amazing phenomenon. A newborn child is suddenly thrust into an alien environment in which he is constantly bombarded from then on by uncountable external and internal stimuli. In the face of this, it is truly incredible that any individual manages to work with himself, others, his experiences, and the world in such a way that he develops into a fairly well-integrated human being who functions in a reasonably adequate fashion.[4]

Influences on the developing individual

This accomplishment, in simplest terms, is made possible by the powers and capacities of the human organism (which are as yet not fully understood) and by the contributions of the Significant Persons who make up the Developing Individual's world. A **Significant Person*** is any person in an individual's life who exerts a substantial influence on him.[5] In other words, a Significant Person is one who "makes a difference" (of whatever kind) in a person's life.

The key functions of Significant Persons are (1) to serve as filters and focusors of the stimuli coming from outside the individual and (2) to teach the individual how to organize, respond to, and manage both internal and external stimuli. Essentially Significant Persons provide the Developing Individual with models of previously experienced ways of integrating one's Self with the environment. In effect, by copying and by accepting or rejecting the directions of Significant Persons, the Developing Individual learns to integrate himself with internal and external stimuli so that he can establish and maintain his dynamic equilibrium.

The influences exerted by Significant Persons, especially during an individual's earliest and most formative years, are incalculable. The important people in a child's life will determine in large part how the child will perceive and respond to the world around him. In essence, Significant Persons are a good part of his reality; thus what they consider to be reality is what he will likely consider to be reality. For example, if a child's parents see the world and life as delightfully interesting and they believe that

---

*This term was coined by Harry Stack Sullivan, the "father" of the interpersonal school of psychiatry, to refer to any and all people who have a marked effect on a person.

most people are basically good, then that is the way the child will likely see life too. If the Significant Persons in a child's world are rigid and closed (especially those who are around him at the beginning), the child will learn to be rigid and closed. If this occurs, it is probable that outside influences and later influences (such as a high school teacher) will have much difficulty intervening and making a difference in the Developing Individual's closedness.

Fortunately, very few people are *so* closed that no one or nothing can make a difference. Most people are at least open enough that a sufficiently strong or meaningful influence can intervene in such a way that the person so affected will probably take another look at his life and himself.

In addition to Significant Persons, other factors contribute greatly to the developmental process. These are **moment-to-moment influencing factors (MIFs)**—phenomena that are potentially present in all moments of living and that influence a person's thoughts, feelings, and actions at a given moment.[6] Although there are more, the following list of ten covers the most important factors. Five of them are "inside operations":

1. Motivation
2. Psychological desires
3. Goals
4. Intent
5. Mood

Three are external matters:

6. Social situation
7. Opportunity
8. Time available

The other two are interpersonal:

9. Societal pressures (collective influences)
10. Significant others (individual influences)

It is important to know two facts about MIFs.

1. All ten moment-to-moment influencing factors are always potentially present in every given situation, but not all ten necessarily operate actively in that situation. For example, the perfect *opportunity* to rob a bank may be present, but a person may not be *motivated* to do so. Or a man may have a strong *psychological desire* to kiss a beautiful female stranger, but *societal pressures* (decorum, the law) and *significant others* (influencing him through his PFLs, for example) probably will restrain him.

2. By and large, MIFs are interlocking and mutually influencing. For example, suppose a mother, Janice Johnson, sharply and unfairly criticizes her daughter Sally. Later Janice realizes (or decides) that she needs to apologize to Sally because she does not want Sally to think ill of her (*intent* and *psychological desire*) and because she believes that an apology will help Sally feel more adequate *(goal)*. But suppose Janice is in a bad *mood* because her husband Harry *(significant other)* has tongue-lashed her for criticizing his favorite daughter. Then Janice's *motivation* to act on her decision may be clouded or blocked by her feelings of anger and jealousy. Or her *motivation* may not be great enough for her to act, since she may think that Sally will still think badly of her even if she apologizes. In addition, suppose the *social situation* is a public one in which Janice would feel embarrased or which makes an apology inappropriate at the *time*. Thus the *opportunity* is not particularly favorable, since *societal pressure* generally dictate that matters of a private nature (such as apologies) be dealt with in private. This one incident then contains and calls forth every one of the moment-to-moment influencing factors; furthermore, the interlocking, mutually influencing nature of the factors is readily apparent.

The developing individual

In addition to societal influences, Significant Persons, and moment-to-moment influencing factors, the Developing Individual himself is an influence on his world and his development. At the outset, he brings with him his core characteristics and his potential and actual functions of thinking, feeling, and acting.

An individual's **core characteristics** are

those natural endowments that form his essential makeup: sex, race, intellectual heritage, biophysiological heritage, and age.[7] Whereas sex and race do not change, the other three core characteristics can and may be or will be affected or modified by influences and circumstances. However, even though some of them are subject to change, all these endowments remain with the person throughout his life, since they are intrinsic to his being.

One core characteristic in particular, his age, is a major determinant of the specific makeup of the Developing Individual's world at any given period of time. For example, in infancy (from birth to 2 years of age) the child's helpless, dependent state limits his contacts primarily to the Significant Persons in his family—especially his mother and father. Thus their influences are likely to be powerful and concentrated. Conversely, when the Developing Individual is an adolescent (from age 13 to 17 or 18 years), his interactions with his peers become increasingly important and often help him to gain new awareness of himself and his family. Through friendships, dating, and meeting others' families, he encounters different PFLs, patterns, and life-styles. All these experiences can help to attenuate the strength of his parents' influences on him. In the process, he is developing his identity—his sense of self.

THE DEVELOPMENTAL PROCESS

The process by which a child develops his identity is always a powerful one, and sometimes (as in the following example) it is an awesome one. A child usually spends the first ten to fifteen years of life in the daily company of at least one parent. Suppose that every day of every week of every month of every year for fifteen long years a child hears, sees, feels, and experiences a pattern of perfectionism: "Don't drop the ball." "Why can't you do better in school?" "What's the matter with you?" "Can't you even understand simple arithmetic?" "How many times do I have to explain to you how to tie your shoes (write the alphabet, cut the lawn, train the dog, etc.)?" "A B+ is pretty good—but how come you didn't get an A?" "When will you ever learn?" He hears it at breakfast, dinner, on weekends, and at night. He hears it on the telephone, when he brings home his report card, when he drops the baseball, and when he tries out for Little League. He hears it when he overhears one of his parents cursing himself or herself for some stupid mistake. If he stumbles, mumbles, cries, falls down, loses a fist fight to the child down the street, hesitates, gives up, hides, if he *fails*—he hears about it; he experiences the weight of disapproval.

How long could an adult, much less a child, hold out against such powerful and massive forces? Every day—*for ten or fifteen years?* What happens, of course, is that the PFLs and patterns which the child is exposed to so steadily for so long gradually become a part of his emotional landscape. Like most objects a person sees everyday, soon he does not see them any more. In the case of PFLs and patterns, they are there when the child arrives on the scene and they are there the whole time he is growing up. They are a part of the emotional landscape that he wanders into; gradually he builds them in without even knowing it, and then they become part of his inner world. In effect, he has developed an identity that shapes the ways he will see and respond to himself, others, and the world around him.

The process in detail

Essentially what enables a Developing Individual to gradually develop his identity is the moment-to-moment interactions that he experiences with Significant Persons in his environment and with the environment itself. The Developing Individual's core characteristics and his thoughts, feelings, and actions provide the initial major stimuli to the Significant Persons; they in turn—through their patterns (undergirded by PFLs)—provide the individual with stimuli. In effect it is this reciprocal exchange of stimuli that, in simplest terms, constitutes the dynamics of developing an identity.[8]

To the influences exerted by Significant Persons, the child responds from moment to moment with his own thoughts, feelings and actions as they are shaped by his core characteristics. As the child receives a steady stream of signals and messages from these important people, as he constantly experiences their PFLs and patterns, and as he repeatedly responds to all of this from moment to moment, he gradually begins to get some "feel" for whatever continuity and consistency exist in these influences. Furthermore, through a long-term process of trial and error, the child begins to learn (consciously and unconsciously) which of his thoughts, feelings, and actions are acceptable or not acceptable to Significant Persons, which ones generate approval or disapproval, and which ones fit the value systems being transmitted to him.[9] In effect the child is learning how to match up his moment-to-moment thoughts, feelings, and actions with the demands, desires, requests, instructions, and directions of the PFLs and patterns of Significant Persons in his world.

In response to how his moment-to-moment thoughts, feelings, and actions "test out" (i.e., how well or poorly they measure up to the demands of Significant Persons and to his understanding of his experiences and his world), the child gradually develops tentative patterns of thinking, feeling, and acting. Now his moment-to-moment interactions with Significant Persons and his world help to test out not only his individual thoughts, feelings, and actions but also his tentative patterns of thinking, feeling, and acting.

As this continual trial-and-error testing-out occurs again and again, the child is slowly forming a concept of his Self. This **self-concept**[10] consists of his **self-image** (how he *sees* and *thinks* about himself) and his **self-esteem**[11] (how he *feels* about himself). As he develops his self-concept, he is learning to "serve two masters"—Significant Persons and himself. That is, he continues to try to match his moment-to-moment thoughts, feelings, and actions and his tentative patterns to the demands and desires embodied in the PFLs and patterns of Significant Persons; but he also tries more and more to suit his moment-to-moment thinking, feeling, and acting and his tentative patterns to his self-image and his self-esteem so that they will support, reinforce, and "prove out" how he thinks and feels about himself. Some of this behavior is **intrapersonal** (how he treats and responds to himself); some if it is **interpersonal** (how he treats and responds to others). ►IE-1, p. 108.

What is occurring is a complex circular process of interaction among various elements, an interaction whose basic aim is to find and maintain stability and dynamic equilibrium. The child's self-concept influences and is influenced by his core characteristics; by his moment-to-moment thoughts, feelings, and actions; by his tentative patterns; and by the responses of Significant Persons to him. At the same time, the child is measuring his core characteristics; his moment-to-moment thoughts, feelings, and actions; his tentative patterns; and his self-concept against the Significant Persons' approval or disapproval and the PFLs and patterns that are influencing him. This constant circular interplay has a cumulative effect. Over a period of years the child gradually learns which PFLs to keep or reject or alter and what patterns of thinking, feeling, and acting tend to help him feel most comfortable *in relation to* the requirements of Significant Persons, to his self-concept, and to reality as he has learned to perceive it.

As he continues to engage in these actions and interactions and as he continues to test out his developing PFLs/patterns, he begins to build in the successful ones (the ones that best enable him to keep his dynamic equilibrium). The PFLs become more firmly established, and his patterns of thinking, feeling, and acting become more and more consistent. He is in effect building in a large number of developing patterns (and the PFLs that underpin these patterns).

As a person continues the process of building in his developing patterns, these patterns (and their PFLs) tend to fall into the identifiable groupings of Child, Parent, and Adult. (See the following section for a fuller explanation of the Child, Parent, and Adult parts and the balance among them.) Essentially these terms are really classificatory tools, which are useful for describing groups of patterns (and their PFLs), their interrelationships, the balance amongst them, the strength and dominance of each, and the quality of each group. For example, suppose a person has the following patterns—outgoing, warm, friendly, gregarious, talkative, spontaneous, impetuous, and disorganized. Probably this person's Child part is quite large, the Parent quite small, and the Adult part rather underdeveloped. If, however, the person's outgoing qualities are tempered by sensitivity to self and others and if the person's spontaneity and impetuous, disorganized qualities are tempered by a sense of responsibility and a regard for others' life "pace," then although the Child part will be fairly large and the Parent part quite small, the Adult part will predominate.

By the time a person's patterns are developed and consistent enough that they are classifiable (both as to content and Child/Parent/Adult balance), they constitute his life-style—his outsides—and his self-system—his insides. (For a discussion of life-style and self-system see pp. 101 to 103.)

The Child, the Parent, the Adult

The largest (and most generalized) component of an individual's insides is the **Child/Parent/Adult balance.** It is the largest because it embodies the teachings and responses based on all the other components—PFLs, packets of PFLs, composite PFLs, patterns, and self-concept. It is the most generalized because each "part" (e.g., the Child) of the balance represents a basic set of overall thoughts, feelings, and actions.

The **Child** in a person is the part of him that thinks, feels, and acts in ways similar to the ways he did as a child.[12,13] For example, if a person has experienced a number of fear-producing incidents during his childhood, he may have a Child part in him that is timid, hesitant, and frightened. Even as a grown person, this individual may still be timid and fearful, afraid to try new things, or take risks. Or suppose a person grew up in a family that nurtured and encouraged curiosity about and spontaneous delight in the world. As an adult, this person will retain a good deal of this inquisitive and spontaneous Child.

The **Parent** in a person is the part of him that thinks, feels, and acts in ways he has learned from one or both of his parents and from other Significant Persons (e.g., grandparents, aunts and uncles, siblings, peers, teachers, bosses, neighbors).[14,15] As a person is growing up, various significant people stand in a "parenting role" and affect his developing personality. The child is exposed to many different influences from parenting figures—societal PFLs, family and personal PFLs, interpersonal patterns, and ways of perceiving and responding to self, others, and life. This exposure comes from direct interaction with others and from what the child observes about and senses from the interactions of those around him. Gradually the developing child internalizes, or builds in, many of these influences; they form what we call the "Parent part" of his self-system. It is this part of him that responds as he believes (whether correctly or incorrectly) his parent figure(s) would respond in similar or similar-seeming circumstances.

For example, suppose a youngster builds in her mother's PFLs and patterns about authority—that people in authority are fearsome, punitive, and threatening; that you should always obey them because they are right; and that if you disobey them, you should feel guilty. Even when this youngster becomes a grown woman, her outsize Parent part will forever be warning her, "Now be obedient—and if you disobey, be frightened and feel guilty." Thus if a policeman stops this woman for barely going over the speed limit, she probably will shake, be extremely nervous, and answer him in scared monosyllables. Later she may give herself a rough time for being so "stupid," and she may even refuse to tell anyone about the incident because she feels guilty and ashamed.

Suppose another youngster grows up around people who are concerned about others, who treat others with kindness and respect, and who cherish the ideal that every human being has a certain inalienable dignity. This person's built-in Parent part will provide him with guidelines for treating himself and others with concern, kindness, and respect.

The **Adult** in a person is the part of him that evolves as he is growing up and hopefully continues to do so throughout his life.[16] The evolution of the Adult part results from the interaction between the growing child's experiences within himself (Child) and with external influences (the influences of Significant Persons, his developing Parent part, and the world around him). When a child is young, one or the other parts (Child, Parent) may dominate at various times, but gradually the growing child learns new positions as a result of the tension and interaction between inside (Child) and outside (Parent and world). He may begin to perceive situations and feel feelings that are both a combination of his Child and Parent parts and something more than that combination. For example, suppose an 11-year-old boy's Child has a venturesome, risk-taking attitude toward physical activities, but he has a Parent built in that constantly cautions, "Be careful; you could fall and break a bone." He may go ahead and take the risks but at the same time be overly cautious and anxious when he does so. Perhaps this overcautiousness hampers him from fully developing his athletic skills. But suppose his sixth grade gym teacher teaches him how to train his body, how to exercise proper precautions, and how to direct his energies. This experience will help the boy develop his Adult part—that part which negotiates between the Child and Parent parts so that neither of them automatically (and therefore inappropriately) dominates. The Adult also evaluates the realities of a given situation and enables the person to respond to reality in direct and appropriate ways. In effect the Adult establishes an appropriate balance between Child and Parent and between them and the realities of a situation. Thus the Adult is the guiding force that helps a person think, feel, and act as a whole, mature, autonomous individual. ►IE-2, p. 108.

THE SYSTEM AND TRANSACTIONAL ANALYSIS: SOME DISTINCTIONS

Because we use the same terms (Child, Parent, Adult) as the transactional school of analysis does,[17,18] it is necessary here to make certain distinctions. Our terms are the same because we can find no other ones that are more apt. However, the concepts to which these terms refer, although related (because we are discussing the same basic human processes), are not identical with those of the transactional analysts.

Our distinctions are as follows:

1. There is nothing static about these "parts"; they do not remain the same throughout life. Rather, the Child, Parent, and Adult are parts of a constantly changing, shifting, dynamic *whole*. For this reason, we have chosen *not* to use the term "ego state" (as do the transactional analysts) because the word "state" carries such static connotations for us.

2. Our term "Parent" refers to the "Parent" defined by the transactionalists but also includes all significant others who have had a notable influence on the growing, developing child.

3. Our concept "Adult" also differs from the "Adult" of transactional analysis. One difference is that our "Adult" includes an active emotional element, whereas the transactionalists define their "Adult" as a computer-like function that processes information and makes realistic decisions but that does not include emotions in its own operations. As a result, the transactionalists attribute all emotions to the Child

and the Parent. This leaves certain types of emotions unexplained—particularly those associated with the higher intellectual/emotional faculties such as the appreciation of nature, of beauty, of the arts, of the works of the mind, and of the wonders of the universe.

Rather than viewing the Adult as an emotionless computer that regulates the Child and Parent parts, we conceive of the Adult as employing all three aspects of human functioning—thinking, feeling, and acting. Moreover we believe that the Adult part contributes its own perspective and functions to appropriately balance the influences coming from both Child and Parent; thus it enables a person to think, feel, and act as a *whole* person. Thus we contend that it is possible, likely, and desirable for a person's Child, Parent, and Adult parts to be operating simultaneously on all three levels of human functioning—thinking, feeling, acting.

In summary, we define the Adult as that part which evaluates, is aware of the many alternatives present in a situation, is flexible, and guides a person's thinking, feeling, and acting in relation to the realities of the situation. The Adult is the mediator between the Child and the Parent; it is the arbiter between responses based on childhood experiences and realities of the present. It is the Adult therefore that enables a person to respond and act in ways that are flexible and appropriate to the here and now. It is the Adult that prevents the past from chaining him to repetitive, automatic, stereotyped ways of thinking, feeling, and acting, which may not be appropriate to the occasion.

DEVELOPING THE ADULT

The Adult part is not "built in" as is the Parent part. Therefore to develop his Adult, a person must become aware of who he is, where he comes from, what forces shaped him, what his parents and family are like, what his PFLs are, what his patterns of dealing with life are, and what his self-concept consists of. As he becomes aware of these things and how they operate in his life, he can begin to evaluate them and see whether he wishes to stay as he is or to change.

Developing the Adult part does not mean, however, doing so at the expense of the Child or the Parent. Both of these parts are necessary and useful. The Child is vital because it is a major source of creative energy, direct and immediate emotional responses, and vivid sensory responses. The Parent is vital because it is the source of knowledge gained from others' living experiences and of patterns of dealing with life, patterns that can save a person from expending enormous amounts of energy in making decisions every moment. Developing the Adult part does mean, however, becoming aware of what is negative and what is positive in the Child and Parent parts and learning how to maximize the positive and minimize the negative. In effect it means learning to achieve a balanced three levels of human functioning—thinking, feeling, and acting. ►IE-3, p. 108.

Self-system

Self-system is the formal term for a person's insides, that is, his internal functioning (thoughts, feelings, and actions). The self-system is therefore comprised of PFLs, intrapersonal patterns, the self-concept, and the Child/Parent/Adult balance.[19]

Life-style

The term "life-style" refers to a person's outsides, that is, his external functioning.

Essentially a person's outsides consist of his interpersonal patterns of thinking, feeling, and acting. Every person tends to have observable interpersonal patterns, which are characteristic of the particular, consistent ways he functions. And these characteristic patterns fit together to form a logical, relatively predictable whole. In effect they form an observable network of interpersonal patterns.

Life-style refers to this observable network of consistent interpersonal patterns, which determine the ways in which a person functions (thinks, feels, and acts) in the interpersonal sphere.[20]

IDENTIFYING A LIFE-STYLE

Because life-style represents the overall thrust of the network of interpersonal patterns, it is possible to identify a style with a one- or two-word name that describes its basic nature. The name given to a particular life-style is arrived at in one of three ways.

1. Often one (or perhaps two) of the patterns in the network is the most dominant and stands out from the others. Then the life-style may be named according to the dominant pattern (e.g., independent, hostile, emotional, impulsive, intellectual).

2. Sometimes it is possible to name a life-style by synthesizing the meaning of all the individual patterns and then giving a name to the synthesis. For example, suppose a person has a network of the following patterns—intellectual, perfectionistic, "nit-picking," nonemotional, moralistic, aggressive, hostile, antichange, strong willed, and motivated by a powerful inner drive. From this network of consistent, significant patterns, it is possible to derive a descriptive name; in this particular case, it would be an "obsessive-compulsive" style.* Some other examples of names determined by a synthesis of interpersonal patterns are extrovert, introvert, hysteric, immature, and mature.

3. Some life-styles are alternating; that is, a person has somewhat opposite patterns, but there is consistency in his style because he alternates between two sets of opposite patterns. A good example of this kind of life-style is the passive-aggressive style. A person with this kind of life-style will alternate between being an aggressive, hard-to-get-along with person and a somewhat passive, easy-going "nice guy." The style is named obviously after its two major conflicting characteristics.

CHARACTERIZING THE QUALITY OF A LIFE-STYLE

In addition to naming the life-style, it is also possible to characterize the quality of a life-style by the terms "open" and "closed." Thus by designating a particular life-style as closed, we indicate that the person's patterns tend to be rigid, inflexible, automatic, and repetitious. (The concepts "closed" and "open" will be discussed in detail later in this chapter.) Thus it is possible by means of a name plus the designation of open or closed to describe in succinct, although general terms, how a person operates: the consistent, public ways he manages his thoughts, feelings, and actions.

Since life-style describes how a person operates (his outsides), it is concerned with phenomena that can be perceived or observed or at least sensed or inferred by others (if not by the person himself.) Even if people cannot state flately that a particular person has a distinct interpersonal pattern of hostility, they are nevertheless conscious of the presence of a pattern because of the vibrations it sends off. They may sense or feel its weight; they may clearly see it in action; they may receive its impact. They may hear it in action; they may cringe from its harshness; they may recoil from its force. In whatever way people may perceive the existence of patterns, what is important is that the interpersonal patterns are indeed perceivable, and often life-style can be identified, named, and characterized.

Life-style then describes a person in terms of his identifiable "major themes"—the quality of his functioning (rigid/flexible, closed/open) and the basic nature of his ways of operating (specific patterns).

*Although we sometimes use certain terms that are drawn from psychiatric nomenclature,[21] we do not employ them to make strict clinical diagnoses of the people we describe. Rather we use these terms because they afford a quick and vivid way of identifying life-styles—they capture in a word or two the essential characteristics of a given personality.

However, although life-style indicates a great deal about a person, it is really only the tip of the iceberg. Underneath lies the self-system.

Relationship between self-system and life-style

For purposes of clarity, at times we separate self-system from life-style and discuss one or both of them as distinct entities. In reality, however, self-system and life-style are not separable. Rather they are two facets of one entity—the whole self. They are intricately interlocked, are interdependent, and exert reciprocal influences on one another. Therefore unless we clearly indicate that we are separating them into distinct entities for discussion purposes, we intend that when you see the term "life-style" you recognize that self-system is implied also; the same holds true for our use of the term "self-system"—you may consider that life-style is implied.

If a person has little awareness of his identity, then his self-system will be translated by his life-style in a largely unconscious, automatic, and repetitious fashion, and the outside translation of his insides may be distorted. His life-style will tend to reinforce and feed the unconscious and often inappropriate workings of the self-system. This kind of personality tends to be rigid, relatively unchanging, and self-perpetuating. It both encourages and is encouraged by its closed nature.

PSYCHOLOGICAL GAMES

Because his closed and dysfunctional life-style and self-system so restrict clear, effective communication and interaction, the closed person tends (whether consciously or unconsciously) to "play" psychological games.

Psychological games* are a person's specific but distorted applications of intrapersonal and/or interpersonal patterns of communication and/or interaction that set up a series of preprogrammed (automatic, repetitious) reactions and interactions to achieve certain psychological ends. In essence these ends are the establishment or reestablishment and maintenance of intrapersonal and interpersonal dynamic equilibrium—no matter how dysfunctional it may be. Thus the ultimate end of games is to serve as a defense against anxiety.[22,23]

Intrapersonal games arise out of and are governed by the player's self-system.[24] For example, Janice Johnson has an interlocking series of games in her repetoire that is based on her negative self-concept. These include such games as "I'm too stupid to do that by myself," "I never quite know what's going on," "What a ridiculous thought (feeling, action)," "Don't be conceited (if she thinks well of herself)," and "Don't be too happy; that's tempting fate and something bad will happen (because I'm not worthy of being happy)." These games interlock with one another into a packet of games just as her patterns and PFLs interlock into packets. These games are consistent with Janice's self-punishing patterns. The psychological ends they serve are those of reinforcing her negative self-concept and of keeping her locked into her familiar positions of undermining self and fostering helpless dependency on others ("bottom dog"). In effect, games are really types of **self-fulfilling prophecies**—beliefs that a person holds which he makes come true because he believes and "feels" them to be true.[25,28]

Similarly, *interpersonal games* arise out of the harmonious or disharmonious interlock between each player's self-system plus life-style. The form or "flavor" of the game reflects the life-style created by the interlock between the players' individual styles, but the psychological ends of the game are determined by each player's self-system. That is, each player plays a particular game to satisfy his own inner thoughts and feelings.

---

*Eric Berne popularized the term "games." For an understanding of his approach to them, see *Games People Play: The Psychology of Human Relationships,* New York, 1964, Grove Press, Inc.

For example, Buck and Terry grew up together and have been friends for a long time. Their friendship has a dominating, independent (Buck)/yielding, dependent (Terry) style. Thus the games Buck initiates have an independent quality, whereas the games Terry initiates have a dependent quality. The psychological ends of Buck's games are to control the relationship and Terry so that Buck maintains his dominance and thereby can come and go and do as he pleases yet not lose Terry's friendship. The psychological ends of Terry's games are to play to Buck's desires to dominate so that Buck "needs" Terry to help him feel independent, decisive, and important. In this way, Terry binds Buck to him in a symbiotic-like relationship.

Following are some of Buck's games: "Okay—if you don't want to do ________, I'll go ahead without you," "Let me decide; you never know what you want to do," "I'm busy; I'll see you around," and "Well, if you can't see it my way, I guess that's it." Terry's games include the following: "It's not important; we'll do what you want," "You decide, Buck; your ideas always turn out better," "You're right, Buck," and "Gee, Buck, you really know where it's at, don't you?"

It is important to note that although we are discussing games as though they are clear cut and readily observable and identifiable, this is frequently not the case. Many games can be (and are) played out so skillfully and subtly that they may not be apparent to even a perceptive observer —much less to the players. In effect, it is frequently easier to *sense* the presence of a game than to identify it. ►IE-4, p. 108.

Psychological games are based on a certain amount of truth or fact (that is, a person plays a specific game because *something* in the reality situation touches him off). Nevertheless, although somewhat reality-based, games are dysfunctional in nature. Like rigid patterns, they are repetitious, automatic, ordinarily inappropriate, and largely controlled by unconscious forces. In addition, games are attempts to manipulate self, others, reality, or all of these. Thus they are dysfunctional forms of interaction engaged in by basically closed persons both as a result of their closedness and as a means of perpetuating that closedness.

Psychological games are a kind of verbal and/or nonverbal interactional shorthand—one signal, one phrase, one look, one move, or one sentence is often so loaded with assumptions or implications or accusations that it sets off a torrent of reactions, involving the other person and the game initiator in an automatic, repetitious, and usually inappropriate series of preprogrammed interactions.

The existence of these games depends on the presence of two interlocking factors.

1. To exist at all, a game must have players willing to play the game. The life of an intrapersonal game depends on the continuing willingness (often unconscious) of an individual to engage in his game.

2. An interpersonal game requires at least two players who are willing to play. If the individual refuses to continue playing his intrapersonal game (by breaking into a pattern, for example), the game will not work because he has changed or removed his side of the game interlock. Or if one of the players refuses to play or stops playing an interpersonal game, it will collapse.

There are, of course, all *kinds* of games that fit all kinds of categories.[29] For example, there are money games; sex games; male/female, husband/wife role games; and Child/Parent/Adult games. There are communication and interaction games, intrapersonal and interpersonal games, verbal and nonverbal games, and conscious and unconscious games. There are intellectual, emotional, and behavioral games. There are games that are mixtures of all of these. There are individual, business, friendship, dating, marital, and family games. The potential range of game possibilities is enormous, since games are what closed people in particular play to achieve psychological ends that are important to them. Whatever the name of the game, games are ways of seeking or reestablishing dynamic equilibrium, no matter how dysfunctional that equilibrium may be.

The more mature a person is the less he needs to employ games to gain or regain his dynamic equilibrium. If a person is fairly mature and is relatively aware of who he is, what he is like, and how he functions, then the interrelationship between his life-style and his self-system will be much more open and flexible. His life-style will accurately and clearly reflect his self-system, since by being in close and constant touch with his self-system, this person is able to adjust his life-style so that it truly reflects his insides. In addition, this person is able to evaluate and use his outside experiences so that he learns more about his insides.

In effect the more mature person's life-style and self-system are available to the influence of new knowledge and information, new awareness of feelings, and new insights, and they are available for renegotiation of thoughts, feelings, and actions. Thus the more mature person is not bound by a life-style and self-system that are rigid, relatively unchanging, and self-perpetuating, and he has minimal needs to play games. Rather he is always involved in the process of change and growth.

UNIQUENESS AND THE DEVELOPMENTAL PROCESS

Since this chapter is concerned with the process of developing an identity—that is, a self-system and life-style—it has focused on the enormous number of influences at work and on their tremendous power to affect and shape the Developing Individual. Because of this focus, it would be easy to get the mistaken impression that each human being's self-system and life-style are simply composite copies of Significant Persons' self-systems and life-styles. However, even when an individual builds in a great deal of other people's influences and seems to be like one or more of the Significant Persons in his life, he still cannot be an exact copy. The developmental process is just not that simple or that systematic. Even if a child grew up around only one Significant Person and they lived in total isolation from outside influences, the child still could not be an exact copy because the child brings to the interaction at least some diversities in his core characteristics. Thus although it is true that the Developing Individual will tend to be like various Significant Persons in his life in certain important ways, at the same time he is not exactly like any other person. Every human being is unique.

What is uniqueness?

What is uniqueness? The answer has to do with two opposites: similarities and differences. People are similar in many ways because there are a vast number of experiences that are common to the human condition. Furthermore, the basic ways of responding to these experiences are common to the human condition. ("Patterns" and "life-style" are the terms used to describe these common ways of reacting.) People also differ from each other in many ways, since each person has his own special, individual qualities that determine how he (and only he) will specifically implement his patterns and life-style in relation to common human experiences. These special, individual qualities result from his background, his core characteristics, certain contributory factors (e.g., religion, occupation), and his self-system. These qualities particularize the general ways he responds to common experiences. Thus a person's **uniqueness** results from the particular manner in which he combines and manages the ways he is similar to and different from other human beings.

What do we mean by **similarities?** In one way or another, all human beings have thought about, felt, and done certain common things.*

*Try checking this out for yourself: talk with others and see if they have thought about, felt, and done (or thought about doing) the things you have.

What common things do human beings *think about?* Birth, death, life, age, love, hate, eternity, immortality, evil, good, suicide, murder, war, peace, God, nothingness, the past, the present, the future, destiny, fate, space, time, other worlds, purpose, free will, order, chaos, identity, nonbeing, and ends and beginnings.

In what similar ways do human beings *think?* All of us decide, assess, weigh things in our minds, ponder, conceptualize, speculate, reflect, dream, reason, muse, deliberate, remember, imagine, reminisce, project, daydream, meditate, rationalize, contemplate, analyze, and synthesize.

Who among us has not *felt* fear, pleasure, anger, joy, depression, delight, sorrow, loneliness, anxiety, annoyance, ecstasy, irritation, boredom, excitement, contempt, relief, anguish, adoration, disgust, glee, pain, euphoria, tension, guilt, hilarity, weariness, awe, bewilderment, and wonder? Who among us has not at some time felt vengeful, tender, frustrated, insane, innocent, horny, wicked, friendly, sinful, sad, tolerant, intolerant, foolish, compassionate, humiliated, wrong, cheerful, impotent, loving, aimless, terrified, rejected, silly, sexy, nervous, kooky, right, proud, self-righteous, "screwed up," inferior, intimate, confused, superior, wronged, spiteful, puzzled, pleased, envious, content, or happy?

What have any of us ever *done* (or else contemplated doing) that others have not done? Been born, grown up, belched, scratched, laughed, cried, screamed, growled, rebelled, stolen, been spiteful, hurt ourselves or another, run away in fear, sweated, cursed, prayed, been sneaky, been brave, thrown rocks, hurled insults, murdered, created, been sarcastic, gotten drunk, gotten high, taken drugs, taken risks, whistled, skipped, hummed, hit someone, made love, giggled, whimpered, masturbated, plotted revenge, jumped to conclusions, forgiven someone, broken the law, been afraid of the dark, tormented an animal or a human being, comforted someone, hated someone, mourned for what is lost or gone, lied, cheated, been honest, followed the leader, led the followers, helped someone, or loved someone or something?

There is then a vast pool of experiences that is common to all of us.

In addition to all these similarities, however, there are all the **differences** that exist among human beings. These are not just the "big" differences like race, religion, nationality, biology, physiology, language, background, sex, age, intelligence, and appearance. There are also the differences that result from my being an inch taller than you and therefore seeing the world from a slightly different perspective; the ones that result from your being an only child and therefore having received more attention than I who come from a family of five; the differences that result from my having a passive father and your having an aggressive father; and the differences that result from your having a sister two years older than you and my having a sister three years younger than I. There are also all the differences resulting from all the different experiences we have had and people we have known. For example, *what* you think about life and death and *how* you think about them is not quite the same as what and how I think about them. You and I have each felt fear. But have we feared the same things? At the same time? In the same way? Probably not. We may have done the same things—but did we do them exactly the same way? Probably not.

We may both be perfectionists. But I may see the world as imperfect, curse its imperfections, and despair. You may see it as imperfect, curse its imperfections, and do your utmost to perfect it. Therein lies the difference. We both have the same pattern, perhaps the same life-style, but we will apply that style differently according to who each of us is as specific, distinct individuals.

Life-style categorizes people in terms of their *general* ways of thinking, feeling, and acting. Uniqueness goes a step beyond. Uniqueness refers to the *specific* way a preson combines what is common to all human beings—general basic experiences and patterns of thinking, feeling, and acting—with what is particular to only him—his background and self-system. In addition, uniqueness refers to the way a person manages that combination of the general and the specific, of the similar and the different.

> There is no one—anywhere—who is totally unlike any one of us.
> There is no one—anywhere—who is exactly like any one of us.
>
> To every person—in every place—in every time,
> There is sound and silence, motion and rest,
> Order and chaos, everything and nothing,
> Time and the timeless, change and the changeless;
> Good and evil, war and peace, dark and light,
> Fire and ice, God and no-god, comedy and tragedy,
> Fullness and emptiness, famine and plenty,
> Sickness and health, pleasure and pain, hell and heaven;
> The conscious and the unconscious, emotion and reason,
> Love and hate, hope and despair, courage and cowardice,
> Concern and indifference, deceit and honesty, sorrow and joy;
> Male and female, adult and child;
> Past, present, future;
> Spring, summer, fall, winter;
> Birth, growth, maturity, death.
>
> And to each person—in each place—in each moment in time,
> There is the singleness of his soul,
> The only-ness of his Self,
> The one-ness of his being.
> He, and he alone—
> In the glory and the terror of his uniqueness—
> Can respond to his experience of Self and Life.
> In that flash of light which is his moment in time,
> He—and only he—may say for himself:
> I am, I choose, I will.

In celebration of uniqueness

In an important sense, one purpose of this book is to celebrate the uniqueness of the individual—of his inner self, of his relationships with other individuals, of his experiences in a world that is aeons old yet ever new. Its other, concomitant purpose is to provide you with knowledge, understanding, equipment, and expertise that will enable you to nurture and celebrate your own and others' uniqueness. This ability to nurture and to celebrate your own uniqueness means getting and being in touch with your insides and allowing and encouraging yourself to change and grow in ways that you determine are appropriate. Ultimately it means becoming more autonomous and being able and willing to accept the responsibilities, the pains, and the joys of openness. Nurturing and celebrating others' uniqueness means being able to reach out to and to share with others without demanding that they be something you want them to be or something they are not.

The problem for many people, however, is that although they would like to nurture and celebrate their own and others' uniqueness, they are not sure how to accomplish this. Their problem is usually compounded by the obscuring presence of restrictive PFLs and rigid, repetitive patterns both in themselves and in others. The remaining chapters in this part are devoted therefore to explaining how to work constructively with the self-system and life-style to become more open. The more open a person is the better able he is to nurture and celebrate his own and others' uniqueness.

Interaction experiences

1. Gaining a better understanding of your self-concept (p. 98)

Your self-concept consists of how you see yourself (what you think about yourself) and how you feel about yourself.

Find a place where you can be alone and uninterrupted for at least 30 minutes. You will need a mirror for this experience, preferably a full-length one.

Stand in front of the mirror and try to get in touch with how you see and feel about yourself. It will probably be helpful if you think in terms of "I think that I am ________________," "I feel that I am ____________," and "I feel ____________."

Now take some of these thoughts and feelings and act them out one by one in an exaggerated manner. For example, if you feel ugly, try to make yourself really look ugly. If you think you are aggressive, then act very aggressive. If you feel that you are clumsy, then act extra clumsy. Watch yourself in the mirror as you do this.

EVALUATION: What did you think and feel as you went through this experience? What and how did you feel as you acted out your thoughts and feelings? This experience can help you get a better feel for your self-concept.

FOLLOW-UP: Ask a friend to tell you how he sees and feels about you. Share your experience with him—your thoughts and feelings and what you discovered about yourself. Also consider what about yourself you would like to strengthen and what you would like to change.

2. Getting in touch with your Child, Parent, and Adult parts (p. 100)

Play a game that you used to play in your childhood (e.g., tag, hopscotch, hide and seek, marbles). Try to let yourself go and play the game as you did in your childhood.

EVALUATION: Could you get in better touch with your Child part? Could you recapture your childhood feelings? Could you feel your Parent part encourage or discourage, approve or disapprove of your Child part? Could you feel your Adult part in operation?

FOLLOW-UP: Draw your Child/Parent/Adult balance. Discuss with others how they see your balance. Share some childhood memories with others. Try to get and stay in touch with your Child part and give it free but appropriate rein.

3. Working with your Child/Parent/Adult balance (p. 101)

Get two or three other people and act out with them (or have them act out for you) your Child/Parent/Adult balance in relation to a particular situation (e.g., a fight with a friend, a disappointment, getting lost). Base your actions on the PFLs and patterns that would apply plus whatever thoughts and feelings you are in touch with.

EVALUATION: Are you surprised at the interaction among the parts? How does it feel to act out the three parts of you?

FOLLOW-UP: Change the balance (that is, if your Parent part is the largest, make your Child or Adult part larger for this experience). Then act out this different balance and experience your feelings about it.

4. "Playing" a psychological game (p. 104)

Since our own games are hard to identify, try this experience with a game that is common: "Yes, but. . . ."

Select a partner. He is to role play the person who tries to help; you are to play the person who asks for help. Ask him to help you solve some problem (e.g., how to study more efficiently, how to handle an unpleasant situation, how to budget your time, how to go about meeting people). Every time he offers an alternative, you are to say, "Yes, but . . ." and give a reason why you cannot.

EVALUATION: What did you think and feel

as you kept thwarting your partner's attempts to help you? Could you sense any frustration or annoyance in his responses? Could you get in touch with the restrictive, automatic quality of the game? Were you aware that you were playing the difficult child to your partner's helpful (and frustrated) parent? In discussing the experience, are you surprised by the thoughts and feelings your partner reports having?

FOLLOW-UP: Role play this game again, only this time let your partner interrupt you after the third "Yes, but . . ." and challenge you to not keep negating his attempts to help. Try then to negotiate some resolution between you and your partner *without* playing the game further. You might also switch roles so that you can experience the other side of the game.

Try also to identify some of your own games (both intrapersonal and interpersonal) and role play both sides of them.

REFERENCES

1. Ackerman, Nathan W.: The psychodynamics of family life, New York, 1958, Basic Books, Inc., Publishers, pp. 57-58.
2. Erikson, Erik H.: Identity: youth and crisis, New York, 1968, W. W. Norton and Co., Inc., pp. 49-50.
3. Erikson, Erik H.: The problem of ego identity, Journal of American Psychoanalytic Association 4:56-121, 1956.
4. Jersild, Arthur T.: In search of self, New York, 1965, Teachers College Press, pp. 10-11.
5. Mullahy, Patrick: A theory of interpersonal relations and the evolution of personality. In Sullivan, Harry Stack: Conceptions of modern psychiatry, Washington, D.C., 1947, William Alanson White Psychiatric Foundation, p. 120.
6. Ruesch, Jurgen: Synopsis of the theory of human communication. In Howells, John G., editor: Theory and practice of family psychiatry, New York, 1971, Brunner/Mazel, Inc., pp. 227-233.
7. Ackerman, op. cit., p. 196.
8. Ackerman, op. cit., pp. 58-62.
9. Sullivan, Harry Stack: Conceptions of modern psychiatry, Washington, D.C., 1947, The William Alanson White Psychiatric Foundation, p. 9.
10. Mead, George H.: Mind, self and society, Chicago, 1934, University of Chicago Press.
11. Briggs, Dorothy Corkville: Your child's self esteem, Garden City, N.Y., Doubleday & Co., Inc., 1970.
12. Berne, Eric: Games people play: the psychology of human relationships, New York, 1964, Grove Press, Inc., pp. 24-26.
13. Missildine, W. Hugh: Your inner child of the past, New York, 1963, Simon & Schuster, Inc., pp. 13-55.
14. Berne, op. cit., pp. 24-27.
15. Missildine, op. cit., pp. 81-280.
16. Berne, op. cit., pp. 24-27.
17. Berne, Eric: Transactional analysis in psychotherapy: a systematic individual and social psychiatry, New York, 1961, Grove Press, Inc.
18. Berne, Eric: What do you say after you say hello? The psychology of human destiny, New York, 1972, Grove Press, Inc.
19. Ackerman, op. cit., p. 53.
20. Symonds, Percival M.: Origins of personality. In Hamachek, Don E., editor: Human dynamics in psychology and education, Boston, 1970, Allyn & Bacon, Inc., p. 580.
21. Committee on Nomenclature and Statistics of the American Psychiatric Association: Diagnostic and statistical manual, Washington, D.C., 1968, American Psychiatric Association.
22. Berne, Games people play, p. 48.
23. De Ropp, Robert S.: The master game, New York, 1968, Delacorte Press, p. 12.
24. Laing, R. D.: Knots, New York, 1970, Pantheon Books, Inc.
25. Drakeford, John W.: Games husbands and wives play, Nashville, Tenn., 1970, Broadman Press.
26. Gillies, Jerry: My needs, your needs, our needs, Garden City, N.Y., 1974, Doubleday & Co., Inc.
27. Mozdzierz, Gerald J., and Lottman, Thomas J.: Games married couples play: an Adlerian view, Journal of Individual Psychology **29:** 182-194, Nov., 1973.
28. Smith, Gerald Walker, and Phillips, Alice I.: Me and you and us, New York, 1971, Peter H. Wyden/Publisher.
29. Berne, Games people play, pp. 67-168.

chapter 7
INTRAPERSONAL COMMUNICATION

THE INDIVIDUAL IS THE STARTING PLACE

The primary vehicle for all human interaction is communication with self and others.[1] For this reason, Chapters 7 through 9 will be devoted to analyzing and explaining the process of intrapersonal and interpersonal communication. The ultimate aim of these chapters is to help you understand and learn to use the communicational process in a conscious, deliberate, and therefore more beneficial manner.

The wellspring of all human communication and interaction is the individual, since it is his insides that provide the content and shape of both intrapersonal and interpersonal communication and interaction. Thus for a person to be able to communicate and interact in a conscious and deliberate manner, he must be in touch with his insides—with his thoughts and feelings and with the actions that result from them. For this reason, this chapter will concentrate on the process of intrapersonal communication—that is, on the process of getting in touch with your insides.[2]

As you will remember, your **insides** consist of your inner (private) thoughts, feelings, and experiences, or your self-system. **Getting in touch with** insides means becoming aware of, identifying, evaluating, understanding, and appreciating your inner thoughts, feelings, and experiences and your self-system. In simplest terms, it means communicating with your inner self.

It is possible to learn a good deal about your insides by *recalling* and *thinking about* your PFLs, by *meditating on* your thoughts, by *observing* yourself in action, by *watching* how you treat yourself and others, and by *thinking about* and *analyzing* your feelings. However, these are all primarily *intellectual* ways of learning about your insides. Getting in touch with your insides means far more than that. It involves not just intellectually understanding your insides but, even more important, *emotionally experiencing* them. It means not just knowing who you are; it means *feeling* who you are.

Intrapersonal communication then is concerned with getting in touch with all three aspects of inner human functioning—thinking, feeling, and acting—so that it becomes possible to achieve a harmonious blend of the three by means of the interactional process. It is by learning to blend and balance these three aspects of human functioning that a person can change, grow, and achieve personal autonomy and greater openness.

The application of the process of intrapersonal communication to all three aspects of human functioning requires more time and space than are available here. But it is possible to teach you this process and how to use it by detailing its application to one of these aspects.

Therefore we will concentrate on feelings because it is our emotions that most of us are ordinarily least in touch with and often least willing or able to reveal to ourselves or others. For example, are you now, as you read these lines, in touch with what you are feeling? If someone asked you right now what you are feeling, could you and would you tell him? Would it not be easier to express either to yourself or to him what you are thinking?

Even though we will focus on feelings, keep in mind that the process of intrapersonal communication can and should be applied to your thoughts and actions. In addition, you will be using your intellect even when you are concentrating on feelings, and you will also be paying attention to the relationship among your feelings and your thoughts and actions.

FOCUS ON FEELINGS

For many of us, our feelings are too often like forbidden, unknown, or unexplored territory, which is unfortunate because feelings are like a dynamo that produces the energy that enables everything else to run. This dynamo operates from moment to moment from birth to death, and it influences (many times controls) what you think and how you act. You cannot *not* feel.[3] Even when you are asleep, your dreams abound with feelings. If you feel as though you do not feel anything, asleep or awake, then you are not in touch with your feelings, but they *are* there—whether you like them and whether you want to or can acknowledge and feel them. Just as your heart beats whether you pay any attention to it or feel it beating, so your emotions operate whether you pay attention to or feel them. The trouble is that if your heart were to stop beating or were to skip beats, you would *know* it, and you would do something about it if you could. But if you block out your feelings or if your feelings are aborted before they have time even to send out recognizable signals, you do not get the same jolt. Some people are not jolted at all. *Most* people are not aware of how blocked or distorted or dulled their emotional signals are or of how out of touch they are with their feelings.

The consequences of such blockage are frightening because the emotions occupy a crucial position in the personality. Although you may act without thinking or think but not act, you cannot think or act (or both) without feeling *something*. Feelings then are the essential underpinning of what you think and do. Frequently, they are the controlling factor in what you think and do. How often do you think one thing and do another? How often do you act one way but *think* you should have acted another? Where does the real conflict lie in both these instances? Is it in what you think or in the way you think? Is it in what you do or in the way you do it? Probably not. Or, at least, probably not as much as it lies in the *feelings* you have in these instances.

For example, suppose you *know* you should write your parents to tell them how you are, but you keep putting it off. Why? Not because you *think* you should not write them and not because you are unable to *act*. More than likely, the strongest influence is your feelings. Perhaps you resent the time it takes. Perhaps you feel angry toward your parents and not writing is your way of "punishing" them. Perhaps you simply *think* they are too possessive and should leave you alone. Such "thinking" is really feeling.

Take another example. Suppose you *act:* you have intercourse even though you *know* you are running the risk of an unwanted pregnancy, because neither you nor your partner has taken the necessary contraceptive precautions. But you go ahead and have intercourse anyway. Why? You are not acting on what you *think*. Indeed you are acting against or in spite of what you *think* or know may be wise. What does motivate your action? Sheer *physical* desire? Probably not. Sexual desire is set off and controlled as much by thinking and feeling as by bodily sensations. The point is that your having intercourse depends not only on your physical desire but also on your *emotional* response to your partner, to yourself, and to the situation.

Feelings then are the key to a person's insides. If you ignore, deny, or block out your feelings, you will not be in touch with the dynamic underpinning of your thoughts and actions. Thus your feelings may control your thinking and acting without your being aware of it. If, however, you can get in touch with, identify, evaluate, and work constructively with your feelings, you will almost always be able to think more clearly and act more appropriately. Often unclear thinking and inappropriate behavior are the result of fuzzy or distorted feelings or of emotional unawareness. In addition, much energy is spent on blocking or avoiding or struggling with feelings on the unconscious level. Thus getting in touch and dealing with your feelings releases energy for thinking and acting and for achieving a balanced blend of these three aspects of human functioning.[4,5]

Hindrances to getting in touch

Since every human being has feelings and since they are so important, why is it so difficult for many people to get and keep in touch with their feelings? A primary reason is that much of the socialization process to which every child is exposed teaches him to control himself—to control what he thinks, what he says, what he feels, and what he does. But far too often, *control* becomes *suppression.*[6,7]

In the course of his socialization, the child learns from his culture (through his parents and other Significant Persons) that he must control (or suppress) many of his emotional and behavioral responses so that he can become a "civilized" human being and eventually a "mature" adult. He learns soon enough that positive feelings (e.g., friendliness, concern, respect) and positive actions (e.g., courtesy, obedience) are laudable and acceptable. He also learns that negative or undesirable feelings (e.g., anger, timidity, cowardice, rebelliousness) and negative actions (e.g., rudeness, disobedience, lying) are not acceptable. Gradually he is trained to gloss over, ignore, suppress, or deny them.

Think of the innumerable suppressive *do* and *don't* PFLs most people have built in at an early age. Be good, be honest, be respectful, be obedient, be quiet, be gentle, be nice, be brave, be loyal, be trustworthy. Think for yourself; be reasonable. Act your age; act like a man (woman). Feel ashamed if you do not obey these PFLs. Feel proud when you are following these PFLs.

Don't *think* "bad" ("mean," "dirty," "nasty") thoughts. Don't think ill of others. Don't think differently from the ways your parents think. Don't *feel* hostility toward those you are supposed to love (your brother, sister, mother, father, grandmother, grandfather, etc.). Don't feel too much pride. Don't feel lustful, angry, petty, weak, envious, or sneaky. Don't *be* aggressive, self-centered, deceitful, stupid, greedy, or hostile. Don't be too curious about your own body or others' bodies. Don't cry in public (and not much in private either). Don't show tenderness except in very carefully defined situations.

This list is staggering. But who among us could not add more *do* and *don't* PFLs to the list? (Try it—make your own additions to this list.) ►IE-1, p. 122.

Somehow the child learns to find his way through this jungle of expectations, rules, and values; somehow he manages to come out on the other side with a part of him still intact. But at what price? Often an enormous one. A child has difficulty making discriminating judgments about what thoughts, feelings, or actions are appropriate or inappropriate in which situations. For example, if he is told again and again that it is wrong to get angry toward his parents, then why is it not wrong to get angry at anybody—no matter what the circumstances and no matter who it is? Unless he is lucky enough to have parents and other adults who can and will communicate with him clearly and honestly, who can and will check out his implementation of the rules, and who can and will help him discriminate amongst different situations, the child may become more and more constricted as he draws back almost instinctively from breaking the rules.

All too frequently, the child does not discriminate and gradually learns to deny not only his negative thoughts, feelings, and actions but many of his positive ones as well. For example, after a while he may not act or (consciously) feel hostile, but he also may not act or feel very loving either. He may learn to be quiet, respectful, and obedient, but underneath he may be seething with rebellion, or he simply may not (consciously) feel much of anything—just gray dullness or vague depression. Or he may feel guilty because he does not feel obedient or respectful.

Of course, many people argue that it is neither wise nor desirable for a person continually to act on whatever comes into his head or heart. And that is true—there is a time, a season, for all things. But too often when the appropriate time rolls around, he who has been so restrictively trained cannot (or does not know how to or does not see the opportunity to) act appropriately. Many people claim that a person should not go around feeling all the time, but the point is that all of us go around feeling all the time—whether or not we know it. The feelings are there; they may be buried under layer on layer of restriction, but they are *there*. And they influence everything we think or do even if we never consciously feel them.

Effects of suppressing feelings

Despite the restrictions placed on freedom of the emotions and despite naivete about and lack of experience with feelings, many people crave more qualitative emotional contact with themselves and others. They long for more fulfilling relationships and for more meaningful emotional experiences. They feel despair and loneliness in a faceless, impersonal, dehumanizing technocracy, and they feel cut off from the real meaning of life—from the joys and hazards of having emotions. It seems evident that this sense of loss and this longing are deeply felt emotional responses, which have led to many of the cultural changes discussed in Chapter 1, such as experimentation with drugs, sex, and personal relationships. This desire for emotional experiences has also found expression in such activities as the human potential movement (e.g., sensitivity training, encounter groups, marathon therapy), alpha brain wave training, yoga, mysticism, Eastern religious philosophies, and the "Jesus Revolution."

Importance of emotional in-touchedness

Although many people long for and seek meaningful emotional experiences, there are many others who contend that deliberately trying to feel feelings which are "beneath the surface" is rocking the emotional boat and thereby risking pain and trouble. They tend to ask, "*Why subject yourself to feelings that are long gone? Why bring to the surface feelings that may be painful, ugly, frightening, or threatening?*"

One major reason for getting in touch with and examining your feelings is that if you do not—if you suppress or ignore your feelings in certain situations or if you suppress certain kinds of emotions (e.g., anger, envy, annoyance)—gradually you will "teach" yourself to suppress most of your feelings. Ultimately you may end up not feeling much of anything. In effect, you may deny a crucial part of your humanity. You may be a brilliant thinker, your actions may be the model of propriety, but you may be a miserably unhappy human being.

Another reason for getting in touch with your feelings is that whether you are aware of them, they are always present. If you are not in touch with them, they control you, since your thoughts, actions, and known feelings will be influenced and sometimes governed by those hidden feelings.

Only when you begin to be aware of and pay attention to your insides, especially your feelings, can you begin to work constructively and wisely with who you are and who you can be. You can begin to understand what you respond to in situations, in others, and in yourself. You can begin to evaluate the appropriateness and validity of your thoughts, feelings, and actions. You can begin to see and to understand how your parents' (and others') PFLs and patterns have influenced and helped to shape your self-system and your life-style (and continue to do so). You can begin to determine how much (or how little) you may be locked into automatic, repetitious patterns of thinking, feeling, and acting. And you can begin to have a sense of, an appreciation of, your uniqueness.[8]

PROCESS OF INTRAPERSONAL COMMUNICATION

Although the idea of communicating with and within yourself may seem rather strange, actually every human being carries on some kind of intrapersonal communication all the time. Each time he thinks to himself, talks to himself, feels a feeling, or acts toward himself in a particular way, a person is communicating intrapersonally.[9] Few people, however, are skilled at communicating effectively with themselves. *But the skills of effective intrapersonal communication can be taught, and they can be learned.* Fortunately the process is a down-to-earth, practical one that can be described, explained, practiced, and utilized step by simple step. The process of intrapersonal communication can be learned so well that you can build it in as a permanent part of your being. As such it can help you experience yourself and life with intense and pleasurable awareness.

If you decide to learn and to utilize the intrapersonal communication process, if you undertake this venture, you will have set out on a life's journey, and like all journeys, the going will not always be easy. You will find that not all your feelings are pleasant ones; they are not always "acceptable" ones (even to you). You will also discover that as you begin to *feel the feelings that you feel at the moment you feel them,* you will often experience discomfort, sometimes anxiety. *That is natural.* It is natural because you will be exposing yourself to newness, difference, and change, and these things naturally arouse a certain amount of anxiety and discomfort. Be assured, however, that if the going gets too rough at any point, you can always back off and rest, or you can completely shut down operations. Or you can block out feelings or defend against them.

If, however, you are willing to risk the journey, the rewards are yours for the asking and the taking. The joy, the thrill, the tremendous excitement of knowing and feeling who you are, and the magnificent sense of power that can flow from being in touch with self are the rewards for those who dare to be.

Overview of the intrapersonal communication process

Following is a list that provides an overview of the process of communicating with self. Remember that, although we apply the process here to feelings, it can and should be applied to your *thoughts* and *actions* also. Only by getting in touch with all three aspects of functioning will you get in fullest touch with your insides. After this overview, the process will be discussed in detail.

LIST OF STEPS

1. Identify your feelings at the moment you feel them.
2. Hold your feelings and allow yourself to really feel them (i.e., do not brush them off as insignificant or trivial).
3. Assess your feelings and their context.
   a. What do your feelings relate to? What is going on around you; what are you, others, doing?
   b. What evoked your feelings? (Was it a touch, an odor, a look, a remark, an action, a thought?)
   c. What do these feelings mean to you? (Are they threatening, depressing, cheering?) How do they serve you? How important are they to you?

4. Evaluate your feelings.
   a. Are your feelings appropriate to the situation?
   b. Is the past involved in your feelings?
   c. Are your feeling responses like those of either or both parents (or other Significant Persons)?
   d. Are they feelings you automatically and repetitively feel in similar or similar-seeming situations? Look for *PFLs* and *patterns* of response.

The process in detail

The detailed explanations of the steps involved in the process of communicating with self follow. Where it is applicable, you are first given whatever information you need to understand and use the step. This information is then followed by instructions on how to implement the step.

STEP 1: IDENTIFY YOUR FEELINGS AT THE MOMENT YOU FEEL THEM

Preparatory information. Your first response to this step may be "But what if I don't feel anything?" Although you may not be aware of feeling anything, remember that you cannot *not* feel.

Your second response may be "Well, I may be feeling something, but what if I don't know *what* I'm feeling?" This response is the most usual one. One reason for this problem is lack of practice. Too often most of us tend to let our feelings slip by us without particularly noticing them. Rarely do we take the time to stop and feel what we are feeling at the moment we are feeling it, and frequently, if a feeling does get through to us, we tend either to shrug it off because it seems insignificant or to squelch it because it is painful or bothersome. Thus we are not accustomed to tapping in on what we are feeling from moment to moment. The "big" emotions generated by crises demand and usually get our attention, but the "little" everyday emotions do not have the same attention-getting power, and therefore they can slide silently by.

The other reason for this problem is that our feelings do not present themselves to us in a neat, orderly, one-by-one fashion, and rarely do we have just one feeling at a time. Even the simplest situation is likely to arouse multiple feelings (although often one feeling will be dominant). When two contrasting feelings are both dominant (e.g., love and hate), we experience **ambivalence.**[10] Whatever the particular combination, the point is that feeling responses are almost always multiple.

For example, suppose you are walking down the street and see a blind man on the corner. He is selling pencils and begging for money. You may respond with an incredible mixture of feelings (depending on many things about you and your background, of course). You may feel *pity* for his blindness and aloneness, *anger* at his lack of initiative in getting work, *guilt* for the fact that you can see and he cannot, *annoyance* because you feel he has put you on the spot, *anger* at a society that does not take care of those in trouble, *annoyance* because you are having these conflicting feelings, and *guilt* because you feel annoyed when you have been taught that you are supposed to pity those less fortunate than you. If a simple event like this one, where you will never encounter the person again and where you do not know him as an individual, can evoke such a variety of feelings, just imagine what kinds and varieties of emotional responses you must be experiencing when you are involved with a person you know and care about personally or with an event or situation that has immediate and direct bearing on your life.

Implementation. How then do you go about identifying your multiple feelings? How do you find out what you are feeling at the moment you are feeling it? *Practice.* Pick a time when a million things are not going on all at once. You might also wish to pick a time when you are not in a situation or with a person that evokes many strong and conflicting feelings in you.

At first, *concentrate on identifying at least one feeling.* When something happens, instead of letting your feelings slip by and disappear, turn off the outside world for a moment and concentrate on what you are feeling. Most of us are not used to doing even this much, but this is the way to start. If you have trouble identifying any feelings and are tempted to say to yourself, "Oh, I don't know; I don't really feel much of anything," *try offering yourself feeling possibilities and alternatives.* In other words, go through a list of possible feelings. The reason for doing this is that it is usually easier to pick one or more applicable feelings from a list than it is to directly identify the particular feeling. A list can help to jog the mind and heart. For example, you might ask yourself the following questions:

Am I	*Am I experiencing*	*Do I feel*
annoyed	pity	ridiculed
angry	sorrow	belittled
hurt	compassion	humiliated
anxious	hostility	cared for
sad	hatred	liked
happy	contempt	loved
delighted	disgust	shunned
pleased	fear	accepted
flattered	joy	put-upon
excited	a sense of well-being	used
?	?	respected
		looked up to
		?

Obviously if you had to go through a long list like this every time you wanted to find out what you are feeling, you would have time for nothing else. If, however, you practice identifying your feelings, soon you will not need any list at all (except maybe in really sticky and complicated feeling matters). The more practice you have in identifying feelings, the more quickly and deftly you will be able to do so. ►IE-2, p. 123.

Although it may seem odd to you that people need to practice knowing what they feel, it is unfortunately true that most of us do not just naturally know how to get or be in touch with our emotions. (If you want to test this out, pick out a number of situations during the next few days and see if you can identify your feelings at the moment you are feeling them. Another thing you can try is asking some of your friends at various times what they are really feeling at the moment. It can be an interesting and enlightening experience.)

STEP 2: HOLD YOUR FEELINGS AND ALLOW YOURSELF TO REALLY FEEL THEM

Preparatory information. This step may seem unnecessary to you. After all, if you are able to identify a feeling, have you not held on to it and felt it? Perhaps—perhaps not. For example, what about the time (or times) you have blurted out something you did not mean to say—a comment, a criticism, a swear word? Most of us in a situation like this have experienced at least a flash of embarrassment, a moment of feeling ridiculous and humiliated, or a pang of feeling stupid and awkward. How many of us, however, are willing to hold on to and really feel any or all of these feelings? Although deliberately holding on to negative feelings might seem masochistic, it does not have to be. Holding on to feelings can be constructive because it enables you to keep them in your awareness long enough to figure out both their importance and meaning.

Implementation. Since feelings can be extremely elusive, once you have identified a feeling, try to stop the emotional action so that you can concentrate on holding the feeling. Holding on to a feeling means far more than just thinking about it; it means letting it register (and stay registered) at the gut level. It means letting yourself feel how your body reacts in response to the feeling. For example, if you identify that you feel scared, can you tap in on and really experience reactions like a dry mouth, the sensation of your skin crawling, your stomach turning over, or a cold sweat?

The value of sticking with a feeling is that experiencing it so vividly helps you to assess its power and to keep it in your awareness. Remaining aware of the feeling then allows you the opportunity to work with it.

For example, suppose you have a repetitive, automatic pattern of blurting out the wrong thing at the wrong time. As long as your resultant feelings of embarrassment, humiliation, stupidity, or awkwardness do not come through to you sharply and last only a moment, you will hardly be aware of feeling them and will probably soon forget them. If you do not catch hold of, hold on to, and *really feel* your feelings, you will not have them around long enough to figure out their relationship to or their part in the pattern they are attached to. And if you are not aware of the relationship between your feelings and the pattern, then your pattern will likely remain intact —as repetitive and automatic as ever. Holding on to feelings is then an important step in breaking up the automatic quality of your functioning.

Being able to hold on to your feelings also gives you the opportunity to process them; that is, it enables you to slow the action down so that not only can you feel multiple feelings but you can also capture your feelings one by one in a given situation and thereby discover the order in which they occur. Learning in what sequence your feelings occur can teach you a good deal about your particular unique ways of responding from moment to moment. For example, when someone criticizes you, do you feel threatened, then angry, then guilty, then despairing? Or do you feel threatened, then guilty, then despairing, then angry? The first sequence (especially if it is one that occurs a number of times) might suggest that your response pattern to criticism is aggressive but underpinned by feelings of helplessness. The second sequence might suggest a more passive response underpinned by frustration, leading to anger. At the least, identifying a specific feeling sequence may indicate your basic orientation to particular experiences (in this case, criticism).

There are, of course, times when it is appropriate to block out or ignore or brush off feelings. But if a person habitually does so, he inevitably cuts himself off from an important part of himself. Not many of us are trained to hold and feel our feelings; thus we start at a disadvantage. How many of us tend to skim over our feelings when someone is rude to us; when someone angers or embarrasses us; or when someone says, "You're fun to be with, you're good-looking, I like you." How often do most of us draw back quickly and nervously when we are suddenly invited or asked or pressured to *feel* life on the feeling level? Why is it that so many of us may reflect on or complain about what happened after it happened, but we can hardly acknowledge the event and the feelings it arouses at the time it is going on? Because we are afraid to do so? Because to do so evokes feelings of discomfort? Because we feel anxious? Because it seems too threatening, too dangerous, or too demanding? Most of these questions and their "yes" answers are all too familiar to many of us. To change that, to learn to be a fuller human being, to be willing to feel takes a lot of courage because too many of us never learned how or were trained not to know how. But it *is* possible to learn (or relearn) how.

STEP 3: ASSESS YOUR FEELINGS AND THEIR CONTEXT

Preparatory information. This step (and the next one) consists primarily of questions you can ask yourself, the answers to which will help you better understand your feelings. As you ask yourself these questions, you need to keep two important things in mind.

1. Try not to ask, "What *caused* me to feel what I feel" or "What (or who) *made* me feel the way I do?" No one and no thing *causes, makes,* or *forces* an adult to feel anything. You respond with certain feelings because you are who you are. This places responsibility for your feelings squarely on you, and that can be uncomfortable. But it provides an advantage too:

if only you are responsible for what you feel, then you and you alone have ultimate control over what you feel.

2. Try not to ask, "*Why* do I feel the way I do?"—at least not in the beginning. Why tends to block the free flow of communication. The reason is that why is the most sophisticated and complex question that can be asked: the answer to why is a composite of the answers to many smaller questions such as *what, who, when, where, how.* Thus why really presupposes that a person already has the answers to all these smaller questions and can give them in the form of reasons.

Most of us when first confronted with *why* simply do not know. We may give a quick answer, but it is likely to be incomplete, since the full answer is only likely to become clear after going through all the communicational steps perhaps several times. So if you want to achieve the clearest, straightest possible communication with yourself (and others), try to avoid asking *why* as an early question.

Implementation. The heart of carrying out step 3 is asking and answering various questions, including the following: *What do my feelings relate to?* In more particular terms, *What is going on around me? What am I doing? What are others doing?* These questions are aimed at eliciting answers to the following key questions: *What am I responding to? What or who (or both), specifically, has evoked the feelings that I feel?*

Here is a specific example illustrating how you could use step 3 (and the ones preceding it). You are sitting in class, and the teacher asks a question. You are fairly certain that you know the answer. You do not know what stops you, but you do not respond. Neither does anyone else. As the teacher looks around the room and the silence lengthens, everyone grows more and more tense. When the teacher looks at you, you avoid his eyes. Finally, the teacher asks someone who says he does not know the answer. You grow even more uncomfortable. Then the teacher asks you. You now feel acutely uncomfortable and wish you were somewhere else. You stammer around for a moment, then say, "I don't know." The teacher stares at you briefly, then asks four other people, all of whom say, "I don't know." By this time, the teacher is really angry and sarcastically comments about "the class's study habits—or lack thereof." Your discomfort is now intense, and although it recedes some as the class moves on, you cannot seem to get rid of your feelings. After class is over, you still feel *upset, vaguely annoyed,* and *dissatisfied*—feelings that stay with you for most of the day, even though you tell yourself it was just an unimportant and passing incident. Finally, the whole matter slips from your mind.

Suppose, however, that instead of letting the incident slip away, you decide to try to find out what you felt at the time you felt it. You also begin to investigate what in the situation called forth your response. Suppose you are able to identify (and to hold and relive vividly) your feelings: you discover that you felt *angry, anxious, embarrassed, humiliated, unsure of yourself,* and *scared.*

Now you start to work on step 3. You ask yourself, "What was I angry about? *Who* was I angry at?" You determine, interestingly enough, that you felt angry even before the teacher got sarcastic, although his sarcasm added fuel to your original anger. If your anger began prior to the teacher's remarks, then who else was there to be angry at but yourself? You focus now on what in the situation evoked your response of self-anger. You begin to realize that you were angry because you knew the answer to the question but were unwilling to take the risk. What risk? The risk of being wrong; the risk of "making a fool of yourself"; the risk of drawing attention to yourself. You were angry at yourself because you felt that you "chickened out." You were angry too because you in effect cheated yourself out of the recognition you so easily and rightfully could have had if you had answered.

You think and feel some more about the incident and discover that your feelings of anxiety, unsureness, and fear were the result of worrying that the teacher might try to force you into answering or might make a nasty comment to you. Yet you were fairly sure you knew the answer, so what aroused these feelings in you? A fear of being put on the spot and of not being able to perform.

If you carry out the rest of step 3, you ask yourself, "What do these feelings *mean* to me? How do they *serve* me? How important are they to me?" Your answers can be highly instructive and helpful to you. In this example, suppose you realize that in a pressure situation, you "play dumb" to protect yourself, that you do not have a great deal of confidence about taking the risk of exposing yourself to possible ridicule or humiliation, that it would be humiliating to you to be wrong, that you lose respect for yourself when you do not do what you are fairly sure you are able to do, and that you get angry at yourself (punish yourself) when you do not live up to your own and others' expectations (in this case the teacher's).

When you first started working with this experience and the feelings it evoked in you, you might have felt like brushing the whole thing aside as trivial and not worth your concern. But as you continue to analyze the incident and your feelings, you probably can begin to see that your feeling responses are important, even if the incident itself is a seemingly minor one. They are important because they operate somewhat automatically, and they point to a number of possible patterns.

Although this is just a small, passing incident, most of life is made up of just such small, passing incidents. The ways that we think and feel and act in response to these incidents are the major ingredients of our lives. To ignore some of these small incidents is natural; to ignore many or nearly all of them because they "are not really significant" is to ignore the real heart of living.

STEP 4: EVALUATE YOUR FEELINGS

This step (like step 3) consists of a number of questions. These questions are concerned not only with the present but also the past. Their answers will help you begin to gain some perspective on how you function in the here and now and on how you learned to function as you were growing up. Ultimately, if you continue to work on achieving better and clearer communication with yourself, you will gain a clearer and more meaningful picture of both your self-system and life-style and a better understanding of how to deal with who you are.

Using the same incident as we did in step 3, let us look at the questions that you need to answer.

Are your feelings appropriate to the situation? In this instance, are your feelings of anxiety, embarrassment, humiliation, insecurity, and fear appropriate to a brief few minutes in a classroom when you might have been put on the spot but were not? In part, these feelings were aroused by your assuming that the teacher *might* force you to answer or *might* direct a nasty comment to you. If this particular teacher's style is to be domineering, to be sarcastic, and to be humiliating to students, then your feelings would seem to be appropriate. On the other hand, if this particular teacher has a reputation for gentleness, respect for students' feelings, and understanding, then your feelings would seem to be inappropriate. Suppose the latter is true; then you need to investigate your responses more fully.

Before you move on to another question, check out the appropriateness of your other feelings. What about your fear of being put on the spot and not being able to perform? In this particular situation, because of the teacher's good reputation, your fear that he will put you on the spot is groundless and inappropriate. As for your fear that you would not be able to perform (e.g., to answer the question), whether this is an appropriate response depends on your past experiences. That is, have there been times when you have been in the "spotlight" and have not been able to answer the question (or do what was required or asked of you)? If that is the case, then your fear has some basis. However, in this *particular* situation, is your fear of failing to perform as expected really appropriate? After all, you knew the teacher would not push you; you also were fairly sure you knew the answer. Obviously there is some doubt about the appropriateness of your emotional response to this particular incident.

One other reaction of yours needs investigation. You were angry at yourself because you did not live up to your own expectations. This particular reaction demands that you look closely at the expectations you have. Are *they* (and the feelings they arouse in you when you do not fulfill them) valid and appropriate and realistic? Is one of your expectations that you *must* answer every time you are fairly sure you know the answer? Is another one that you must always be sure you are right before you will risk public exposure? Is another that you cannot afford (or bear) to be wrong—ever? These expectations are not realistic; they place almost impossible demands on you. And since your expectations are unrealistic, it is inevitable that when you do not fulfill them, your feelings will be unrealistic and inappropriate also.

Is the past involved in your feelings? Many of your feelings in the present can be traced to influences from the past. So that the past will not tyrannize you or exercise undue (and usually unrecognized) control over your present responses, you must search out and understand the extent to which your past still influences your present.

To do that, you must go PFL hunting, since you need to know what PFLs are influencing you and who you got them from. For example, did your father (or your mother or both) say, feel, or act as though he had to say something every time he believed he was probably right? Did he believe he had to be right before he would commit himself publicly to something? Or did he feel that he could not be wrong? Were these *expectations* also passed on to you in the form of *rules* and *values* (e.g., "don't make mistakes")? Did one (or both) of your parents disapprove if you gave a wrong or stupid answer? Were you raised in an atmosphere in which your parents *stressed* correct performance and *ridiculed* failure? Did you see one (or both) of your parents get angry at himself for failing to meet his own standards? These PFL-hunting questions lead naturally to the next one.

Are your feeling responses like those of either or both parents (or other Significant Persons)? To complete your answers to this question, you will need to reach back in your memory. How have I seen my parents (or other Significant Persons) feel and act in similar (or similar-seeming) situations? To get at similarities, try to see the basic likenesses in a situation (e.g., a question asked by a person in authority). To get at what your parents' feeling responses might have been, try to remember not just what your parents said but also their tones of voice, their movements, and the ways they looked. If you find that certain of your feeling responses are like those of one or both parents (or other Significant Persons), then you can be sure that you are dealing with feelings of yours which are not just of the moment and not just of the present. If you are copying them, you may be responding automatically. But whether you are copying others or are responding strictly from your own position, you need to evaluate the degree of spontaneity in your reactions. The way to do this is to find the answer to the following question.

Are your feelings repetitive and automatic? Do I tend to feel much the same way each time I get in a similar (or similar-seeming) situation? For example, when you feel pressured to perform, do you *consistently* experience a fear that you might fail? In addition, ask yourself—Do I respond *automatically* without forethought, without conscious intent to do so, and almost without conscious control over my emotional reactions? Was I even *aware* of how I responded? For example, when the teacher asked his question, did I automatically and without conscious awareness feel feelings of fear and anger? If you discover that your feeling responses are indeed repetitive and automatic, then you can be sure that you have identified patterns of thinking, feeling, and acting.

If you look back over these four steps, you can appreciate the complexity and richness of your insides. You are probably also aware that you may not always get all the answers to all these questions. But that is natural, and continued practice will enable you to increase your chances of succeeding. Although you may not always know all there is to know about your insides, even a little knowledge can be extremely useful. ►IE-3, p. 123.

When you are able to recognize what you feel at the moment you feel it and to see the relationship of your feelings to the past and the present, then you can begin to gain insight into the dynamics of your self-system and life-style. Once you gain that insight, you are in a position to alter, to modify, to expand, to add to, or to change how you think and feel and act. You are now on the road that leads to personal autonomy. Not that the process is an easy or simple one; indeed it is extremely complex. But once you begin to see how and why you function as you do, you have a chance to make freer, more appropriate, and more meaningful choices and decisions about how you will live your life.

Possible reactions or problems

You are bound to have had some thoughts and feelings as you read this explanation of the step-by-step process of communicating with yourself. You may have had some of the following reservations, doubts, or questions.

1. You may feel resistant toward trying the process. If you do, it is a natural reaction. Your culture and your background have encouraged you (by and large) to ignore or avoid or hide your feelings. Now you are being urged to examine and feel your feelings as intensely and as fully as you can. You are being encouraged to try and to practice a process that is new and unfamiliar to you, and newness and unfamiliarity arouse anxiety and resistance.

2. You may feel that this process is unrealistic because it must be done piecemeal and because it would tend to isolate you from people and events around you. Admittedly to use this process you must focus on what is going on inside you and temporarily separate yourself from things around you to achieve that focus. At the start, you will have to pay extremely close attention to what you are doing. But as is true of most things you learn by practicing, soon you will find that you can move through these steps rapidly without really interrupting whatever else you are doing. Eventually the process will become second nature to you. In addition, as you begin to discern patterns in your responses, certain sets of feelings will begin to stand out. Thus you will not always have to go through every step of the process every time you have a feeling.

3. You may feel that this process is artificial, almost unnatural, because it must be carried out in conscious, step-by-step detail. It is artificial in that it is not a process which you instinctively know all about and can apply with ease. What is unnatural, however, is not the artificiality of the process but the very fact that most of us have to be taught and have to relearn how to get in touch with this precious natural resource—our feelings.

4. You may feel that the communicational process is too complicated, too difficult, and too time-consuming. To the beginner, yes, but to someone who is accustomed to applying the process, it is actually a fast, simple, and direct way to get at feelings and deal with them. To verify this, try it, practice it, and give the process and yourself time and a fair chance. You are the only person who can convince yourself of its value.

BENEFITS OF THE PROCESS

What benefits can you hope to gain by getting in touch with your insides? The benefits are numerous, and they will have significant impact on your life.

1. Since the intrapersonal communication process applies to all three aspects of functioning—thinking, feeling, and acting—using the process can enable you to get in touch with the roots and the full range of your functioning. In effect you will be in touch with your self-system and your lifestyle and therefore with your past and present.

2. This process will enable you to use the Interactional Therapeutic System in a conscious, deliberate, and constructive manner. By being in touch, you can find out what PFLs are at work in your life. You can begin to determine how and from whom you got them and whether you wish to keep them, alter them, or get rid of them. Being in touch can help you to determine what your self-concept is (how you really see and feel about yourself). And if your self-concept does not please you, you can begin to change it to suit you. Being in touch can help you to realize what your intrapersonal patterns are (i.e., how you treat yourself both in terms of your self-concept and in terms of what others think and feel about you). If you do not like the ways you treat yourself or if those ways seem inappropriate, then you have the opportunity to intervene in and alter your intrapersonal patterns if you choose.

Being in touch with your insides allows you to investigate and discover which part —Child, Parent, or Adult—operates most strongly in you. If there is an imbalance among them, you are in a position to work on freeing or calming the Child, curbing or encouraging the Parent, or giving vitamins and penicillin to the Adult or just cheering it on. Being in touch with your insides also gives you the chance to understand the dynamic underpinnings of your interpersonal patterns. And once you gain this kind of understanding, you can interrupt, alter, modify, or keep these patterns as you see fit.

3. Once you develop this kind of in-touchedness, you can evaluate and work with the ways you come across to others nonverbally (i.e., even before or at the same time as you are speaking).

4. Being in touch with your own insides puts you in the best possible position to communicate effectively and meaningfully with others; qualitative interpersonal communication depends ultimately on two (or more) people's sharing and negotiating about their insides. And qualitative interpersonal communication is the golden key to more qualitative interpersonal relationships—friendships, dating, living together, marriage, and the family.

Interaction experiences

1. Working with a restrictive PFL (p. 112)

Using one of the PFLs listed on p. 112 or drawing on your memory, pick a PFL that restricts the way you think or feel or act. When you have chosen the specific PFL, then *act contrary to* what it prescribes. For example, if you have a PFL that says, "Don't think dirty words," try thinking some dirty words. If you have a PFL that says, "Don't feel envious," try allowing yourself to envy another person. If you have a PFL that says, "Don't show too much interest in another person," go out of your way to show and express interest in another. Try to feel what you are feeling at each moment in the experience.

EVALUATION: Could you get in touch with your feelings? How did it feel to go against the PFL? Could you feel the power of the PFL? Were you aware of more than one feeling? Could you identify any sequence of feelings?

FOLLOW-UP: Try doing this same experience with other PFLs you have so that you can practice identifying your feelings and practice feeling the force of your PFLs. Share your experience of going against your PFLs with another person. You might also want to encourage him to try going against one of his PFLs and then sharing his experience with you.

2. Getting in touch with moment-to-moment feelings (p. 116)

Find a quiet place where you will not be disturbed for a while. Close your eyes and recall an event that evoked strong feelings in you, or fantasize an event that would do so. Examples of such events are a wedding, a death, a separation, a shocking revelation, an accident, being pushed around, being embarrassed or humiliated, or receiving an unexpected compliment. Make your experience as vivid as possible. Try to get in touch with what you are feeling from moment to moment as you relive or experience this event.

EVALUATION: Were you able to identify at least one feeling? Could you identify more than one? Were you surprised at what your feelings were, by their strength or weakness, or both? Did you try offering yourself alternative feeling positions? (See p. 116.) Could you feel different stages in your feeling responses—that is, did you experience and *feel* a sequence of feelings?

FOLLOW-UP: Try this experience with other events. You might also have a friend recall the same kind of event and then share and compare your feeling responses.

3. Practicing the intrapersonal communication process (p. 121)

Follow the instructions given in Interaction Experience 2 but now go through all four steps of the intrapersonal communication process.

EVALUATION: Were you confused by dealing with a number of emotions? That is natural and will ease up as you gain more practice. Were you able to get in touch with your feelings, hold them, assess them and their context, and evaluate them? How did it feel to deliberately try to become aware of and work with your feelings?

FOLLOW-UP: Try this approach on other feelings and on your thoughts and actions also.

REFERENCES

1. Satir, Virginia: Conjoint family therapy, Palo Alto, Calif., 1964, Science & Behavior Books, Inc., pp. 63-64.
2. May, Rollo: Man's search for himself, New York, 1967, The New American Library, Inc., p. 91.
3. Birdwhistle, Ray L.: Expressions of the emotions in man, New York, 1963, International Universities Press.
4. Duffy, Elizabeth: An explanation of "emotional" phenomena without the use of the concept "emotion." In Candland, Douglas K., editor: Emotion: body change, Princeton, 1962, D. Van Nostrand Co., p. 27.
5. May, op. cit., pp. 91 and 100.
6. Freud, Sigmund: Civilization and its discontents, translated by James Strachey, New York, 1961, W. W. Norton & Co., Inc.
7. Fromm, Erich: Beyond the chains of illusion: my encounter with Marx and Freud, New York, 1962, Simon & Schuster, Inc., pp. 71-134.
8. Ibid., p. 129.
9. Ruesch, Jurgen, and Bateson, Gregory: Communication: the social matrix of psychiatry, New York, 1951, W. W. Norton & Co., Inc. pp. 278-279.
10. Ruesch, Jurgen, and Bateson, Gregory: Therapeutic communication, New York, 1961, W. W. Norton & Co., Inc., p. 327.

chapter 8
NONVERBAL COMMUNICATION

Chapter 7 was limited to a discussion of the individual and his intrapersonal communication and interaction. It focused on how he can get in touch with his insides, what he can learn about and from his insides, and how he can benefit from his "in-touchedness." For the most part, the physical, nonverbal aspects of intrapersonal communication and interaction were not considered.

This chapter will be devoted to the pivotal role of **nonverbal communication,** that is, to its effects on both intrapersonal and interpersonal communication. Becoming aware of, understanding, and learning to interpret body language—the physical, nonverbal means of communication—are important in many ways. In the most general terms, these skills are important because they contribute to personal and interpersonal competence. Thus gaining fluency in the language of the body means acquiring further abilities to use the Interactional Therapeutic System in a deliberate and constructive manner.[1,2]

The ability to interpret your own body language is extremely important. Being in touch with what your body "says," feels like, and does enables you to understand the part it plays in your self-system. For example, if you determine which parts of your sensory responses are least operative, you may be able to track down some suppressive PFLs. If, for example, you have trouble maintaining eye contact with others, you may have PFLs that warn against trust, intimacy, or curiosity. Furthermore, being able to "read" your body's language can help you get in touch with your *physical* self-concept, which exercises a strong influence on your overall self-concept.[3,4] And, of course, the ways you treat yourself (intrapersonal patterns) are partly physical and nonverbal. In addition, your body reacts to what is going on inside you and, subtly or not, expresses its comfort or discomfort with your inside operations.

It is also necessary to know what your body says so that you can evaluate how appropriately your body language reflects your insides. Is your body a clear and undistorted mirror of your inside operations? Or is it a fun house mirror that twists and distorts the reflections of you?[5]

Being aware of and understanding body language are of equal consequence to your interpersonal communication and interaction for four reasons.

1. Since the body and its language are the outside expression of insides, you need to realize what your body says to ascertain what nonverbal signals you send to others. Only then can you determine whether you are transmitting accurate or distorted signals about yourself to others.
2. You need to be aware of other people's body language because it exerts a major influence on your impressions of and responses to them.
3. You need to be able to read others' body language so that you can evaluate whether you misinterpret their signals or whether they send distorted signals.
4. You need to understand body language so that you can realistically assess its influences on the spoken word—both your own and others'.

SIGNALS, VERBAL MESSAGES, AND METAMESSAGES

All human communication consists of sending and receiving messages of one kind or another. Essentially there are three kinds of messages: signals (nonverbal messages), verbal messages, and metamessages.

Signals

It is the body that conveys almost all nonverbal communication. Since the body is a talented instrument of expression, the variety of signals it can send and give off includes a vast range of possibilities.

A **signal** is a brief, nonverbal message (conscious or unconscious) that is limited to a few comparatively simple and specific meanings, which are determined by their context.[6-8] For example, when a winner of a track event raises his clenched fist, it can mean victory. When a black speaker at a black power rally raises his clenched fist, it can mean anger and power. A signal does not need many, if any, qualifications to make its meaning clear. Frequently, it is crudely symbolic and is relatively unambiguous (e.g., thumbs down; a sneer). Generally, it has an agreed-on meaning ascribed to it by the group or culture in which it is used.

Although a signal is a quick, direct, nonverbal communication that carries only one or two meanings in a given context, it may suggest more complex meanings (e.g., a raised eyebrow may indicate sexual interest and suggest that the receiver of the signal should make the next move). Nevertheless, because a signal's meaning content is limited, a signal cannot in and of itself convey a complex message, since it can neither express nor explain the relationships between various factors. For example, crossed fingers signals that "I hope something does (or does not) happen." But the crossed fingers alone cannot express or explain relationships between the hope and such matters as time or cause; that is, crossed fingers cannot indicate that "I hope something happens" *tomorrow* or *because my job depends on it.* To express relationships, a person would have to send many other signals and probably would have to transmit a verbal message as well.

Road signs are good example of signals; they convey simple direct, immediate, and unambiguous meanings: *Stop! Detour. One Way. Curve.* However, signals given by human beings are often not so easy to read or interpret because people tend to give off series of signals (a number of signals occurring one after another) or sets of signals (groups of interrelated signals given at the same time). If the signals in a series or set all convey essentially the same meaning or if they reinforce one another, there will be little difficulty in interpreting their meaning. But if, as is frequently the case, a person transmits a series or set of signals, some of which conflict with or contradict one another, then interpreting what the person means can be difficult and confusing and sometimes impossible. For example, suppose your advisor calls you in to talk about what you should do about your poor academic performance. He tells you he wants to come to a joint decision about the matter, one that is based on reason and that is agreeable to both of you. As he talks, you note the set of signals he is sending: his voice is calm and controlled, but his tone is annoyed and his manner distant. Although he smiles from time to time, his eyes are cold. Although he reassures you that he is not annoyed, that he really cares what you think, how are you to read his set of conflicting signals? This example may provide some idea of the difficulty of interpreting conflicting signals.

Verbal messages

Verbal messages are all those communications which employ spoken words to convey meanings.* Verbal messages can be of

*In intrapersonal communication, the words may not be spoken aloud, but the person does (whether consciously or not) conceptualize the meaning of the verbal message.

any length and of any degree of complexity, and they can have unlimited meanings. These messages may be literal, symbolic, or both; they can range from simplicity to great refinement and sophistication. They may, and frequently do, have numerous meanings, which can be either personal or general or both, and they can be open to many interpretations.

A verbal message may be a lengthy or brief setting forth of meanings. It can be sustained for as long as necessary and elaborated as much as necessary to convey and clarify complex meanings. It can ask about, suggest, explain, and express intricate, delicate, and complicated relationships. It can convey multiple meanings at the same time.

Metamessages

Metamessages are meanings that either reinforce, expand on, or undermine the meaning of the spoken message. These metamessage meanings can result from the combination of signals (nonverbal messages) and verbal messages transmitted (whether intentionally or unconsciously) by the sender of the communication. Or these meanings can result from the ways the receiver interprets the combination of signals and verbal messages that he hears. A metamessage may convey exactly the same meaning(s) as the verbal message does. This reinforcement of the verbal message occurs when signals and verbal messages are congruent with each other: the sender says what he means and means what he says.[9] For example, Wayne tells Sally, "I really admire the way you treat your parents; you're so pleasant and friendly to them." As he says this, Wayne looks directly at Sally, his eyes light up, he smiles, and his tone is warm and sincere.

By means of the signals accompanying the spoken words, the metamessage may expand on the verbal message. For example, Walt and Marcia are about to part after having dinner and going to the movies. As they pause at her door, she enthusiastically says, "Thanks a lot, Walt; I *really* enjoyed being with you." With that, she throws her arms around his neck and kisses him. The metamessage expands on the spoken message by saying, in effect, "I really like you and would like to go out with you again soon."

Conversely, a metamessage may convey meanings that are different from those of the verbal message. Such a difference is a form of distorted communication. This difference can occur because one verbal message contradicts or undercuts another. For example, suppose a wife asks her husband to help her decide what color to paint the living room. He suggests white walls, and she replies, "Yes, but white gets dirty so quickly." Then he says, "Well, how about off-white?" and she answers, "Yes, but off-white looks dirty to begin with." He may suggest four others, and she may answer, "Yes, but . . . " to all four. The following is one metamessage she may be sending (whether or not intentionally): "You can't really be of any help to me. Your suggestions aren't any good."

The meanings of the verbal message and the metamessage can also clash because the signals (or some of them) and verbal messages in some way conflict with or contradict one another. For example, if you say firmly to yourself, "I'm not really afraid of the dark," but your body signals you with fear and anxiety, then the metamessage might be, "Let me out of here!" Examples and explanations of metamessages in interpersonal communication will be given in detail in Chapter 9.

CULTURAL TEACHINGS ABOUT THE BODY

A primary reason for distorted metamessages is our lack of in-touchedness with our bodies and their language. Why does this problem exist? One likely reason is that many of us in this culture are "trained" from childhood to ignore or at least courteously avoid taking much notice of the human body—others' or our own. Early on, children are taught in a number of ways that it is not nice or it is evil to touch certain parts of their own or other people's bodies. It is not nice to sniff and smell others; it is not nice to pick your nose or scratch private body parts; it is not nice to listen to (or at least show that you hear) the noises other people make. It is not nice to kick or bite or lick or sniff or touch or pat or stare.

Expose children to those dictates for any length of time and, although they may not like it, they will catch on to the PFL: *That which has to do with the senses—the physical—is either off limits or very restricted.* It must seem to many children that only adults are allowed to have any fun with their bodies. The trouble is that for many an adult it is often too late. He has learned his childhood lessons all too well and has turned off or at least radically checked his natural tendencies to use his senses in the richest and fullest possible way.[10]

In our culture, not only growing up but adulthood as well is a time for receiving confusing signals and teachings about our bodies. Look at the mass media and the ways it reflects what we as a culture accept and reject. On the one hand, the media is loaded with suggestive materials: the stunning, eye-catching centerfold pictures in *Playboy;* pictures in magazines of handsome, virile young men in tight bathing suits; stacked women and well-built men on television and in the movies. But the philosophy underlying all this is sexual voyeurism: Worship from afar, but *don't touch!*

It is important also to note that for the most part the media plays down physical imperfections. The media—and the media's public—does not seem to want to notice that which is less than ideal. Thus we tend to be so bombarded with sexual and sensual ideals that if a person's body is less than perfect, we become conditioned to feel that it is not worthy of our attention. Yet if we are trained to look away in the presence of imperfections, we lose contact with the larger part of our experience, since most of us are hardly perfect physical specimens.

In addition, our culture seems determined to avoid the physical realities of our existence. Granted, halitosis and some body odors are not particularly pleasant. Granted, filth and sewage and garbage are ugly and unpleasant. Granted, it may not be esthetically pleasing to look at dirty or oily hair or to smell stale sweat. But if a Martian were to base his evaluation of our culture *solely* on our advertising, he would surely report back to his fellow Martians that Americans are obsessed with controlling, purifying, and neutralizing their bodies and their physical environment and are thereby busily denying the natural state of their physical being.

Look at the ads that assault us during our waking hours. Don't have bad breath; eliminate body odor and stay dry all day; disguise genital odors. Be clean, shiny, bright, silky, nonoily, nonflaky, hairless, odorless, tasteless, sleek, smooth, and clean-shaven. Smell exotic, erotic, lemony, lime-y, spicy, woodsy, springlike, and outdoorsy. Don't let your house smell like you have ever cooked anything in it. Don't even let your dog or cat smell like a dog or cat.

The point is that advertising and the mass media are rather accurate reflectors of our cultural orientation toward the physical—that somehow the human body must be made as perfect as possible before it is acceptable to us. The ways to make it perfect are to envelop it in a protective casing—in an aura of perfume and sprays, in a halo of cleanliness, in a covering of cosmetics, and in a film of lotions. The end result of this envelopment is to divorce us from our bodies as they really are. Our commercials reflect a kind of national lifestyle that consists of being out of touch with ourselves as *physical* beings.

This is not to say that we have no awareness; we do, however, severely limit and restrict our awareness and our physical behavior to certain times, situations, and people.[11,12] We have all kinds of rules to govern all kinds of exigencies. For example, it is all right for a boy to kiss his father when the boy is young (until he is about 7 or 8 years old), but after that age, too often we teach him that there is something unusual or unmanly about kissing his father. Another example is that women may hug and kiss each other, but men may not. Another is that women and children may cry, but boys over 10 years old or so may not. Gradually most of us learn not to look at or maintain eye contact for any length of time with most people and certainly not with a stranger unless we are sexually interested. We also learn that except in limited situations, reaching out and spontaneously touching another person can and often will be misinterpreted.

Most of us are finished products of this system of limitation: we tend to ignore, avoid, or not be aware of many of the signals that our own bodies send or give off or many of the signals that others' bodies send or give off. So we tend to miss a lot of what is going on. However, the way that we handle and use our bodies is a key way of communicating and of expressing ourselves.

Our everyday verbal language attests to the way we rely on and readily accept body language. Even more, many familiar phrases are a startling testament to the way we make assumptions about each other on the basis of nonverbal signals.[13,14] If someone looks you "straight in the eye," he is someone you can trust. If we say a man has a "roving eye," we mean he is likely to be unfaithful or at least very active sexually. When we say that a person goes around with her "nose in the air," we are saying she is acting superior and condescending. If we think someone has really worked well and constructively with a problem, we say that he "sank his teeth into the problem." If someone is "sharp-tongued," he has a tendency to make harsh and punitive remarks to others. The number of expressions we have in the language is enormous and fascinating: "Don't give me any lip." "You've got a big mouth." "I'm all ears." "He just elbows his way in." "I'm all thumbs." "Keep a tight rear." "Stand on your own two feet." "Don't turn your back on me." "I'm all choked up." Not only do these metaphors describe in physical, nonverbal terms how a person feels or acts, but they also convey the assumptions we make about others when we receive certain nonverbal signals from them.

Our nonverbal actions and reactions are reflections of our inner states; they are the outer, observable expressions of our insides. They are the sometimes subtle, sometimes not-so-subtle clues to and signals of what is going on inside of us. All the nonverbal signals that a person sends therefore (some of which he knows about and sends deliberately, some of which he does not know about and sends involuntarily) are expressions of his self-system and life-style. In fact, they both express and make up a part of his self-system and life-style. If there is a gap between a person's inner world and what he wants it to be like or if he is unaware of his insides, some of the signals he sends may be distortions of what he is really feeling. For example, suppose a person feels vulnerable and inadequate and is anxious about his ability to "deliver the goods." He may present a nonverbal front consisting of aloofness, coolness, and determination. He may be tight-lipped, frowning, and jut-jawed. These would be false signals; that is, they would not be expressions of what he is really feeling inside. In another sense, however, they would be true signals, since they would reflect his efforts to appear adequate and able and perhaps to persuade himself that he is. But his interpersonal pattern of coolness would be a distorted expression of his self-concept.

Whatever the individual case may be, each of us is constantly sending, giving off, and receiving nonverbal signals. Part of learning to communicate more clearly with oneself and with others therefore involves learning what to look for on a nonverbal level and becoming more aware of and sensitive to nonverbal signals. ►IE-1, p. 139.

TRIDIMENSIONAL ASPECTS OF NONVERBAL COMMUNICATION

The body's language then can reveal much information about a person—both to other people and to the person himself *if* he can tune in on it. In learning to apply this process of tuning in, it is vitally important to realize and remember that through his senses, nonverbal signals affect every person on all three levels of functioning—intellectual, emotional, and behavioral. For example, suppose you are driving along the highway and suddenly a car swings into your lane and heads directly for you. By swerving your car onto the shoulder, you narrowly avert a head-on crash.

An "instant slow-motion replay" of this event makes clear how many sensory inputs occur and how your responses are tridimensional in nature. You receive a signal through your visual sense: a car is speeding directly toward you. This is both a *physical* (sight) and intellectual perception. Your *intellect* (memory, evaluation, judgment, spatial perception) tells you that if you do not get your car out of the way, a crash will inevitably result. In addition, you *feel* the emotions of fear, terror, perhaps despair, anger, and aggression. In response to both your sensory/intellectual perception and your emotions, you react involuntarily and voluntarily. Your body receives a shot of adrenalin (among other things that occur automatically), and you swerve the car off the road out of danger (*behavioral*).

Then as you *think* about what almost happened and what it could have meant (crash, injury, pain, maybe death), you *feel* more terror and horror and perhaps imaginatively "feel" the pain. You also feel anger. Your body reflects these emotions in its *behavior:* shaking, sweating, teeth chattering, tension, and rigidity. You also use your body and your intellect to vent your emotions; you swear and you think ugly thoughts.

Although this particular example is an intrapersonal one, the same truths apply to an interpersonal situation. Hopefully, this example underscores the importance of paying attention to your sensory responses and to all three levels of functioning when you work on becoming aware of nonverbal signals and their effects.

BODY LANGUAGE

Following is a list of various body language signals that provides you with clues about what kinds of factors to look for. The meanings of these signals are not discussed, partly because a signal's meaning may change according to the series or set it is in and partly because many of them are self-revelatory. As you go through this list, try to decide what each signal alone could mean and what each might mean in combination with others. In addition, try to think of other signals you have both seen and sent. Keep in mind that although the signals are presented from the third person point of view (interpersonal), the first person point of view (intrapersonal) is also included by implication.[15]

Physical appearance

Physical appearance constitutes a specialized category of body language because it does not refer to what a person does with his body to send signals. Rather it refers to what a person looks like and what he does (or does not do) *to* his body to make it look a certain way. Physical appearance then is a form of body language that presents stimuli, which act as signals both to self and to others. In effect a person's appearance provides stimuli, which are read as signals indicating who he is and what he is like.[16] For example, skin color is a signal. Depending on many factors, a black person might read his own skin color as a signal of pride in his race or of inferiority. A white person might (depending on many factors) read the black person's skin color as a signal that the black person feels hostile toward him. Or the white person might simply read it as a signal that here is someone who is different from him or who is strange and exotic.

SKIN

What color is the person's skin? What is his skin tone? Flabby? Muscular? Drawn? Is his skin dry and scaly, flaky, oily, or in-between?

HEAD

What is the size and shape of his head? What color is his hair? What is its texture? What about facial hair? Are the eyebrows thick and bushy, average, or sparse?

Do the person's ears lie flat or stick out? Does he have a low forehead or a high one? What color are his eyes? Is his nose straight or crooked; large or small; or pug, upturned, hooked, aquiline, or squashed? Is his mouth large, medium, or small? Are the lips thin or full or turned somewhat inward or outward? Are his teeth white, yellowish, or discolored? Is his chin square, rounded, jutting, or receding? Is his whole face proportioned or not?

BODY

Is his neck short or long, skinny or thick? Does he have a short or long torso? Long or short arms and legs? Large or small hands and feet? What about height: short, average, tall? What about weight—is he thin, average, overweight, or obese? What about body development? If the person is male, is he weak and underdeveloped, well muscled, or muscle-bound? If the person is a female, is she skinny, of average size, well rounded, or too heavy? Is the body poorly or well proportioned?

PHYSICAL PROBLEMS OR IMPAIRMENTS

Does the person have any physical impairments? Does he have a harelip or a clubfoot? Is he deaf? Blind? Paralyzed? Does he limp? Are his eyes crossed? Does he have a noticeable, perhaps disfiguring birthmark? Does he have noticeable acne? Does he have bad teeth? Does he has disfiguring scars?

PERSONAL GROOMING

Is the person clean? Has he got black grime under his nails, or are they clean? Are they smooth, ragged, or bitten to the quick? Are his teeth clean, or do they look fuzzy or greenish? Are his clothes reasonably clean and neat?

STYLE

How does he dress? Conservatively? Mod? Far out? Are his clothes flashy, dull, or gaudy? Are they too big or too small? Does he slavishly follow the fads? Or does he dress with an individual touch? Does he wear his hair the same way everyone else does? Is he up with, ahead of, or ten years behind the times?

Silent body language

Silent body language consists of any signals a person sends with his body without using words or sounds. Basically it includes facial expressions, positions, movements, and (to some extent) odors.

FACIAL EXPRESSIONS

Consider the possibilities of signals from just the face. What about the eyebrows? Raised? "Scrooched" together? What about the forehead? Is it full of wrinkles or smooth? What about the eyes? Are they keen looking, unfocused, or dreamy? Does the person maintain eye contact, or does he constantly look off into space or shift his gaze? Does he wrinkle his nose or turn up his nose? Does he look down his nose?

What about the mouth? Is the person tight-lipped? Is his mouth turned up in a smile or down in a look of sadness or disappointment?

What about the jaw and chin? Does his jaw jut forward as though he is angry with the world? Does his chin tremble as though he were fighting not to cry? What about the throat? Does the person swallow constantly as though nervous or afraid?

How does the person's whole face look? Is he smiling, frowning? Is his face closed and aloof? Does he look fierce, gloomy, unhappy, sad, mischievous, angry, compassionate, contemptuous, or loving?

POSTURE, OR WAYS OF HOLDING THE BODY

The way a person holds his body can provide certain information about him. Is the person tense, stiff, and rigid? Is he loose, sprawling, and relaxed? Does he slump or slouch? Is he awkward and uncomfortable looking? Does he hold himself in check, aloof, and above those around him? Are his fists clenched? Do his hands hang loose and relaxed? Does he hold his head up, or does he let it hang down? When he sits, does he cross his legs? Does he sit sprawling, with his legs apart? Does he sit with his feet on the floor, with his legs together? Do his arms hang comfortably at his side? Does he put his arms and hands behind his back? Hands in pockets? Arms akimbo?

WAYS OF MOVING OR HANDLING THE BODY

The way a person moves and handles his body often says a great deal about how he feels about himself and the world around him. Is he a "toucher" or a "nontoucher"? Are his movements smooth or awkward, confident or hesitant, or reassuring or threatening? Is he tense and restless (always moving), or is he able to be still and relaxed?

What about the hands? Do his hands twitch? Does he wring them or clench them together? Is the person forever scratching or picking at or pulling on something—his nose, his earlobe, his chin, his hair? Does he wave his hands about or chop the air when he is talking? How does he use his hands when he is talking? Is he a thumb-twiddler, a knuckle-cracker, a nail-biter, a hangnail-picker?

What about his breathing—is it rapid and shallow or slow and deep? What about his legs and feet—does he shift from foot to foot or does he stand still? Does he shuffle along, or does he lift his feet when he walks?

Audible body language

Audible body language consists of any signals a person sends by making (or by refraining from making) nonverbal sounds.[17] Is the person usually silent? Is he a throat-clearer, a hummer, a yawner, a belcher, a grunter, an "um-er," or an "ah-er?" Does he tend to whimper, chuckle, laugh a lot, groan, snort, whine, or cry (or sound like he is about to cry)? Does he snarl? Does he choke up when he is speaking?

Another factor that influences the meaning of what is said is *the way a person says it.* Does he speak fast or slow? Does he hesitate? Does he stutter? Is he positive, aggressive, questioning, self-assured, or arrogant? Is he calm and low-keyed?

• • •

This list of nonverbal signals is vast. However, the purpose of this list is not to provide you with innumerable signals to memorize but, rather, to raise your consciousness of the tremendous number of possibilities for nonverbal communication. In addition, the purpose is to heighten your awareness of the enormous number of nonverbal signals that can act as influences on us and that we are constantly having to evaluate and respond to in some way.

Nevertheless, you probably will never catch all the nonverbal communication that is occurring at a given time. You may spot only a little of it, but awareness of even a little can be helpful to you. If you practice, you can expect to significantly improve your ability to spot signals. Thus this list can serve you in another way: use it as a checklist to remind you of signals to look for.

Interpreting signals

Since signals abound and can exert significant influences on both intrapersonal and interpersonal communication and interaction, you need not only to be aware of them but also to develop the ability and means to interpret them accurately. One important method for evaluating signals and the appropriateness of your response to them is to check them out in reference to whatever moment-to-moment influencing factors (MIFs) are present in a given situation. As was discussed earlier (p. 96), MIFs include the following: motivation, psychological desires, goals, intent, mood, social situation, opportunity, time available, societal pressures, and significant others. Some MIFs, if not all, are always operating in any given situation.

For example, suppose you encounter a person whose face is grimy and sweat-streaked, whose hands are dirty, whose fingernails have black grease under them, and whose clothes are greasy and dirty. How you read these signals will depend on the relevant MIFs. If you meet him at the garage where your car is being fixed and he is the mechanic who is going to work on your car, these signals may mean to you that he is a hard-working mechanic who really gets in there and tangles with the problems. If, however, a friend brings him by your house on her way to the movies and introduces him as her new boyfriend, you will react differently. In this situation, you might size him up as an uncaring slob or as someone who is so egotistical and contemptuous of women that he does not even have the courtesy to clean up before going on a date. Obviously then those MIFs that are relevant play an integral role in determining the meaning of signals that are sent and received. Therefore to evaluate the meaning of signals and the appropriateness of your responses to them, be sure to check out whatever MIFs are operating.[18]

EFFECTS OF NONVERBAL SIGNALS: YOURS AND OTHERS'

Many factors affect the ways a person will interpret or misinterpret nonverbal signals, including his self-system and lifestyle, the degree of his awareness of signals, and the extent of his in-touchedness with his insides. In turn, the ways a person consciously or unconsciously interprets or misinterprets nonverbal signals determine how he will perceive himself and others. For the sake of clarity, the following discussion will be divided into perceptions of self and perceptions of others.

Your signals

The way a person perceives himself depends on his nonverbal signals, the degree of his awareness of them, and his interpretations of them.[19,20] For example, suppose at the age of 13 years, Steve grew seven inches in an 8-month period and, as a result, was gawky and awkward. His family and friends made fun of his awkwardness, and this, added to his earlier doubts about his athletic abilities, contributed to Steve's developing a poor physical self-concept. He saw himself as awkward, ungainly, and uncoordinated (and to a degree he was correct). He felt ill at ease with his body and despaired of ever being any different. As a consequence, Steve tended to stoop and slump to minimize his height, he kept his hands in his pockets to keep from swinging them wildly, and he shuffled because walking fast tended to trip him up.

Now at 16 years of age the rest of Steve's body has caught up with his height so that his body is well proportioned and he is well coordinated. But he continues to go around stooping and slumping, keeping his hands in his pockets, and shuffling. He continues then to send himself distorted "awkward body" signals, and these tend to perpetuate his earlier perception of himself.

Suppose, however, that Steve's older brother Luke notices all this about Steve and talks to him about it when Luke is home on vacation from college. Luke asks Steve if he realizes how he moves and looks; perhaps he gets Steve to shoot baskets with him and points out that Steve really is pretty well-coordinated. With just this kind of minimal intervention, Steve may become aware of his body language, change it so that it is more appropriate, and begin to experience the effect of positive signals on his self-concept.

Another example of the relationship between signals and perception is as follows. Suppose you were raised with a strong PFL that says, "Always be cheerful; nobody likes a sourpuss." You have built in this rule so thoroughly that you are known for your cheerful nature—always smiling, joking, making remarks in a light-hearted tone, and always on the go, and you treat yourself in this same cheery way. There are times, however, when it is inappropriate to be cheerful, such as when you fail a test, when you are worried about your mother or father who has to have major surgery, or when you have a serious falling-out with your closest friend. But you merrily proceed to act cheerful—even to yourself. The problem is that your body is thoroughly trained to automatically send cheerful signals, no matter what. The result may be that you are unaware of your negative feelings because you are trained to deny them. One possible effect of these denials might be as follows. You might go through one of these unhappy events and experience anxiety or fear or disappointment only on an unconscious level. If that is the case, any signals from your body to you about these feelings will likely be unconscious also. However, if they occur often enough without your dealing with them, they may deviously signal their presence through psychosomatic symptoms such as gastritis or nausea or, more seriously, an ulcer.

Another possible effect might be that you become aware of your negative feelings and the clash between them and your cheerful mien. In this case, you might begin to feel that you are being hypocritical, or you might begin to feel confused and anxious because of the paradox between your positive actions and negative feelings. Whatever effect you experience, however, your perception of your self will be affected.

The two examples just given illustrate strictly intrapersonal nonverbal communications. These signals are those that the person sends to himself, interprets, and then uses as guides to perception of self. There is another realm, however, that needs consideration. This realm has to do with the intended or unintended signals about himself that a person sends to others. They may or may not reflect his perceptions of himself, just as they may or may not reflect who he really is. But they most certainly will affect others' perceptions of him. Thus if you want to have some idea of the ways you come across to others, you will need to become aware of and get in touch with the signals you send and what in you generates those signals.

Some signals you send to others may deliberately be misleading. For example, have you ever felt really turned on by someone but acted as though you were not the least bit interested? Have you ever felt tremendously silly but acted calm and pleasant? Have you ever felt hurt by something someone said or did to you and wanted to cry or be sarcastic but instead played it cool and pretended you were not affected by the remark or the action? Your body language would be misleading to others, since your actions do not accurately reflect what you really feel. Presumably in these instances, you are intentionally sending these false signals: you do not want anyone else to know what you are feeling so you act in opposite ways. At various times for various reasons, probably all human beings deliberately send false signals; on rare occasions, it may be appropriate to do so. For example, if your best friend's sister dies and you are worried about him because he is so upset, you might hide most of your worry and instead send signals of calmness and reassurance. However, if you find that frequently you intentionally send false signals, then it is important to evaluate your reasons for doing to. Furthermore, it is a good idea to check whether your doing so is appropriate and whether it is automatic. If you discover that you deliberately send false signals a good deal of the time and that they are inappropriate and automatic, then you would be wise to investigate your motives, your perceptions of you, the effects on others' perceptions of you, and the kinds of interactions and relationships you have with others.

A more serious problem occurs when an unintentional disparity occurs between the signals you assume you send and the ones you really do send. In other words, you may feel one way but act another without being aware of the disparity: not only may you fool others, but you may also fool yourself. For example, suppose you have been raised with various PFLs that insist that competence, adequacy, and a degree of knowledgeability are some of the best qualities a "good" human being can have. You have gradually developed patterns of acting competent, adequate, and knowledgeable. In situations in which people seem indecisive, you automatically tend to take the lead, make decisions, and tell others what to do. You are cool under stress: you look unworried, unflustered, and determined; your tone is commanding and steady; your movements are calm but unhesitating. These are the ways you automatically act, and your actions are signals to others that you are competent, adequate, and knowledgeable.

But suppose you do not always feel this way? Suppose that you deny other emotions that you have such as feeling weak, dependent, scared, lonely, and unsure of yourself? All you may be aware of is that at times you feel weary and slightly irritated by people's "demands" on you. Even though it may be *extremely* difficult for you to get in touch with or admit to these feelings, they are there inside you. But because it is *automatic* and repetitive, your body language is sending you false signals and is falsely reflecting your feelings. You are so used to acting this way, however, that it may never occur to you to hold or move your body in other ways, ways more expressive of your real feelings. Your automatic patterns of body language tend to help obscure—even from you—what your true feelings may be.

Consider also the following example, which illustrates another problem: the confusion created by a disparity between a faulty perception of self and signals that accurately reflect real feelings. Suppose you perceive yourself to be a mild-tempered, easygoing, relaxed kind of person. Yet you keep getting indications from other people that they are not comfortable around you. Now suppose you look more closely at your body language and find that much of the time you chew on your lip, clamp your teeth together, clench your fists, and hold yourself tensely. Is your body language appropriate to your perception of yourself? No. If you investigate matters in greater depth, you may discover that your body is expressing your real feelings; you may discover that you have talked yourself into feeling that you are easygoing and accepting of others because that is what you were taught to value as a child. In fact, you may find that many people irritate you and that you do not accept them as easily as you thought you did. When you make this discovery, then you are in a position to make decisions about whether you wish to stay the same or change.

This kind of experience points up the need for paying attention to other people's responses to your body language and for checking to see whether your perceptions and signals match. It should be clear then why it is so important that you become aware of or get in touch with your body and its language. Being aware and in touch enables you to know better what your true feelings may be. It helps you find out whether you are throwing up a smoke screen around your real feelings. Intouchedness helps you detect what kind of nonverbal messages about yourself you are sending to yourself and others and what kind of image you are projecting to yourself and to them. Such knowledge helps you to determine whether you are projecting a distorted image. Knowing these last two things is especially important to your interpersonal relations because people respond to you partly on the basis of nonverbal messages (signals) you send. Thus knowing how you come across to others nonverbally can be extremely valuable to you in learning how to communicate more honestly and openly with others.

HOW TO GET IN TOUCH WITH YOUR BODY

Knowing that it is important to get in touch with your body and the ways it expresses you is one thing. Knowing *how* to get in touch is another.[21] It is simple enough to say, "just stop everything and feel what your body is doing and the way it is doing it." Such directions would be fine if you were practiced in or accustomed to feeling what your body is doing, but most of us are not. To help you practice getting in touch with your body and its language, try one or all of the following experiences, or think up your own comparable ones to try.

1. Imagine (or remember) yourself in a situation in which you are extremely angry but are prevented for one reason or another from verbally expressing that anger. Let yourself really feel angry. How does your body feel? What is it doing? Experience; feel your body. Now exaggerate the physical reactions you are aware of. If your mouth is tight, make it tighter. If you are scowling, scowl harder. If your fists are clenched, clench them harder. If your body is tense, increase the tension. Now experience and feel your body. Check out the various parts of your body that you are aware of—your mouth, forehead, face, jaw, neck, torso, hands, feet, etc. How does each one feel? How does your whole body feel? What does your anger feel like physically?

2. Try assuming an opposite feeling position. Imagine feeling happy or content or passive. Follow the instructions given in the first experience.

3. At some point in your day today (or tomorrow or whenever you choose), catch yourself for a moment and freeze (at least, inside yourself). Check out the following: What is the situation? What are you feeling? What is your body doing? How does it feel? Are what you are feeling and what your body is doing congruent or contradictory? Is your body language appropriate? Did it occur automatically?

As you probably realize, the process described here is an abbreviated version of the process of intrapersonal communication described in the previous chapter. In effect, getting in touch with your body's language involves essentially the same procedures as getting in touch with your thoughts and feelings because your body language is the expression of your insides. Therefore to acquire the most thorough practice in getting in touch with your signals, go back to the detailed presentation of the intrapersonal communication process on pp. 115 to 121 and apply it in step-by-step fashion to your body language.

Others' signals

The signals that other people send to us are extremely important; in fact, they are just as important as the ones we send to them. Signals are powerful stimuli, and human beings simply cannot *not* respond to stimuli. So powerful are signals that often we form strong impressions on the basis of signals alone—before one word is exchanged. Even after verbal communication occurs, our impressions of others may continue to be based primarily on the nonverbal rather than the verbal messages. It would be safe to say that at least 50% of what influences us in initial and early encounters is the signals we receive. Unfortunately these early signals may discourage us from seeking further contact or from trying to establish a meaningful relationship, which might occur if we stuck with the person and really got to know him.

In addition, of course, signals continue

to influence our responses to and evaluations of others throughout the course of our relationships with them. And the quality of our relationships depends in good part on whether we correctly interpret or misinterpret their signals. It also depends on what means and skills we have for checking out our interpretations and for determining and correcting our misinterpretations. (Those means and skills that are intrapersonal in nature will be discussed later in this section; those that are interpersonal will be analyzed and explained in Chapter 9, which focuses on the process of interpersonal communication.)

FIRST IMPRESSIONS

The importance and the influence of nonverbal messages can best be illustrated by an example. Suppose you and a friend go to a rock concert, and your friend sees someone he knows (Ed) and introduces you. Then your friend wanders off to the men's room, leaving you to talk to Ed for a while. When your friend pointed Ed out from across the room, this is what you saw: Ed is about five feet nine inches, of average weight and build; his hair is sandy-colored and cut fairly short. He is pleasant looking, but there is nothing outstanding about him. He is neatly dressed in a dark blue shirt and jeans and boots.

As your friend makes the introduction, Ed stands there tense and rigid; he holds his arms stiffly at his sides. When he shakes hands with you, his grip is tentative, and his hand is clammy. The two of you talk about the coming concert and about the weather. As the two of you talk, Ed looks down at his feet as he shifts restlessly from foot to foot. Rarely does he meet your eyes, and when he does, he seems startled and immediately drops his glance. His mouth stays in a turned-down position, and his lips—when he is not talking—are pressed tightly together. He swallows frequently. His breathing is somewhat shallow and rapid, and he often clears his throat. He is pleasant enough, but he speaks hesitantly, almost in a whisper. His tone is rather flat and colorless. When your friend returns and you part company with Ed, he mumbles "so long" and drifts off like a shadow.

Since the content of your conversation with Ed was so shallow and your encounter was so brief, you have necessarily formed your impressions of him almost totally on the basis of the set of nonverbal messages he sent. What are your impressions of Ed? Prior to meeting him, your response to his appearance may be that he looks nice enough, but he never would have attracted your attention. After you meet and talk with him, you may decide that he is a person who is miserably uncomfortable in a social situation, especially one in which he is meeting someone for the first time. You may also assume that he is not a happy person, that he seems to feel inadequate, and that he is nervous and tense. In addition, although you may feel sorry for him because he seems so ill at ease, you may feel that he is dull, colorless, and probably boring. With impressions and feelings like these, if you should meet him again, would you go out of your way to strike up a conversation with him, much less really try to get to know him? But who knows—underneath his nervous and shy exterior, Ed may be a great person. He may be bright, interesting, humorous, loyal, compassionate, strong, gentle, and loving, but because nonverbal signals can exert such a powerful influence, neither you nor many other people may ever give yourselves and Ed the chance to find out. ►IE-2, p. 139.

INTERPRETING OTHERS' SIGNALS

Correctly interpreting the signals of others is a threefold process and involves (1) being aware of the signals that the other person sends and of the MIFs that are operant in the particular situation, (2) checking to make sure that because of your insides you are not distorting the other person's signals, and (3) evaluating the nature and style of the other person's signals.

An example will help to illustrate the

need for this threefold process. Suppose you ask a teacher to explain a math problem to you. She agrees and begins to explain. After you have gone home, you think back and realize that you hurried through and did not ask all the questions that you needed to because you felt she was impatient and annoyed. Because you are no longer with her and therefore cannot verbally check out your impression, you must rely solely on the nonverbal messages you received at the time. If the teacher kept looking at her watch, moved restlessly around the room while she was talking, looked at the door every few minutes, and answered your questions in an irritated, sharp, abrupt tone of voice, your interpretation that she was impatient and annoyed is probably an accurate one. If, however, the teacher sat and quietly waited for your questions, asked you several times if you had other questions, and answered in a calm, unhurried way and in a quiet, relaxed tone of voice, then your interpretation that she was impatient and annoyed is probably not accurate.

AWARENESS OF OTHERS' SIGNALS

Obviously the first step in evaluating another person's signals is to become aware of them. Essentially this step requires paying close attention to the other person's body language and the situation. Once you become aware of these, then you can begin to assess how appropriate the person's signals are to the situation, and you can begin to determine the accuracy of your interpretations. (How to become more aware of others' signals will be discussed later.)

THE INFLUENCE OF YOUR INSIDES

When you become aware of and identify another person's signals, you need to check out your interpretations of the signals. In the example given previously, if you misinterpreted the teacher's calm signals as ones of impatience and annoyance, then look to your own insides. Do you have PFLs about people in authority that might lead you to distort their signals? Suppose by using the intrapersonal communication process, you discover that you have a PFL that says, "People in authority are busy, important people and don't like being bothered by details or questions." Suppose you find another PFL that teaches, "Adults get annoyed when children ask them silly questions." This discovery may lead you to examine your *Child/Parent/Adult balance.* Do you hold yourself in a distorted child's position of awe and fear of all people who have any power whatsoever over you? What about your *self-concept?* Do you see yourself as being unworthy of attention from an adult? Do you view anyone in a position of authority as being superior to you? Do you feel that you are silly or stupid for not understanding and having to ask questions? Do you have a *pattern* of perfectionism, which requires that you know all the answers? And if you do not know all the answers, then you are a failure and people have a right to be annoyed with your stupidity?

You may not be this thorough with every person and situation you encounter, but when you find that you are grossly misinterpreting signals, then you ought to try to be this thorough. From the previous list of questions, it is probably clear to you that being this thorough means using intrapersonal communication to carry out the process of gathering information, identifying feelings, and acquiring insights. In effect you will be applying three basic steps of The System. Until you are willing and able to do this kind of checking out, you are vulnerable to the possibility of your insides' causing you to misinterpret others' signals.

WHEN OTHERS SEND DISTORTED SIGNALS

After becoming aware of another person's signals and checking out whether you have misinterpreted them, suppose you ascertain that you have not read them in a distorted fashion, but something does not jibe. Then you need to evaluate the other person, his signals, and the situation. Look first for repetitiveness of the signals. If you discover that your math teacher consistently acts impatient and annoyed in various situations, you may be seeing a pattern of hers, which governs the signals she sends. There are three criteria to apply when evaulating others' signals: Are the signals repetitious? Are they automatic? Are they appropriate? If you find that the other person's signals are repetitious, automatic, and inappropriate and if you want to clarify and straighten out your relations with that person, you will have to rely on verbal communication with him. We will consider that process in detail in Chapter 9.

HOW TO BECOME AWARE OF OTHERS' BODY LANGUAGE

Since the crucial first step in evaluating other people's signals is becoming aware of them, you need to learn how to do so. One of the best ways is to practice observing how people use their bodies. It also helps immensely to try to put yourself in another person's shoes—to try to *feel* his body language. Following are three suggestions for getting such practice:

1. If you can recreate how someone looked during a moment that was fairly emotionally charged, do so. Try to remember sharply and accurately what his face looked like, how he held and moved his body, and what sounds he made. Now try to "be" him. Put your body in the position he took, make your face take on his expression, move your body the way he moved his, and try to catch the sound and intonations of his voice. (You may feel silly the first few times you try this. In that case, just make sure you are alone when you try it. But silly as you may feel, try it anyway. It is one of the best ways to appreciate what another person's body language feels like to him.)

2. Get together with a friend (or a stranger) and try to communicate nonverbally some strong feeling to him. Let him try to do the same with you. Watch each other closely; observe and feel your feelings. (DO NOT TALK!) Now trade: you become him (mimic him as exactly as you can), and let him do the same for you. Really try to put yourselves in each other's places. After it is over, you can discuss the accuracy of what you assumed the other person was trying to communicate and the accuracy of your portrayals of each other.

3. Get two friends, and let them talk to each other about something that is important to one of them. You take the role of "mirror" to one of them—mimic this person's *nonverbal* actions as clearly and as exactly as you can. Discuss the experience afterward. This is excellent practice in observing and experiencing the style of another person's body language; it also gives the mimicked person a good look at how he comes across to another person.

BLENDING THE NONVERBAL AND THE VERBAL

The physical, or the nonverbal, is an area of human experience that none of us can afford to ignore. Body language plays an important and significant role both in our relations with ourselves and in our relations with others. However, body language is only one means of communicating and interacting. Our other means—the verbal—is equally important. Ultimately it becomes imperative that we treat the nonverbal and the verbal together as a sum that is greater than the two parts. Each alone means something; together they may influence or completely alter the meaning of the messages sent and received.

Interaction experiences

1. Experiencing the power of nonverbal communication (p. 128)

A good way to experience the power of nonverbal communication is to "eyeball" another person. An "eyeball-to-eyeball" encounter can help you get in touch with your feelings by pressing you to *look,* to *see,* to *feel,* and to make genuine contact with another person without the distraction of words. In this way, you may experience the truth of the old adage that "the eyes are the windows of the soul."

Select a partner and sit facing him. Look (and keep looking) directly into one another's eyes for 5 minutes. Do not talk at any time during the experience. Try to tell your partner something important with your eyes. Try to receive his message(s) to you. Afterward share with each other what you were feeling and what you were trying to communicate.

EVALUATION: What did you think and feel during this experience? Were you embarrassed, anxious, bored, or excited? Did you learn something about yourself, your partner, or both?

FOLLOW-UP: Try this experience again with someone you are close to, but this time gently explore the person's face with your fingertips. Share with each other what you thought and felt.

2. Increasing your awareness of body language signals (p. 136)

Using the list of body language signals as a guide (pp. 130 to 131), observe a stranger for a period of time and try to get in touch with your feelings about this person. Try to let your senses open up so that you can become aware of as many signals as possible.

EVALUATION: What was your first impression of this person? What were your thoughts and feelings about the person? Did you like or dislike him? Did you feel attracted or repulsed? What was the person communicating about himself that evoked whatever you were feeling? Did he remind you of someone you know? How aware were you when you were carrying out this experience? Were you able to notice many signals, or did you focus on just a couple? Could you see the interrelationship among various signals? Could you feel the power that nonverbal communication has to influence your responses to other people? What signals influenced you the most? Which ones did you notice first? Second? Third?

FOLLOW-UP: Try this experience with a friend. That is, both of you observe the same stranger and then share your observations, feelings, and responses with each other. Did each of you respond much the same way to the person, or did you each feel different things? Did you each notice different or similar signals? Did you interpret the same signals in different or similar ways? What did you learn about yourself? Are your perceptions and value judgments essentially the same as or different from your friend's?

REFERENCES

1. Kahn, M.: Non-verbal communication and marital satisfaction, Family Process **9**:449-456, 1970.
2. Schutz, William C.: Joy: expanding human awareness, New York, 1967, Grove Press, Inc., pp. 25-50.
3. Fast, Julius: Body language, Philadelphia, 1970, M. Evans & Co., Inc.
4. Ruesch, Jurgen, and Kees, Weldon: Nonverbal communication, Berkeley, Calif., 1956, University of California Press.
5. Birdwhistle, Ray L.: Kinesics and content, Philadelphia, 1970, University of Pennsylvania Press.
6. Howells, John G., editor: Theory and practice of family psychiatry, New York, 1971, Brunner/Mazel, Inc., p. 26.

7. Ruesch, Jurgen: Therapeutic communication, New York, 1961, W. W. Norton & Co., Inc., p. 453.
8. Satir, Virginia: Conjoint family therapy, Palo Alto, Calif., 1964, Science & Behavior Books, Inc., p. 75.
9. Ruesch, op. cit., pp. 423-436.
10. Callahan, Sidney Cornelia: Parenting, Garden City, N.Y., 1973, Doubleday & Co., Inc., p. 173.
11. Fast, op. cit., pp. 64-82.
12. Schutz, op. cit., pp. 36-50.
13. Allport, G. W., and Vernon, P. L.: Studies in expressive behavior, New York, 1967, Hafner Publishing Co.
14. Scheflen, A. E.: Non-language behavior in communication, Address to New York Chapter of American Academy of Pediatrics, New York, N.Y., Sept. 2, 1969.
15. Argyle, Michael: The psychology of interpersonal behavior, Baltimore, 1967, Penguin Books, Inc., pp. 105-110.
16. Montague, Ashley: Touching: the human significance of the skin, New York, 1971, Columbia University Press.
17. Hall, E. T.: The hidden dimension, Garden City, N.Y., 1966, Doubleday & Co., Inc.
18. Nierenberg, Gerald I., and Calero, Henry H.: How to read a person like a book, New York, 1973, Pocket Books, pp. 13-26.
19. Jourard, Sidney M.: The transparent self: self-disclosure and well-being, Princeton, 1964, D. Van Nostrand Co., pp. 91-98.
20. Morris, C. W.: Signs, language, and behavior, New York, 1946, Prentice-Hall, Inc.
21. Howard, Jane: Please touch: a guided tour of the human potential movement, New York, 1970, McGraw-Hill Book Co.

chapter 9

INTERPERSONAL COMMUNICATION

Each of the three types of communication (intrapersonal, nonverbal, and interpersonal) is essential. Without intrapersonal communication, we could not get in touch with what we think and feel and intend to do and with our inner responses to the external world. It is the pipeline to all our inner thoughts, feelings, and actions. Nonverbal communication is one of our two means of expressing our insides and of receiving signals and messages from others. In conjunction with the verbal, it influences the meanings and implications of our messages. Both intrapersonal and nonverbal communication contribute directly and significantly to interpersonal communication: the intrapersonal provides the content; the non-verbal serves as one means of expressing this content.

Of the three kinds, interpersonal communication (both verbal and nonverbal) is perhaps the most important in a personal sense to most of us; it is the master key to all social interaction and to all personal relationships. Interpersonal communication is the way we establish and maintain contact with one another; it is our means of reaching out to and of experiencing one another. Through interpersonal communication we have the opportunity to share our differences and our similarities. As a result, we can decrease our aloneness and isolation, assert our identities, and validate our existence. In effect, interpersonal communication is our way of sharing our humanness with one another.[1,2]

Not only is interpersonal communication tremendously important, but it is also complex. Why? Because two (or more) human beings are involved with each other. No matter what the subject, each person brings to the exchange all the complexities of his personality. Each person brings with him his *insides:* his PFLs, his intrapersonal patterns, his self-concept, his Child/Parent/Adult balance, and all his thoughts and feelings about the external world (which includes the other person). Furthermore, each person communicates his insides to the other person(s) by way of his *outsides:* that is, he sends signals and verbal messages through his interpersonal patterns. Thus each person must work with his own insides, his own outsides, and the other person's insides and outsides. In addition, each of them must deal with their relationship and with the world around them.

On the one hand, the complexities of interpersonal communication increase the possibilities for misunderstandings, misinterpretations, and misassumptions. On the other hand, these same complexities greatly increase the potentials for fascinating and worthwhile interchanges that reach far beyond superficialities and greatly increase the potentials for deep and meaningful relationships.

As you consider the complexities of the interpersonal communication process, you may be feeling that it is a difficult process to learn to do with skill and ease. Although it is true that learning to communicate well requires a lot of hard work, it *can* be learned—and learned well. Remember one important fact: you already know how to use most of the skills involved in this process and you already use most of them. We are trying to help you become much more aware of what you already know and use; awareness coupled with motivation and practice will enable you to become far more skilled at communicating honestly, openly, clearly, and effectively.

SIGNALS, VERBAL MESSAGES, METAMESSAGES

Since their sensory responses are so intricately interrelated and so diverse, people are capable of transmitting and receiving a great number and variety of signals and messages. One possible result can be rich and rewarding communication with self and others. But another possible result can be a tangled web of distorted communication based on misunderstandings, misinterpretations, and misassumptions. For example, if a person has a passive life-style, he may present even his most important messages in such a dull and lifeless voice that the hearer may assume that the messages are not important or that the speaker just does not care about much of anything. Or another person may state many of his messages in a dry, ironic manner and thus lead others to assume he lacks much feeling about what he says—even though he may in fact care very deeply.

These are only simple examples of distortions and misassumptions that can occur. Matters can and do get even more tangled when people try to communcate without being in touch with or honest about their insides or without being in touch with how they use their senses. They may say things they do not mean, transmit contradictory double messages, and/or undercut the real meaning of their messages with misleading or contraditory signals.

To understand how interpersonal communication can get distorted, it is first necessary to consider both the ingredients of the process and the interplay among them. During interpersonal communication, each person sends and receives signals (brief, nonverbal messages transmitted through body language) and, ordinarily, verbal messages (communications that employ spoken words to convey meanings) as well. The combination of signals and verbal messages produces metamessages, the meanings that either reinforce, expand on, or undermine the meaning of the verbal message. The meanings of metamessages can result from the actual combination originating with the sender or from the ways the receiver interprets the combination.

In clear, undistorted communication, all three elements—signal, verbal message, and metamessage—are congruent with one another.[3] They do not conflict with, clash with, or contradict one another. In distorted communication, however, these three elements in some way do not match up with each other.[4]

Let us give you an example of clear, undistorted communication. In this example, both Mr. Amiable and Ms. Friendly are sending (and receiving) signals and messages that are completely congruent. In his *verbal message,* each says what he means ("It's good to see you") and means what he says. Each backs up his message with matching, reinforcing *signals* (smile, friendly tone of voice). Thus their *metamessages* ("I feel friendly toward you") are congruent with their spoken messages.

Problems occur, however, when the signals and messages clash and the metamessages therefore belie or negate either the signals or the messages. Distorted communication is the result as the following two examples illustrate.

1. Bill has just told Andy that he took the liberty of borrowing Andy's car for a few hours while Andy was gone over the weekend. Furthermore, Bill reveals that he had a slight accident in which a fender was damaged and a headlight broken. Apologizing profusely, Bill says he will have the car fixed, but he cannot do so until next week because he does not have the money. Bill now says to Andy: "Andy, I'm really sorry. I sure hope you don't

mind too much." Andy replies, "It's okay, Bill. It wasn't your fault" *(verbal message)*. But Andy's eyes are distant, his mouth is set in a straight line, his voice is cool, and his body is tensed *(signals)*. If we could fluoroscope Andy's heart and gut, we would see this: "I really think you're an s.o.b. for taking my car without asking me and then racking it up. But I don't want trouble, so I'll be nice to you. But if I had the guts I'd smack you one in the face" *(metamessages)*.

Bill's reactions are the following: he says, "Good, I'm glad. Thanks, Andy. I was afraid you'd really get mad or something" *(verbal message)*. By his verbal message, Bill implies that he believes Andy. With a questioning look in his eyes, Bill peers nervously at Andy. Bill is tense and holds himself aloof—a wait-and-see reaction *(signals)*. Thus although Bill's verbal message says that he is relieved by Andy's reassurance, Bill's signals send a conflicting metamessage, which is "I'm not sure whether I really believe what you're telling me." This is hardly clear and honest communication.

2. Don and Kathy are in the same chemistry class. She has asked him if he will explain some things to her before the final exam, and he has agreed. They have had some trouble finding a time that is convenient for both of them but now are meeting according to their agreement. Kathy is uptight because she is nervous about the exam and because she is not sure whether Don minds helping her.

Don has just finished explaining an important and complicated concept to her. He asks if she understands.

Kathy: "Yes—I–I think so" *(verbal message)*. She stammers slightly when she says this, her tone is hesitant and doubtful, and she looks upset *(signals)*. Her metamessage is that she is not at all sure she understands and that she is scared.

Don: "Kathy, are you sure you understand? If you're not sure, just say so, and I'll go over it again" *(verbal message)*. His tone is slightly doubtful and concerned. He gives her a questioning look *(signals)*. His metamessage is "I'm worried that you don't really understand but are afraid to say so."

Because of her uptightness, her fears, and her insecurity, Kathy interprets Don's message and signals as conveying a different metamessage. She reads it as saying, "I don't believe you understood the explanation at all. I really doubt that you're smart enough to catch on. Maybe we're wasting our time." Kathy's interpretation of Don's metamessage is distorted, and unless she carefully checks out what he means and feels, the rest of what happens is likely to become more distorted as it builds on this initial misinterpretation.

INTERPERSONAL COMMUNICATION: DYNAMICS OF THE PROCESS

A primary way to deal constructively with interpersonal interactions and to build healthy relationships is to communicate clearly and honestly. Being able to do so requires an understanding of the way the whole process of interpersonal communication works.

Basic underpinnings of the interpersonal communication process

Three procedures—giving and receiving responses, checking out, and giving and getting feedback—underpin the whole process of interpersonal communication. The major steps of this process, which are discussed later, are the specific applications and results of these three procedures.

GIVING AND RECEIVING RESPONSES

This procedure forms the basis of all human communication and interaction. Every person at all times is **giving and receiving responses:** taking in and registering in-coming stimuli and sending out or giving reactions to stimuli. In effect, as a person meets with inner and outer stimuli he responds to them and they to him, and as this occurs and reoccurs, it generates further responses. In this manner a person maintains a "dialogue" with himself, with others, and with his physical and emotional environment. It is the interaction of his thoughts, feelings, and actions with self and others. In the specific terms of communication, giving and receiving responses consists of transmitting and receiving signals, messages, and metamessages. This procedure may take place on either a conscious or unconscious level or both, but on whatever level it is occurring, it is going on all the time. A person cannot *not* communicate; he cannot *not* respond.

If a person is closed, he tends to give and receive responses in a selective manner that tends to reinforce and perpetuate his closedness. His communication tends to be distorted because he consciously and/or unconsciously communicates in ways that fit his view of himself, others, and the environment. Although it is true that no one can communicate without *some* distortion (since no one can be in total touch with himself or others), the more open a person is and tries to be the more he will work to prevent distortion.

CHECKING OUT

The basic method for preventing or cutting down significantly on distortion is checking out. **Checking out** entails the following various procedures:

1. It means asking questions to make sure you really do understand and know what the other person thinks, feels, and means.
2. It entails asking the other person whether he understands and knows what you think, feel, and mean.
3. It involves giving and getting feedback about anything that may need clarification or verification.
4. It means really listening to the feedback, taking it in, and letting it make a difference. (For example, if you ask a question, do not just listen politely and then go ahead as though you had never asked.)

Checking out is not a one-shot procedure, to be done once and then be put aside. It is a procedure that should be carried on almost continuously, from moment to moment if necessary. The basic (and cardinal) rule underlying checking out is—*do not assume; ask.* Do not assume that you know what the other person is thinking, feeling, or meaning or that you know what his actions mean. And do not assume that he knows what you are thinking, feeling, or meaning or that he knows what your actions mean. Instead check it out.

For example, suppose you ask your friend Dave if he minds if you borrow his tennis racket for the afternoon. Dave says, no, he does not mind. But he scowls when he says it. You *assume* that he does indeed mind, and, according to whatever your life-style is and what your relationship with him is, you may get annoyed with him, or you may get upset. Maybe you even say in an irritable tone that you have changed your mind and will not need it—because you assume he does not want to lend it to you. You are, of course, feeling and acting on the basis of an assumption. The problem is that your assumption may not be correct.

Suppose instead of assuming that because he scowled Dave does not want to lend you the racket, you check out what his feelings are and ask for feedback.

You: "Dave—when I asked if I could borrow your tennis racket for this afternoon you said I could but you scowled and looked ticked off when you said it. Are you angry I asked to borrow it?"

Dave (looking slightly startled): "I didn't realize I'd scowled. Sorry. No. I'm not angry about that. I want you to borrow it."

You: "What *were* you feeling, then?" (You laugh.) "That was one ferocious scowl."

Dave: "I guess your question made me

aware of how disgusted I was with myself at that moment. I realized I couldn't go play tennis myself because I have to study for a test. If I'd studied earlier in the week, I could be out there playing. I guess I was scowling because I'm really annoyed at myself for not planning ahead." (He grins.) "If I can't play, at least you can use the racket. Go on and have fun. I'll see you later."

Simple? Yes. Effective in clearing up a potential misunderstanding? Very. Necessary to good communication and interaction? Extremely. But too often, too many of us rely on the assumptions we make, frequently on the basis of incomplete or poorly understood or misinterpreted information or signals or messages. The example we gave is not about a crucially important matter; however, if a large part of a relationship between two people is based on assumptions (many of which may be incorrect) and on little checking out, the relationship is likely to be plagued by distortions, misunderstandings, misinterpretations, and hard feelings.

Checking out and giving and getting feedback are interlinked, interdependent parts of a procedure that is essential to the success of good communication. It is this procedure that enables each person to get in touch (and stay in touch) with himself and with the other person. And it is this procedure that underpins every other step in the process of effective interpersonal communication.

Major steps in the process

Interpersonal communication consists of two (or more) people who are simultaneously engaged in *intrapersonal* communication, the fruits of which they share with one another. Giving and receiving responses, checking out, and giving and getting feedback are the means by which this sharing is carried out. Thus the steps described in the following explanations are specific applications of these means, procedures that are intended to achieve particular goals (e.g., gathering information, negotiating).

What follows are explanations of each of the major steps in the process of interpersonal communication. As you will see, most of these steps have the same names as do those in the explanation of The System in Chapter 10. Since communication is the vehicle by which a person carries out The System, it stands to reason that the steps would be essentially the same. We are willing to run the risk of some repetition, however, because communication is a specialized form of interaction and deserves its own specialized treatment. In addition, you will also note that some of the terms used are the same as those used in the explanation of the intrapersonal communication process (Chapter 7). This is inevitable because interpersonal communication consists of sharing and working with the results of intrapersonal communication.

The purpose of these explanations is to identify, conceptualize, and analyze each step so that you will understand it and be able to make *conscious, deliberate* use of it and the whole process of which it is a part. When you learn to do this, you are well on your way to becoming an effective communicator, which in turn can enable you to utilize The System in ways that will help you change and grow more open and autonomous.

As you read these explanations of the steps, keep in mind that they are *not necessarily sequential* and that interpersonal communication is a complex process involving two (or more) unique people. Each person goes at his own speed; each functions according to his own life-style. Thus it is possible that one person may be dominant or that one person may be doing most of the work. And it can easily happen that each person is involved with different steps. For example, when you are ready to negotiate, the other person may be wanting to gather more information. When one person is available for implementing, the other may be cautiously holding back. Thus although we have tried to present these steps in an orderly fashion, real, live, on-the-spot communication is not nearly so orderly. Communication can make sense, and it can be consciously directed by the participants, but it will not necessarily follow a smooth, straight, and orderly path.

GATHERING INFORMATION

What is the subject? What are the facts? What is the issue? What, where, when, who? What has happened? What is happening? What did "X" do? What is he doing now? What will he do? What do each person's terms mean? Basically much information is usually given and received early in the communication, but pieces of information will continue to be inserted when needed at any time in the process. The fuller the amount of information and the clearer it is to each person the better the communication. Obviously if vital information is not available or is held back, then clear communication is not really possible.

For example, suppose Al wants to know if his friend Jerry will be mad if Al dates a girl Jerry has been dating from time to time. But suppose Jerry does not tell Al that he (Jerry) and the girl have decided to live together, that they are in love. Even if Jerry tells Al that he has no objections to Al's asking the girl out, obviously there is little if any real communication between Al and Jerry. And there is potential trouble ahead.

Take another situation: Carol and Nadine start talking about whether or not they believe in "power to the people" and the need for revolution to change the miseries of our society. Carol means power to all the people who are oppressed and means revolution that would destroy the existing governmental and cultural structure. Nadine means power to people who know how to use power effectively and who would use it responsibly, and she means revolution that would be nonviolent. Unless these two people clarify what each one means by her terms, they cannot communicate in any clear way.

These two examples point up the need for plain, accurate information; they also underscore the dangers of *assuming* something to be truth or a fact without checking to see if that is indeed so.

IDENTIFYING FEELINGS

It is not just what a person thinks and means and knows that is important. Feelings are at the heart of whatever a person thinks and does and means. Feelings are the generator that makes the dynamos run as they do. Thus to have real communication—communication that deals with who he really is and where he is really at—a person must try to find out what his feelings actually are. To do that, a person must try to *feel the feelings that he feels at the moment he feels them.*[5]

To communicate and to interact with maximum satisfaction and meaning, each person needs to go through the same steps that he follows in communicating with self. But, in addition, he will be sharing some or much or all that he discovers about his feelings with the other person and will be incorporating or dealing with the other person's feelings as they are reported to him. Note that the following are general instructions; thus your application of them will need to be tempered by whatever specific considerations are relevant. For example, it is not always appropriate to share all your feelings. How much, when, where, and with whom to share depends on your evaluation at the time.

1. Identify what your feelings are at the moment you feel them.
2. Hold them and feel them.
3. Verbalize and report these feelings to yourself—and to the other person. Unless you do, neither of you will get far in achieving good communication.
4. Ask for and try to get feedback both from yourself and from the other person about your feelings. Listen to the feedback and try to let yourself let it make a difference to you.
   a. What do your feelings relate to? (What is going on around you;

what are you and/or others doing? What has the other person said or done? How does he react to you and to what you say and do?)

b. What evoked your feelings?

c. What do your feelings mean to you? To the other person? (Are they threatening to him or you? Are they depressing, cheering, hostile, or kind?) How do your feelings serve you? How important are they to you?

5. Check out your feelings against what you know about yourself and against what the other person has to say.
   a. Are your feelings appropriate to the situation? Does the other person think your feelings are appropriate? Is he puzzled by your emotional responses, or do they make sense to him?
   b. Is the past involved in your feelings? Are you reacting to yourself, the situation, or the other person as you have reacted in the past—even if the present is different?
   c. Are your emotional responses like those of either or both of your parents (or other influential adults)?
   d. Are your feelings ones that you automatically and repetitively feel in similar or similar-seeming situations? Look for patterns to your responses. Does the other person see you as reacting according to a pattern?
6. What effect are the communication and interaction having on your feelings? What do you feel toward the other person? How do you react toward what he tells you about *his* feelings, thoughts, and reactions? (For example, if he tells you that he is hurt by something you just said or did, how do you react? Do you automatically get upset? Do his hurt feelings make you nervous? Do you expect him to get angry? Do you get defensive? Do you try to placate him? Do you apologize?) How do you feel about the developing relationship?
7. What do you expect from yourself in this situation? What do you expect from the other person? (For example, do you expect to like the other person? Do you expect him to treat you well and to like you?)
8. How do you feel about whatever MIFs are relevant (such as other people, your situation, the amount of time you can spend)?

In addition to each of you going through these steps to get in touch with your feelings and to share them, try to help one another by offering alternative feelings. For example, if the other person is having trouble identifying what he feels, try suggesting possible feelings from which he can choose.

All these questions and the honest answers to them are helpful in understanding yourself and in fostering good communication both with yourself and with another person. Granted, there may not always be time to ask and to answer each and every one of these questions, and there may be times when to ask would be inappropriate. But this list can at least serve as a guideline for getting in touch with and evaluating your own and the other person's feelings and also the development of your relationship. ►IE-1, p. 155.

ACQUIRING INSIGHT

Insight is personal understanding that results from being able to put things together in conceptual form. **Acquiring insight** is realizing what is going on and what things mean; it is suddenly "getting the feel of" things. In the conversation given previously about the tennis racket, your insight might be that you tend automatically to assume that negative signals (e.g., Dave's scowl) are directed at you. Dave's insight might consist of the realization that he sent you a distorted message and that he is mad at himself.

Both your and Dave's insights are primarily *intellectual* ones; they are realizations. But there are other kinds of insight, too—*emotional, physical,* and *social.* If you were to get in touch with the feelings that you tend automatically to feel in response to negative signals, this would be an *emotional* insight. If Dave were to get in touch on a gut level with the chain of physical reactions he experiences when he gets annoyed or disgusted with himself, that would be a *physical* (and emotional) insight. And if he were to see how his signals touched off by his inside feelings turned people off in situations that had nothing directly to do with what the people were doing, that would be a *social* (and intellectual/emotional) insight.

NEGOTIATION

It would be entirely possible and perfectly logical to treat negotiation and decision-making as two interlinked steps of one process. Ordinarily negotiation leads to decision-making, and decision-making is the outcome of negotiation. We have, however, chosen to separate these two steps to outline more sharply what is involved in the operation of each one.

Negotiation takes place both intrapersonally and interpersonally. Interpersonal negotiation builds off of intrapersonal negotiation.[6,7] In both types of **negotiation,** a person gets in touch with his insides to determine what his thoughts and feelings are, to evaluate them, to ascertain what alternatives exist, and to evaluate those alternatives. He does these things to figure out what he thinks and feels and what he might do in relation to whatever is under consideration at the moment. Essentially a person is negotiating within himself all the time. However, much of the time the negotiation is so quick that the person is not aware of doing it.

A simple example of **intrapersonal negotiation** is as follows. You negotiate with yourself when you think whether you will sleep for another fifteen minutes in the morning. Do you really want to sleep longer? Can you afford to? What will happen if you do? Will you have to skip your shower? How dirty are you? Will you have to skip breakfast? How hungry are you? Will you be late to class or work or your appointment or whatever? Will you get in trouble if you are late?

Interpersonal negotiation occurs when two (or more) people interact with each other to develop some kind of outcome—to find out how each stands in regard to the other, to the matter at hand, and to their relationship. Negotiation between two people follows the same steps as intrapersonal negotiation, but it becomes more complicated and delicate because two people plus their relationship are involved.

In this kind of negotiation, each of you needs to be available to listen to and to hear and to understand the other person's insides. Each person tries to present his insides as openly and as clearly as he can to the other person and to encourage and help the other to present his. You both need to state and have a clear idea about the issue or problem or circumstance. You need to check each other out and to give and to get feedback so that you are sure you understand one another. You need to have some awareness of how this negotiation relates to your total relationship and some awareness of how you evaluate your relationship. You need to determine what alternatives are available and to assess their appropriateness. And you need to evaluate the alternatives in terms of your insides and your relationship.

Consider the following example of interpersonal negotiation. Kate and Arnie have been living together for a little over a year. They are negotiating about an imminent week-long visit from Kate's parents who know only that Kate and Arnie date each other. The problem they are negotiating about is what to tell Kate's parents about their relationship.

Arnie: I think we should just tell them straight out.

Kate: Arnie, I think it would be a mistake to tell them the truth. My parents wouldn't understand and they wouldn't approve.

Arnie: I think that's being hypocritical.

Kate: Well, maybe so—but I'd rather be hypocritical and not hurt them.

Arnie: I get the feeling you don't want to tell them because you're ashamed of our relationship or maybe of me. If that's so, I don't like it.

Kate: Well, it's not so. But my parents are old-fashioned. What I *am* afraid of is that they'd turn against you. And I want them to like you. Because I love you.

Arnie: Well, then, I feel better. Though I still feel a little like the local monster. But I can see how you feel.

Kate: And, to be honest, Arnie, I'm also afraid they might turn against me. I couldn't stand that. I mean—I want time for our relationship to grow even stronger before I'm willing to risk telling them. And if we should break up, it would be easier if they never knew.

Arnie: Okay. I'll buy that. I thought maybe you were really saying you valued them more than our relationship. That would really hurt. Now that I know how you feel, I agree with you. Let's not tell them.

This is a fairly clear-cut example of interpersonal negotiation. Both Kate and Arnie share their inside thoughts and feelings, and they give and get some feedback from each other about the issue, their insides, and their relationship.

This example is, however, a "clipped" one; that is, we did not portray all the possible "ins and outs" of the negotiation. Kate and Arnie do a fairly good job, but their negotiating would be even more qualitative if they stopped and dealt more fully with their insides. (For example, what does Arnie mean when he says he still feels a little like the local monster?) Nevertheless, they negotiate fairly effectively, and they manage to fulfill the basic aims of interpersonal negotiation. They try to develop an outcome that is acceptable to both of them. Even if they do not necessarily like the outcome, they can feel that they have worked together and done their best to consider openly and honestly their individual and joint thoughts, feelings, actions, and desires. Hopefully, both the outcome and their shared efforts will be satisfying to each of them, but whatever the outcome, their negotiation helps them to build on their relationship in positive and constructive ways.

Ultimately it is fair to say that although good communication and a satisfying outcome are devoutly to be desired, perhaps what is even more important is that two people care enough about themselves and each other and their relationship to be willing to try their best to communicate honestly. The risks, the possibilities for growth, the excitement, and the joys result from the doing—not so much from the getting. (Although the getting can be extremely rewarding too.)

DEVELOPING ALTERNATIVES

Although some alternatives ordinarily become evident or naturally arise out of moment-to-moment negotiating, to prepare for the most constructive kind of decision-making, it is often necessary to develop alternatives. **Developing alternatives** means consciously and deliberately trying to discover, identify, and evaluate all the possible alternatives. This procedure consists of examining those alternatives that have become evident during negotiation, determining what additional ones exist, and evaluating the desirability, the feasibility, and the appropriateness of all the possible alternatives.[8]

In the previous example of negotiation between Arnie and Kate, two alternatives are evident and, in fact, form the basis of the negotiation: to tell or not to tell Kate's parents. One reason that the negotiation is, in a sense, incomplete is that Arnie and Kate do not go on to develop other alternatives; thus they limit themselves to just two, one of which Arnie finally agrees to. Suppose, however, that rather than simply agreeing, Arnie asks Kate what she thinks they might do.

Kate: Well, we could do various things. We could tell them the truth—flat out.

We could lie and say we're married, but I don't want to do that. We could say we're going steady, and you could stay at Vince's apartment while they're here. That way they could get to know you and could get to know us in our relationship without having to deal with sexual questions. We could also play it by ear. I might be able to hint to or tell my mother. She's more liberal. Then maybe she could tell Dad. Or we could tell both of them about Michelle and Dan—their living together, I mean—and see how they take it.

Kate responds by suggesting various possible alternatives and some of their possible consequences. If, however, Kate and Arnie are going to do a thorough job, they need to see if there are any other alternatives. In addition, they need to evaluate all these alternatives and negotiate about and decide which course they will follow.

DECISION-MAKING

Decision-making (which is both an intrapersonal and an interpersonal process) consists of *choosing* one or more of the possible alternatives produced by negotiation.[9] That is why evaluating the appropriateness of alternatives is so important in negotiation.

Each of us makes decisions all the time: from moment to moment each of us—whether consciously or unconsciously—is deciding what to think or say or feel or do. Because we make so many tiny, step-by-step decisions constantly, we tend to not be aware of many of them as separate and distinct decisions. Even many of our larger decisions seem to occur "out of nowhere." This can happen because the negotiation leading up to the decision has taken place on an unconscious level and is thus not apparent. Or it can happen because there is such good rapport and agreement inside a person or between people that the negotiation occurs rapidly and smoothly; thus the negotiation may go unnoticed and unappreciated. The point is, however, that negotiation is a prerequisite to true decision-making, which involves choosing among alternatives.

The variant of this process, which looks like on-the-spot decision-making (but which is not), involves actions and reactions based on automatic, repetitious patterns of thinking, feeling, and acting. In these instances, whatever negotiation may have taken place occurred long ago. Now the pattern is short-circuited. There is little if any consideration of the alternatives in the here and now.

Intrapersonal decision-making draws on a person's life-style, his background, his uniqueness, his insides, his inner negotiations, and his insights. *Interpersonal decision-making* draws on all these individual components of each person's inside operations plus all the things they share with each other—information, feelings, insights, negotiations, mutual and individual goals, and their relationship.

Decision-making may take one of three forms. Two of them, *power-playing* and *compromising*, are not constructive ways to make decisions. They either short-circuit or subvert honest and open negotiations; in effect, at least one person's insides will be ignored or neglected. The third way, *respectful settlement* by means of negotiation, is constructive. Two people work together to negotiate about their insides, their relationship, and the issue at hand. They then make a decision based on a real respect for one another's positions. Thus their settlement may or may not mean they agree. They may agree to disagree. They may agree to go do their own thing. They may make a mutual decision. Whatever they decide, however, that decision is based on their appreciation of and respect for each one's uniqueness and for the nature and meaning of their relationship.[10]

If you go back to the last part of Kate and Arnie's negotiation (p. 149), you can see that they are ready to make a decision about how to deal with her parents. If Arnie were to insist that they tell her parents they are married and if he will not agree to do anything but that, then if they decide to tell the parents they are married, the decision is the result of a power play. If Arnie were to argue forcefully that he would feel very uncomfortable saying they were going steady and that he really would prefer to tell Kate's parents they are married and if Kate yields to assuage Arnie's feelings even though she is against this alternative, the decision is the result of compromise. If, however, they feel that telling her parents they are going steady is the most appropriate alternative even though neither Kate nor Arnie feels entirely comfortable with this alternative, then their decision to do so and to work with their feelings would be the result of respectful settlement by means of negotiation. ►IE-2, p. 155.

IMPLEMENTATION

Implementation means acting on a decision (no matter how large or small); it means putting the decision into effect. Implementing a decision entails being willing to take risks and actually taking them. For example, if Kate and Arnie decide to tell her parents the truth, they risk incurring her parents' disapproval. If they say they are going steady and play the rest of it by ear, they risk having her parents find out by accident or they risk the false assumptions and inevitable distortions and strains resulting from covering the truth.

Actually *risk taking* permeates the whole process of communication and interaction: you take risks when you implement any part of the process.[11] You take risks when you reveal your true feelings; you take risks when you reveal what is going on in your insides; you take risks (and invite others to take them) when you check things out and when you give and ask for feedback. You risk hearing and learning and feeling things that you may not like or may be fearful of. You risk leaving yourself open to criticism, ridicule, rejection, or other negative experiences. You also risk opening yourself to friendliness, intimacy, caring, concern, love, laughter, and joy.

If you try to minimize risk by avoiding making decisions or implementing them or if your life-style is one that screens out or protects you from decision-making and implementation, then you are probably running even greater risks. One is that you will not control what happens in your life; life will happen to you, and you will be acted upon. The other risk is that you will live a life of emotional sameness.

BUILDING IN

Building in refers to a process that is the outcome of both intrapersonal and interpersonal communication and interaction. **Building in** means taking whatever you learn and making it an integral part of your life. Although it is true that we all learn things from moment to moment, what is meant by "whatever you learn" are things that are repeated enough times over a long enough period of time so that they achieve a significance and meaning for you and so that you can conceptualize them and thus make them your own.[12]

Building in then is ordinarily the result of long-term experience. Over a period of time, as two people communicate and interact repeatedly, they come to know a good deal about each other's insides and outsides and how they mesh in terms of the relationship. These two people establish a relationship marked by durability, consistency, and reliability. For example, Jed and Glenda develop a long-term friendship. When they first knew each other, Jed really did not trust anybody. As he and Glenda come to know each other, as they share their thoughts and feelings and insights, as they negotiate and decide and implement things, Jed consistently experiences Glenda as a trustworthy person. When she says she will do something, she does it. She is honest with him. If she assures Jed she will not repeat something he tells her, she means it. She does not act friendly one minute and aloof the next; she is consistently open and caring.

These are the values of a *long-term relationship* based on good communication. Time, repetition, and consistency enable us to validate the truth or falsity of what we may think or feel or assume at a given moment. There are times and opportunities to check out and to give and get feedback and thereby adequately evaluate the reliability and the quality of the relationship. Thus a long-term relationship based on good communication considerably lessens the risks and problems of anxiety and defensiveness. For example, as Jed experiences trust over a period of time, he begins to build in a feeling of trust—specifically for Glenda. He no longer has to constantly check out whether he trusts her; he has built in his trust. (And, of course, she has earned that trust.) In addition, he has built in the *possibility* of trusting others; he has built in an alternative to not trusting.

This example illustrates a central difference between the short-term and the long-term relationship (both with self and with others). In the short term relationship, there simply is not much time or opportunity to validate your feelings. Thus much depends on luck (good or bad), on appearances, and on the degree of openness each person brings. The long-term relationship, however, offers numerous opportunities to validate your experiences and learn things worth learning and building in. In our view, this is one of the big payoffs of the long-term, carefully tended relationship. It is this kind of significance and meaning that people hunger for and seek from their relationships.

BACKSLIDING AND BACKING OFF

Let us remind you of two safety valves that are available. **Backsliding**[13] is the unconscious and **backing off** is the conscious process of pulling back from that which is new, unknown, and unfamiliar and temporarily returning to that which is old, known, and familiar. It is perfectly natural to retreat at times, since taking chances on thinking, feeling, and acting in new and unfamiliar ways can arouse great anxiety. It is extremely important, however, to realize that retreating does not have to be a permanent matter, and it does not signal failure. It is a natural human response to stressful situations. Any time you want to pull out and rest or regroup or take a breather, you can do so.

APPLYING YOUR KNOWLEDGE

Up to this point, we have presented explanations of the major steps in the process of achieving clear, effective communication. In Appendix B, we provide some examples of distorted, not-so-clear, ineffective communication.

We have three reasons for doing so.

1. Since most people's communication and interaction skills are somewhat less than ideal, these examples are more in keeping with most people's experiences.
2. Examples of problems in communicating and interacting can make you more aware of the pitfalls to watch out for.
3. These examples can serve as models for dealing with the kinds of problems that often complicate or prevent clear communication and meaningful interaction. ►IE-3, p. 155.

Guidelines to better communication

In Chapters 7 and 8, in this chapter, and in Appendix B we have analyzed and explained different kinds and qualities of communication: intrapersonal, nonverbal, interpersonal, and distorted communication. There is much that we have not covered. We have kept our treatment of the communication process fairly basic because we are not attempting to provide you with a theoretical view so much as a practical understanding of the subject. What we have tried to give in these chapters and the appendix is a working knowledge of communication so that you can put that knowledge to use.

In keeping with our approach, this last section is as brief, common-sensical, and useful as we can make it. What we present now is a practical guide to better communication. These are ground rules that are essential to good communication. They will not answer all the possible questions that can arise about particular situations and communications. They will not exactly fit or solve every problem that arises in trying to communicate well. But they will serve you as clear and simple ways to check out your communicational skills and methods.

These guidelines are presented to you as an individual, to you as one person, since even though communication usually involves more than one person, what most frequently happens is that one person has greater skill (or maybe more courage or initiative) than the other. It is a relatively rare occasion when two people of approximately equal communicational skills get together. So we present these guidelines directly to you because if you have read this far and have taken in even a part of what you have read, *you* are likely to be the person who has the greater skill.

The guidelines to better, clearer, and more meaningful communication can be broken down into two large categories: (1) your attitudes and approach and (2) your methods.

ATTITUDES AND APPROACH

1. Never try to *force* a person to communicate. On the other hand, do not give up too quickly or easily. Many people need to be coaxed or nudged or encouraged before they will try a new and different experience.

2. Take it easy: try not to go at communicating with too much intensity. If you are too intense or move too quickly, you may scare off the other person. Go at it slowly, gently, and caringly.

3. Try not to get turned off before you even have a chance to get to know a person as an individual. At first you may feel someone is stupid or dull, but people are really anything but stupid or dull once you get past the facades, cliches, and patterns that they may have erected to defend or protect themselves.

4. Try not to get turned off if it is slow going and you feel bored. Most people are not used to communicating on a meaningful level; many simply do not have the vaguest idea of how to go about it. Thus you will frequently find that you have to teach people even the simplest and seemingly most elementary things so that they can begin to communicate with you.

5. Be as honest as you possibly can (within, of course, the bounds of what is appropriate). Dishonesty destroys the very foundations on which good communication depends.

6. Try not to be hostile. It is one thing to be really angry at someone; it is another to be hostile toward him. Telling another person that you are angry with him may or may not cut off the communication. Being hostile—humiliating him, laughing at him, being sarcastic or cutting—will most surely undermine the chance for good communication.

7. Try to maintain your sense of humor. It tends to help you keep your perspective.

METHODS

1. If necessary, explain your motives, your reasons, and your feelings *before* you begin to ask the other person how he feels. Preface your communication with whatever is necessary to set the communication on a solid course.

2. Always try to work with feelings. This is not to say that communication does not or should not try to deal with ideas and behavior also, but real communication *cannot* occur if feelings are ignored, pushed aside, or left out.

3. Check out your own feelings and get feedback from yourself—if possible, every step of the way. Keep in touch with your insides and selectively report your insides to the other person.

4. Check out with and get feedback from the other person—if possible, every step of the way. Listen carefully to the feedback: be sure you understand what

that feedback means both to you and to him.

5. If the other person has trouble giving you feedback, if he has trouble getting in touch with his insides, by all means help him. One way to do this is to reassure him. Another key way is to give him alternatives from which to choose. For example, if you ask him how he feels about something (checking out) and he says he does not really know (feedback), then give him alternative feeling possibilities. It is often easier to choose from a list than to start from scratch and think up the words to describe how you feel.

6. *Never* assume. If you assume something, you are in effect saying that you know something to be true without having checked it out. You cannot know unless and until you have checked it out. The wildest and sometimes the saddest distortions, misunderstandings, and other faulty communications are the direct result of faulty assumptions.

7. Try to avoid asking *why*. Ask what, how, when, where, who, how much, how long, and how little—but try *not* to ask why. (See p. 118 for the explanation of this.) Incidentally you will find that frequently you instinctively tend to ask why. You will also find that asking questions without using *why* (or "how come") sometimes leads to awkward-sounding phrasing. It is worth a little awkwardness to avoid *why* because it is the question that can stop communication dead in its tracks.

8. Remember—if things get too hot, too uncomfortable, or too anxious (for either or both of you), you can always rest: pull back, back off, or stop. Do not wait until "the lid blows off." If you are upset and do not want to continue, *say so*. If you sense that the other person is upset, *ask him*. Check it out. You can also negotiate with each other about stopping so that neither of you ends up feeling that the other person has deserted him or lost interest in him. You can negotiate at a later time about whether you wish to go back to your communication.

9. *Practice!* The more practice you get the better you will be at communicating. Practice your communication techniques and skills in any situation—at parties, at home, in class, at work, in your fantasies, in your dreams, and on past events in your life. Practice them on anybody—the dog, the cat, the Good Humor man, the bartender, strangers, parents, teachers, relatives, classmates, friends, lovers, colleagues, enemies—anybody. We urge you to involve others in communicating with you but not to exploit or to manipulate them. Granted, the practice will help you enormously, but it can also help them enormously. Everybody needs more practice in clear, effective, open communication. In this sense then people can be good for people. And you and they will probably have some fun and excitement along the way. Even the cat.

Our belief

When we speak of communication, we are talking about both a means and an end. Trying to live as a sensitive, aware, and striving human being can be an awesome experience: the changing and growing that come about through communication can sometimes be painful processes, full of conflict, struggle, and often very real suffering. But they are also processes that carry within them the seeds of joy and exhilaration, freedom and fruition. Communication as a means of changing and growing and achieving healthy interaction is also the means for achieving greater involvement with and commitment to life.

Effective, healthy communication and interaction *are* involvement; they *are* commitment; they *are* life.

CONCLUSION

This chapter completes our discussions of communication. The procedures and techniques described and explained in Chapters 7 through 9 can enable you to communicate more effectively. And the ability to communicate effectively is the vehicle for using the Interactional Therapeutic System to change and grow.

Interaction experiences

1. Practicing methods of interpersonal communication (p. 147)

Have a conversation with another person, using the ideas and methods presented on pp. 145 to 154.

EVALUATION: How and what did you feel as you tried to get at and to share feelings during this conversation? How did the other person respond to this process? Was he aware of what was going on? Were there times when the conversation almost "died"? Can you identify these times and what the causes might be? Can you see what helped and what hindered the communication?

FOLLOW-UP: Practice these methods whenever you get a chance and with whomever you can. Try to become aware of what you are doing and how you can improve your skills.

2. Practicing more conscious and deliberate negotiation and decision-making (p. 151)

Negotiation and decision-making lie at the heart of the interpersonal communication process. Select a partner and then negotiate and make a decision about a particular issue (e.g., what movie to go to, where to eat).

EVALUATION: Did you experience difficulty negotiating? Did you have any trouble developing alternatives? What form did the decision-making take—power play, compromise, or respectful settlement? Did you enjoy the experience? How might you have made it more qualitative?

FOLLOW-UP: Try to make your negotiations and decision-making more conscious and deliberate. Practice these processes as much and as often as you can. Try teaching these conscious methods to others.

3. Improving interpersonal communication (p. 152)

Choose a partner and then select one (or more) of the situations in Appendix B to role play. Incorporate as much nonverbal and verbal communication as possible into your role. Feel free to add to the "script" anything you feel is relevant to the situation. Really try to get "inside" the person whose role you are taking. Feel his or her feelings, actions, thoughts, conflicts, and risks. After you have done this, discuss your experience with your partner, the class, or both.

EVALUATION: Try to report how you felt and what evoked your feelings; try also to analyze and explain the dynamics of the communication/interaction that occurred.

FOLLOW-UP: Try making the communication less distorted and more open in one of these situations.

REFERENCES

1. Howells, John G.: Theory and practice of family psychiatry, New York, 1971, Brunner/Mazel, Inc., pp. 25-26.
2. Satir, Virginia: Conjoint family therapy, Palo Alto, Calif., 1964, Science & Behavior Books, Inc., pp. 63-64.
3. Howells, op. cit., p. 26.
4. Rabkin, R.: Uncoordinated communication between marriage partners, Family Process 6:10-15, 1967.
5. Fromm, Erich: Values, psychology, and human existence. In Hamachek, Don E., editor: Human dynamics in psychology and education, Boston, 1968, Allyn & Bacon, Inc., pp. 671-673.
6. Nierenberg, Gerald I.: The art of negotiating, New York, 1968, Hawthorn Books, Inc.
7. Satir, op. cit., pp. 13-18.
8. Satir, op. cit., p. 13.
9. Maslow, A. H.: Self-actualization and beyond. In Hamachek, Don E., editor: Human dynamics in psychology and education, Boston, 1970, Allyn & Bacon, Inc., p. 177.
10. Satir, Virginia: Symptomatology: a family production. In Howells, John G.: Theory and practice of family psychiatry, New York, 1971, Brunner/Mazel, Inc., pp. 664-667.
11. Rogers, Carl: On becoming a person, Boston, 1961, Houghton Mifflin Co., p. 173.
12. Ibid., pp. 156-158.
13. Ibid., p. 115.

chapter 10

THE INTERACTIONAL THERAPEUTIC SYSTEM

concepts and process

Drawing on all the previous material presented in Part II, this chapter explains how a person can use the Interactional Therapeutic System (ITS) to change, grow, and become more open. Whoever he may be, every person is constantly and continuously engaged in the most basic and universal of all human processess—the process of human interaction. No person can avoid interacting with self and others. What is so important is *how* a person engages in this process. The **Interactional Therapeutic System** is a deliberately designed, systematic approach that teaches how to consciously use this process of human interaction in constructive ways. Learning to do this enables a person to better understand himself, others, relationships, and interactions and to use this understanding in ways that can open up exciting opportunities for personal and interpersonal growth.

Specifically, The System analyzes the various steps inherent in the process of human interaction, explains the meaning of each step, and, ultimately, teaches how to use each step in order to change and grow. By helping him get in touch with the steps and the dynamics of this process, The System helps a person use it for his own benefit rather than be unaware and at the mercy of the energy and forces that are always present in human interaction.

The essential purpose of this chapter therefore is to help you gain a basic understanding of what The System is, how it works, and how it can work for you. Thus you will be able to see and feel *ITS in action.* First, we will orient you to the figure illustrating the process and explain the steps of the process. Second, using specific examples of a closed and an open person, we will explain how each utilizes the process.

The closed person's interactions illustrate unconscious use of the process, the kind that produces minimal, if any, growth. The open person's interactions illustrate conscious use of the process and therefore of *our System of developing greater personal and interpersonal competence.* It is by means of these two examples as they are used to explain the process of interaction that we will try to help you understand how utilizing The System—that is, consciously and deliberately applying the interactional process—can enable a person to develop greater personal and interpersonal competence.

WHAT EVERY PERSON BRINGS TO THE PROCESS OF INTERACTION

Every person brings his whole Self—his universal human functions and experiences—to the process of interaction, and this Self significantly affects the impact and meaning of his interactions. Whether his involvement in the process of interaction is advantageous for him depends on how he engages in the process. If he does so in a primarily unconscious or unaware manner, whatever advantages he may gain are likely to be haphazard and sporadic. If, however, he chooses to employ this process in a conscious and deliberate manner (i.e., if he uses The System), then he is likely to receive benefits that are significant, far reaching, and long lasting.

Specifically, every person brings to his every interaction his past; his present; his thoughts, feelings, and actions; his responses; and his psychological defenses. Depending on how closed the developmental influences on him have been, his past will at least partially control and influence his present. Thus his current self-system and life-style will reflect and be partially governed by his past and will affect the content and quality of his interactions.[1]

The three functions of thinking, feeling, and acting are also fundamental to the process of being alive and interacting (both intrapersonally and interpersonally), and their effects on the person's interactions will depend on the particular balance existing among them (see pp. 69 to 71).

As a person engages in the process of living, of interacting, he is continually encountering internal and external stimuli, which he must deal with in some way.[2] We have designated the major groupings of internal and external stimuli as moment-to-moment influencing factors (MIFs). At least some MIFs are operating in every moment of experience. For example, what is the social situation (public or private)? What societal pressures are present? What influences from significant others are operating? (See p. 96 for a full discussion of MIFs.)

As a person encounters MIFs and other stimuli, he is **giving and receiving responses**—communicating with both his inner and outer environment. As he meets with inner and outer stimuli, he responds to them and they to him; as this occurs and reoccurs, it generates further responses. In this manner, the person maintains a "dialogue" with himself, with others, and with his physical and emotional environment. This communication is his way of achieving and maintaining in-touchedness with his inner and outer environment.[3]

As the person gives and receives responses to MIFs plus other assorted internal and external stimuli, he utilizes the components of his self-system and life-style to maintain his dynamic equilibrium. You will recall from the discussion of dynamic equilibrium in Chapter 5 that a person uses PFLs and patterns (undergirded by his self-concept and Child/Parent/Adult balance) as ways of organizing and managing internal and external stimuli so that they do not overwhelm him and upset his emotional balance. In effect he employs his **psychological defenses**—his particular ways of thinking, feeling, and acting that he (consciously and/or unconsciously) employs to protect himself against anxiety.[4,5]

These kinds of defensive operations are ones that to one degree or another most of us use fairly frequently. These are what we call "first-line defenses." Everyone has available other defenses that back up this first line, but ordinarily circumstances are not so laden with anxiety that the stronger defenses are necessary.

As you read about the process of interaction in detail, keep in mind that all these universal human functions and experiences (the past; the present; thinking, feeling, and acting; giving and receiving responses; psychological defenses) are present in the process of interaction and are constantly affecting the way a person engages in this process.

INTERACTIONAL THERAPEUTIC SYSTEM: THE PROCESS

The closed person who engages in the process of interaction does so, by definition, largely on an unconscious level. As a result of his lack of awareness and his closedness, his experiences tend to be limited and not ordinarily growth producing. Basically he engages in the process in a manner that selectively reinforces his self-system and life-style; his interactions (both with self and others) tend therefore to limit or block rather than encourage growth. In other words, because of his closedness, the ways he experiences the process of interaction tend to support and perpetuate his closedness.

The System itself

For the aware and open person (or the person who is open to becoming more aware and open), the process as presented in Fig. 1 represents the ten steps (not necessarily sequential) of the Interactional Therapeutic System. It is The System that identifies, conceptualizes, and explains the process of human interaction so that the person who wishes to do so can learn to use the process to his best advantage. In effect, the Interactional Therapeutic System provides a person with knowledge, understanding, and equipment, which can enable him to make conscious, deliberate use of the process of interaction and thereby change and grow.

STEP 1: GATHERING INFORMATION

Because it is absolutely basic to all other steps, **gathering information** is depicted as the foundation of the process. Every person is always gathering information both consciously and unconsciously about many

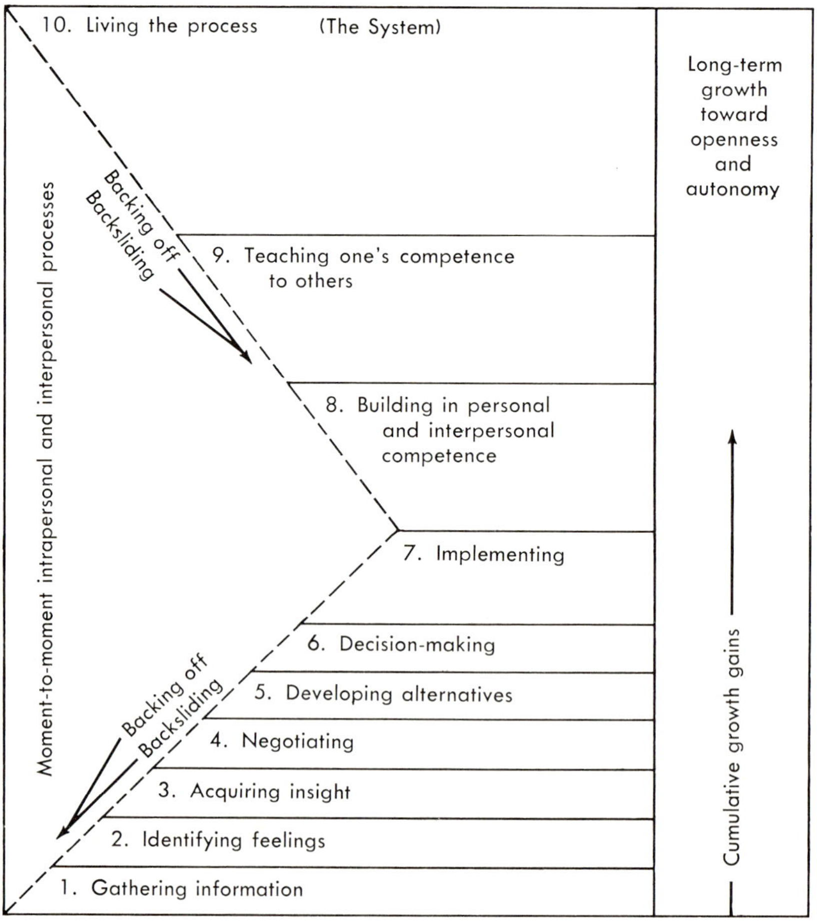

Fig. 1. The Interactional Therapeutic System: the process.

things. If a person is consciously working to acquire insight, he is trying to gather as much information as he can about who he is now, how he got to be the way he is now, and where he may go in the future. He is trying to gain information about how he relates to himself, how he relates to others, how they relate to him, and how he relates to his environment. He is trying to gather information about his PFLs, his patterns (both intrapersonal and interpersonal), his self-concept, his Child/Parent/Adult balance, his ways of maintaining his dynamic equilibrium, his life-style, and his uniqueness in terms of both the past and the present and with an eye to the future. He is in effect trying to learn all he can about himself and the influences on him so that he can put the information together, evaluate it, and arrive at meaningful and useful insights about his personal identity.[6]

STEP 2: IDENTIFYING FEELINGS

Every human being feels feelings, but some people are more aware and better able than others to identify their feelings. The person who intentionally engages in the process of interaction to gain some self-awareness and insight will inevitably pay a good deal of attention to **identifying** his **feelings.** Such close attention is necessary, since feelings lie at the heart of whatever a person thinks and does. Thus although it is helpful and necessary to gather information, it is equally important to identify (and be willing to *feel and work with*) emotions; otherwise the process of interaction tends to stay on an intellectual level, or it may be "acted out" but not "felt out." Those insights that come out of these self-exploratory procedures will be limited if the person does not identify the feelings attendant on his thoughts and actions and on the information he gathers.[7]

STEP 3: ACQUIRING INSIGHT

In the fullest sense, acquiring insight demands that a person not only gather information but also that he identify feelings. At the same time, he evaluates the information and feelings to determine their meaning, significance, and interrelationships. As he does so and as a result of his doing so, he often **acquires insight**—personal understanding that results from putting together in conceptual form his thoughts, feelings, and actions. Acquiring insight then is gaining a grasp of what is going on and what that means; it is suddenly "getting the feel" of situations. Acquiring an insight is sometimes called an "a-ha!" experience. It occurs at that moment when a person suddenly "sees" the meaning of something, when the meaning and significance of something are crystallized and become clear to him.

STEP 4: NEGOTIATING

Although negotiating is placed immediately after acquiring insight, it actually could go anywhere in the process, since a person is negotiating all the time, whether consciously or unconsciously. It is put after acquiring insight, however, to emphasize the importance of negotiating *about* and *on the basis of insight.*

Essentially **negotiating** consists of trying to assemble, identify, and examine all the thoughts, feelings, and actions that are relevant to whatever is under consideration (e.g., an event, an insight, a circumstance, an issue, a situation, a thought, a feeling, an action, a goal, a task, a change, a decision). This assembling, identifying, and examining of relevant thoughts, feelings, and actions has four purposes.

1. It enables the negotiator to better understand and appreciate what is going on, where he is at emotionally, and what options may exist.
2. As a result, the negotiator can evaluate the appropriateness and workability of the relevant thoughts, feelings, and actions.
3. The negotiator can evaluate those alternatives that have become evident in the course of the negotiation and can attempt to develop alternatives.
4. As a result of these three previous procedures, the negotiator can decide whether to make a decision.

Thus the negotiator obviously draws on

any or all of the preceding steps of the process—gathering information, identifying feelings, and acquiring insights—to determine what his thoughts, feelings, and actions are and what they mean; to evaluate their validity and appropriateness; and to consider what possible alternatives and decisions exist. The more open a person is, the more he negotiates, the greater are his alternatives, and the more conscious and appropriate is his decision-making.[8,9]

STEP 5: DEVELOPING ALTERNATIVES

Potential alternatives are present all the time as a natural part of living. During the course of moment-to-moment negotiating, some possible alternatives become evident, and some are developed. Even though developing alternatives may be considered a part of negotiating, at the same time it can be considered as a logical and specialized extension of negotiation. In this sense then **developing alternatives** means making a conscious, deliberate attempt to discover, identify, and evaluate all the possible alternatives.

Although one reason for setting developing alternatives off as a distinct step is that it is an extension of negotiation, there is another, equally important reason. In any person's long-term use of The System to change and grow, developing alternatives becomes extremely important because it takes on far-reaching significance. In this sense, developing alternatives means investigating, considering, and at least experimenting with major alterations or changes in PFLs, patterns, self-concept, and Child/Parent/Adult balance.[10]

STEP 6: DECISION-MAKING

In the simplest terms, **decision-making** means making a choice (or choices). Since choice presupposes the existence of at least two alternatives, decision-making depends on a certain amount of prior negotiation (whether conscious or unconscious).

There are two types of decisions. Both depend on a person's putting together all the material that is available to him from negotiating—information, facts, ideas, opinions, feelings, sensory impressions, reactions, and behavior—and making a choice. One type of decision-making consists of reaching a conclusion about the material by selecting from possible alternatives.[11] Following are some examples of conclusions: "I feel sad (rather than happy or angry)," "I shouldn't have done that (rather, I should have done this)," "I believe what this person says (rather than what another says or what I read)," and "I disagree with this idea (rather than that idea)."

The other type of decision-making consists of selecting from among various alternatives with the intention of implementing or putting the chosen alternative into action. For example, a person might negotiate with himself about what he is going to do on the weekend. Suppose he determines that he has four viable alternatives: stay home, visit friends, go skiing, or spend his time with his girl friend. Depending on further negotiation, he may decide to stay home part of the time and spend part of his time with his girl. Both decisions are made with the intention of putting them into effect.

There are three basic ways of making decisions: the power play, compromise, or respectful settlement by means of negotiation. All decision-making, whether intrapersonal or interpersonal, rests on some negotiation or interaction between at least two entities.

On an interpersonal level, in a **power play** the "stronger" person wins and makes the decision in terms of what he wants or what he thinks or feels is best or right. In a **compromise**, one of the people gives in and agrees even though he may not be pleased or satisfied with the decision. Obviously power playing and compromising are not the most constructive ways to make decisions. They either short-circuit or subvert honest and open negotiations; in effect at least one part or one person's insides will be ignored or neglected.

The third way is that of **respectful settle-**

ment by means of negotiation. *Intrapersonally,* the Adult mediates between the conflicting desires and demands of the Child and Parent and then negotiates about the issue at hand. The Adult gathers information, identifies feelings, acquires insight, puts all this together and evaluates it, develops alternatives, evaluates them, and then decides. This decision by the Adult is made with respect for the wishes of the Child and Parent but is based ultimately on what is most appropriate and constructive for the person as a whole.

Interpersonally two people work together to negotiate about their insides, their relationship, the issue, and the relevant moment-to-moment influencing factors. They then make a decision based on respect for one another's positions. Thus their settlement may or may not mean they agree. They may agree to disagree. They may agree that each will go and do his own thing. They may make a mutual decision. Whatever they decide, however, that decision is based on their appreciation of and respect for each one's uniqueness and for the nature and meaning of their relationship.

Clearly, respectful settlement by means of negotiation is the method that an open person will most often use when he is making decisions.[12]

STEP 7: IMPLEMENTING

Implementing means putting into effect or action. Like decision-making, implementing goes on all the time and can be applied to any other part of the interactional process. For example, if a person gathers information about how to build a cabinet, then building it would be implementation. If a person feels angry, he may implement his feeling by reporting his anger and demanding an apology or by hitting the person who evoked his anger. Suppose a person has the following insight: "In social situations, I have a pattern of being overly intellectual, which often drives people away from me." His implementation of this insight might consist of trying to identify and share his feelings with others and of attempting to be more sensitive to their feelings. Suppose a person's Adult negotiates a reasonable settlement between his Child and Parent: his Child wants to buy five records; his Parent says, "No, that's foolish; you need your money for food and clothes." His Adult negotiates between the two positions and develops a workable alternative: that it would be appropriate to buy one record now and start putting money aside to buy other records later. When the person buys one record and starts saving for others, he is implementing the outcomes of his negotiation, implementing a decision reached by means of reasonable settlement.

From these examples, it should be obvious that decision-making (which occurs in all these examples) and implementation frequently go hand in hand. In fact, without implementation, no amount of decision-making will produce results. It is all well and good to decide something, but not until it is implemented will there be much change or growth.

Some words of caution. Following this discussion of implementation, it is appropriate to pass on some words of caution.

Experimentation that results in a person's changing from one psychological position to an extreme opposite position (e.g., from passive to aggressive) does not ordinarily constitute growth or even movement toward growth. *Change and growth are not synonymous.* If experimentation is to lead to constructive change and growth, you must guide it by exercising judgment, controls, moderation, and responsibility; using these four as guides is as much a part of moving toward autonomy as is the experimentation itself.

STEP 8: BUILDING IN PERSONAL AND INTERPERSONAL COMPETENCE

The next step in the process is that of building in personal and interpersonal competence. Every person, whether closed or open, **builds in** what he learns from his moment-to-moment experiences; that is, he takes what he learns and through repetition and practice incorporates it into his self-system and life-style. Thus he builds in his insights, his implementations of these insights, and all the procedures he uses to acquire and implement his insights (e.g., communication, negotiation, decision-making, taking responsibility for self). What he learns and builds in becomes an intrinsic part of the ways he functions both intrapersonally and interpersonally. He has then gained competence in using what he has learned and has made that competence an integral part of him. Even though some growth occurs every time an open (or partially open) person experiences and learns from newness and difference, *long-term growth* begins occurring when a person gains even a small amount of competence.

STEP 9: TEACHING ONE'S COMPETENCE TO OTHERS

A further step in The System is that of a person's **teaching** his **competence** to others, whether intentionally or unintentionally.

The open person intentionally and unintentionally teaches PFLs to others—his children, his spouse, his friends, and his colleagues; but the kinds of PFLs he teaches are not flat, rigid rules or sweeping values but guidelines for living. It is true that he teaches his patterns to others, but they are not the automatic, inflexible, unchangeable patterns of the closed person. Rather they are patterns that are more flexible, more appropriate, and more responsive to change. However, perhaps the most important lesson he teaches is a whole approach to life. He teaches others both by instruction and by example his way of approaching life with openness, with availability to newness and change, with flexibility, with eagerness and vitality, and with a willingness to experiment.

He also teaches others the methods by which he successfully carries out his approach. Essentially he shares with and teaches people the techniques and skills of clear communication. By employing the techniques and skills himself and by directly instructing others, he teaches them how to work with their defenses, how to gather information, what to look for in self and others, how to get in touch with one's inner life, how to arrive at insights, how to communicate effectively, how to negotiate, how to seek possible alternatives, how to arrive at decisions, and how to implement insights and decisions. In essence he teaches people how to use the process of human interaction consciously and deliberately to promote constructive growth and to develop autonomy. He teaches them The System.

STEP 10: LIVING THE PROCESS

As we stated earlier, living means interacting with self and/or others all the time; thus every human being constantly engages in some way in the process of interaction, which has just been described. But when a child is developing his life-style, he does not "live" the process of interaction. Although he is engaged in interaction all the time, he is learning how to interact in particular ways, ways that do not yet come naturally to him. In like manner, the person who tries to learn to use the process of interaction consciously and deliberately to change and grow does not acquire expertise in the use of The System overnight. Both the child and the seeker of change and growth must gradually learn effective ways of interacting. Both must work at it.

If the child develops a closed life-style, then living the process of interaction will amount to interacting in ways that are automatic, repetitious, and self-perpetuating of closedness. Few different or new positions will be interjected into his style of living the process; therefore few modifications or alterations will occur in his style, and little change or growth will occur.

For the person who is open (or who is attempting to change and grow and thereby become more open), **living the process** means something different. Learning to use The System to change and grow and become more open is a slow, gradual, step-by-step, sometimes laborious procedure that requires a lot of psychological work and a great deal of practice. But as he works and practices, gradually the balance shifts away from old, not-so-constructive ways of interacting with self and others to newer, healthier ways. Gradually, as this person practices and builds in this newer, healthier life-style, he acquires expertise in healthy humanness and expertise in interacting. Over a period of time, he becomes so familiar with and practiced in the techniques of The System that they become second nature to him. Then he is living the process of interaction; he is living The System.

PROTECTIVE PSYCHOLOGICAL MEASURES

In addition to the various steps of the process that have been described in this chapter, there are two particular protective measures that a person may employ while engaging in interaction. They are backsliding and backing off, designated by the broken line in Fig. 1.

Backsliding and its companion phenomenon, backing off, refer to the ways a person protects himself from being overwhelmed by the anxiety or discomfort attendant on anticipating or trying new and different activities.[13] Under the pressure of such anxiety, the person may, without having much control over his actions, slide back to a psychological position that prevents the arousal of so much anxiety. Consciously or unconsciously he returns to earlier, more familiar, more comfortable defensive positions.

For example, suppose you have an insight about yourself: you realize that you have a pattern of smiling politely or even laughing when you feel angry or irritated or hurt. Furthermore, you discover underlying PFLs that say, "Don't embarrass yourself or others by showing your irritation or hurts in public"; "People won't like you if you show your negative feelings"; and "Don't let others see that you're angry or hurt because they'll take advantage of you." You decide that your PFLs and your resultant pattern do not suit you; they are not appropriate, and they stand in the way of greater openness. You decide to implement your insight: you will try not to smile or laugh under these particular conditions and instead will try to feel your feelings and express them to others. You put your new resolve into effect. But suppose the going gets too rough: you find that you feel intense, almost unbearable anxiety when you reveal your true feelings. Maybe someone you report your feelings to treats you coldly or puts you down. As a consequence, you experience fierce anxiety. It is at a point like this that you may backslide. In this case you might backslide to your original defensive pattern of smiling and laughing to cover and to manage your negative feelings.

Backing off is the companion phenomenon of backsliding. The difference between them is that whereas backsliding is usually unintentional and not really under your control, backing off is an intentional, controlled, and deliberate process. Backing off is a matter of your *choosing* to rest, to take a breather, or to take a vacation from newness and anxiety because you are tired of the pressure. It is choosing to move away from what is new and unfamiliar and anxiety (and growth) producing. It is deciding to give yourself time to relax and an opportunity to regroup your self-system. Backing off is a reaction to the stress of changing and growing but to stress that is not as strong as the anxiety eliciting backsliding. Backing off can have a variety of motivations such as being scared, not understanding something, not being sure of a message you are receiving, or deciding it is not a good idea to experiment in a particular way. In terms of the example given before, backing off could mean choosing to return for a while to your original defensive pattern of laughing to cover your negative feelings, or it could mean deciding to implement your insight only around trusted friends. It could also mean deciding not to implement a new pattern right now but instead to work on gaining more insight about the underlying PFLs.

Remember that backsliding and backing off are natural protective measures that all of us use from time to time. They serve as important emotional safety valves and allow us to let ourselves off the emotional hook when the going gets too rough. But it is important to remember that if you backslide or back off, this does not mean that you have lost the ground you had gained or that you have failed or that you will forget what you have learned. Learning The System is like learning to swim or to ride a bike: you may forget some of the fine points, but once you have acquired the basic skill, you *never* really lose it.

Long-term growth toward openness and autonomy

Up to this point the discussion has focused on moment-to-moment interaction with self and others. This discussion has explained the ways such interaction can be consciously used so that a person can grow and develop personal and interpersonal competence in interacting as an autonomous individual, one whose functioning is essentially healthy, mature, and responsible and whose blend of thinking, feeling, and acting is appropriately balanced.

Now it is time to look at the cumulative effects of the moment-to-moment "growth gains," which occur again and again over a long period of time. As you use the System, moment-to-moment experiences of difference, newness, and change occur and reoccur, and short-term progress takes place. As this kind of growth happens over and over again, it is gradually translated into **long-term growth toward openness and autonomy.**

Obviously what counts over the long run is the slow but steady accumulation of the small gains that occur from moment-to-moment use of The System. There is also a strong factor of interrelationship amongst the various parts of the self-system and life-style, both in moment-to-moment and in long-term activities. That is, if you gain and implement a number of insights about a variety of PFLs, you are bound to learn something about and to influence your self-concept. Similarly, if you make significant long-term growth gains in working constructively with PFLs and patterns, these gains will influence the development of a more autonomous Adult. In addition, although gains in moment-to-moment interaction obviously affect and, in fact, cause long-term growth, what is perhaps less obvious but just as important is that long-term gains affect and influence moment-to-moment growth. For example, suppose your self-concept slowly moves from one of self-doubt to one of greater self-confidence. This greater confidence will then influence the ways you think and feel and act from moment to moment. You now are freer to try ways of thinking, feeling, and acting that you were doubtful you could try before. In effect, confidence breeds courage, which breeds implementation, which breeds success, which breeds more confidence, which breeds more success. Over the long haul, as your PFLs become less harsh, your patterns less automatic, your self-concept more positive, and your Adult more autonomous, you become more and more free to work on yourself with more confidence and with less anxiety. Consequently, you become less defensive. In effect your growth gains help to release you to use The System to grow even more. ►IE-1, p. 170.

TWO EXAMPLES OF THE USE OF THE PROCESS OF INTERACTION

To distinguish sharply between that use of the process of interaction which produces little if any growth and that which does, we now will describe how a closed person (Harry Johnson) and an open person (Stan) utilize the process. When the process of interaction is utilized in the manner that Stan does it, then the process may properly be termed the Interactional Therapeutic System. In other words, for him "ITS is in action."

Gathering information, identifying feelings, and acquiring insight

The first three steps of gathering information, identifying feelings and acquiring insight in the process of interaction can be best understood by examining them in relation to one another. The outcome of this part of the process is frequently the acquisition of insight. By gathering information and evaluating it and by identifying his feelings, a person often acquires some kind of insight.

THE CLOSED PERSON

If a person is closed, he gathers and evaluates information, feels feelings (although he does not necessarily identify them), and acquires insights in rather "specialized" and restricted ways. He gathers his information selectively so that it supports and reinforces his self-system. As he takes in and receives information—whether it be about thoughts, feelings, or actions—he sifts and shapes the information so that it fits his predetermined self-system and views of the world. In this way, he maintains his dynamic equilibrium, and he goes to considerable lengths to maintain that equilibrium. For example, he blocks out thoughts, feelings, and actions that might rock his emotional boat. He distorts situations. He sees what he want to see, hears what he wants to hear, and feels what he wants to feel. Thus his insights most often take the following forms: "Aha! It's just as I thought." "I knew that's the way things are." "All along I felt that those ________ were no-good bums." "Now I see I was right not to trust ________. It's just as my father warned me." By and large, the closed person does all this unconsciously, automatically, and repeatedly. Thus he reinforces his sameness and, by doing so, cuts himself off from the possibilities for significant growth.

As an example of how the closed person follows this procedure, let us look at Harry Johnson. (See Appendix A.) He is strongly against women's liberation. Suppose Harry is talking to an attractive, intelligent, well-informed woman at a cocktail party; and they begin talking about the women's liberation movement. She belongs to the movement and tells Harry about its belief that day-care centers for children of women who have to work are urgently needed. She goes on to describe how her particular organization has sought to apply political pressure to influence pro–day-care legislation. If you recall Harry's personality and style, you can imagine his reaction. Harry gets hot under the collar and says that women should stay home where they belong, that women were not meant to work outside the home, and that he thinks day-care centers will undermine family unity.

By this time, Harry has probably worked himself into a self-righteous lather about the matter. If you notice, he has managed to *not hear* the key qualifier—mothers who *have* to work. But Harry's PFLs about women's and men's roles have risen up so strongly that it is almost as if he cannot hear. Even if he does hear the qualifier, he has a difficult time responding with any openness or equanimity; women's liberation constitutes a threat to Harry's traditional, comfortable, familiar ways of thinking, feeling, and acting. So he cuts himself off from what might have been an interesting, perhaps enlightening, conversation because he automatically defends his entrenched position.

THE OPEN PERSON

What about the *open* person? How does he engage in the procedure of acquiring insight? He consciously seeks and finds information and identifies his feelings to acquire insight about himself so that he can know himself better and perhaps grow as a result of that knowledge. He tends to let the information—whatever it is about—take its natural, realistic shape. He does not try to fit the information to preset, predetermined views about himself or the world. Instead the open person uses, to the best of his ability, the methods and techniques of intrapersonal and interpersonal communication. Thus he is usually checking out his insides, sharing them with others, evaluating information, considering alternatives, negotiating with self and others, and making decisions as he goes along. His participation in this process of gathering information and acquiring insight is active, vital, and ongoing. As often as not, he is not fully sure where his inquiries and information gathering will lead him or what his feelings will be. However, he is willing and able to take a certain amount of risk—even the risk of not knowing what his insight may consist of. He knows that he may not always like his insights, and that they may not always be comfortable or comforting. But he also knows they will be interesting and exciting, since they will help him to become more aware of who he is. He knows that this awareness is what enables him to grow.

In some ways it is difficult to give an example of how the open person operates while gathering information, identifying his feelings, and acquiring insight because he will be engaged in many interactional activities at once. Suppose Stan is at the same party that Harry is attending. He meets the same woman that Harry has talked to, and she makes essentially the same comments about day-care centers. Stan is about the same age as Harry, from the same cultural background, and of the same social status, but there is one crucial difference—Stan is an open person.

The conversation can go in any number of directions. Stan may simply say, "Tell me more, I'm interested and I don't know much about the matter." Or perhaps he catches himself feeling slightly uncomfortable, a little annoyed, and realizes that he is about to argue with the woman. He may stop and try intrapersonally to identify his feelings and their source. He may say to the woman, "You know, when you talk about working mothers and day-care centers, I get to feeling uncomfortable and annoyed. I wonder why that is. Maybe I'm more of a male chauvinist than I realized." He and the woman may talk about his feelings, her feelings, the women's liberation movement in general, or PFLs about women that Stan learned from his parents. The list is fascinating and practically endless. What is most important is that Stan does not try to force what he hears into his mold, nor does he turn off because the information arouses discomfort in him. Notice also that Stan has many alternative ways of moving within this procedure. The payoff for Stan will more than likely be some kind of insight into his thoughts and feelings about women and their roles or about men's roles (or both) or insight into some of his PFLs and perhaps into his patterns in regard to women. Whatever the insights may be, however, Stan has increased and enhanced his opportunities for learning about himself and therefore for growing.

Gaining insight means shifting your perspective. If you can shift your perspective, you are likely to see with new eyes something that originally puzzled you or did not make sense. Suddenly it will become clear to you. And it will take on new and different meanings.

The open person is willing and able to risk some anxiety to gain new perspectives so that he can grow. By being willing to take the risks, he ends up lessening his risks in the long run. The reason is that gaining new perspectives and insights means becoming more aware of unconscious material. When unconscious material is brought into the light of consciousness, a person has less need to defend himself against it. Thus the open person releases some of the energy he has spent on defending himself for the more constructive activity of growing.

Not only do new perspectives and insights result in growth at the moment, but they also become the basis for further growth. For example, suppose Stan realizes that he has a societal and personal PFL that says, "A woman's place is in the home." He takes this insight, and knowing that PFLs come in packets, he looks for other, related PFLs. He soon finds that he has others such as "women should not work outside the home," "women should run the household for the convenience of their husbands," and "the wife should have the evening meal ready when her husband gets home from work." Stan undoubtedly has many other PFLs about this, since the whole subject of female/male roles is a large and complex one. But these few will suffice for this example. When Stan thinks about these PFLs, he realizes that he can trace them back to his father's verbal and nonverbal teachings and to the relationship between his mother and father. He remembers how his father would follow a pattern of getting angry and then sulking when dinner was not ready on time.

As Stan and the woman at the party talk some more, if she is receptive and communicative, Stan may share his discoveries with her. Suppose he also shares with her that he feels a certain rush of anger when she expresses her opinion that a wife's having to fix dinner on such a rigid schedule is really a subtle form of psychological bondage.

Now Stan takes the various pieces of information he has been gathering—the discovered PFLs, his memories of his father's anger and sulking pattern, and his own feelings of anger about the whole subject—and he puts all this information together. Stan realizes that he feels anxious because his old, familiar, comfortable PFLs and patterns are being challenged.

In spite of his anxiety, however, Stan stays open enough to continue to work with his insights. He thinks about how he treats his own wife if dinner is late: it dawns on him that like his father, he gets angry and sulks to "punish" her. He thinks about this more and decides that he acts like a petulant, spoiled child: he never discusses the matter directly with his wife (although they may quarrel), and he does not accept her apologies readily. Stan's further insight is that in this behavior, his Child part (copied after his father) dominates.

As you can see, Stan's series of insights cover a lot of significant territory: his thoughts, feelings, and actions; his PFLs; his patterns; his Child/Parent/Adult balance; and his past, present, and future. With this series of insights, Stan has already grown in terms of awareness about his personal identity. He is also ready to develop some alternatives to his current behavior and to make some important decisions about his future. (Incidentally, "future" does not necessarily mean some hazy, far-off time. Rather it means something much closer and more specific like tomorrow or next week or next month.) When Stan starts trying to make these decisions, he will have to deal with whatever MIFs are relevant and with his own defenses (as is true always during every moment of this process). For example, he will have to deal with his motivation about continuing to work with all this material in the face of his own anxiety, with his mood, with his time, with his opportunity, and with significant others (such as his mother and father in this case).

Negotiating, developing alternatives, decision-making, and implementing

The steps in the interaction process of negotiating, developing alternatives, decision-making, and implementing are also best illustrated by viewing them in relation to one another. These steps are directed at implementing the insights that have been gained. To do this in a constructive way, a person must be willing to negotiate with himself (and others); to recognize and develop alternative ways of thinking, feeling, and acting; to make decisions; and, finally, to implement those decisions and insights.

THE CLOSED PERSON

The closed person will tend to negotiate in the same old ways with the same old patterns of thinking, feeling, and acting. Thus he usually is unaware that he is negotiating. His alternatives are limited because they are the same ones that he has always felt were available to him, and they tend to fall into rather rigid categories of black and white. He is not likely to make many new decisions. Rather he tends to automatically make decisions on the basis of his PFLs and patterns, which activate preprogrammed thoughts, feelings, and actions. Finally, instead of implementing new insights, alternatives, or decisions, he usually reimplements responses that were set long ago. Thus he ordinarily does not engage in relationships, situations, or activities that are new and different. As long as this is true, he will experience little or no anxiety because his dynamic equilibrium will remain unchallenged and unshaken. However, he will also experience little or no growth.

For example, Harry's insight from talking to the woman at the party is that women liberationists and women who support them are troublemakers; he came to this conclusion because the woman dared to challenge his set views and to argue with him. The way Harry implements this insight is to carry it around inside of him and fit it onto every woman who shows any signs of favoring the women's liberation movement. He looks hard for signs that these women are indeed troublemakers. (And he will find or unconsciously manufacture such signs, since he will be looking for any indication whatsoever.) In effect, such women do not have a chance with Harry; they already stand prejudged and guilty in Harry's mind and heart. When he reads the newspaper, when he watches television, or when he goes to parties, some part of him will be alert to women and women's liberation. Unconsciously Harry will be watching and waiting for the "troublemakers" to tip their hands.

Obviously the closed person does not stand much chance of growing by seeing new alternatives and implementing his insights. He is too busy reinforcing his sameness and maintaining his dynamic equilibrium to allow for difference and newness. Only significant intervention by someone or something outside the closed person (a therapist, a life crisis) is likely to enable him to experience newness in ways that could lead to change and growth.

THE OPEN PERSON

The open person implements his insights in a different way and gets different results. He tends to take his new insights and negotiate with himself about them. He then puts them together with other things he already knows and feels and does and begins to develop alternatives. His implementation process is thus much more complex than the closed person's. Since he is working with difference and newness he experiences some anxiety as he deals with the particular MIFs of the new situation. But he risks the anxiety most of the time, figuring that at the worst he can always back off and take a breather if he feels he has to.

The open person may implement his insights partly from plain curiosity and partly from a desire to modify or alter or change his old ways. In one sense, his implementation is based on the age-old idea that you cannot know what you want or do not want, what you will like or will not like, or how you will feel until you have tried something or at least have become aware of and seriously considered the alternatives. Furthermore, to understand what the alternatives really mean and involve, you need to have had some actual experience with them; you need to test them out. A quick example of this is the person who says, "I don't like foreigners" on the basis of having briefly met and talked to maybe two or three people from other countries. First, this person is responding in terms of predetermined attitudes. Second, since he has had little meaningful experience with foreigners, he is not in a position to make an informed decision based on *real* alternatives. He has in effect cut himself off from alternatives.

Stan, however, is an example of the open person who gives himself greater access to more alternatives. Suppose Stan negotiates with himself, comes up with some alternatives, and decides that he will implement his series of insights about himself and his feelings and attitudes toward women's roles. His *negotiations* might run something like this: "I'm not a child, yet I get angry with my wife and sulk and act like a child. I don't like this particular child quality in my makeup, so I will try to act differently next time she doesn't have dinner ready when I think it should be."

The next time dinner is not ready, Stan implements his insight further. Using the techniques of intrapersonal communication (and perhaps interpersonal communication too if he shares all or some of this with his wife), he lets his thoughts and feelings through and reports them to himself, he holds them, he thinks about them, and he *feels* them. He *checks out* his thoughts, feelings, and actions against his memories of his mother and father's quarreling at dinner time. He feels how unpleasant those quarrels were; he remembers the feel of his father's contempt and anger and sulking. As he does this, Stan decides he does not like these same responses in himself. He also decides that they are not really appropriate to what is going on in the present (and were not appropriate in the past).

Stan may also try to understand his wife's point of view. He may ask her, without being accusing, what prevented her from having dinner ready, and he may be surprised to hear her reasonable answer. He may ask her how she feels when he gets angry and sulks. He may explain his whole group of insights to her, an action that may set off a long series of constructive communications between them about women's and men's and husbands' and wives' roles. He may ask her help in implementing his insights, in developing alternatives, and in altering his PFLs and patterns. She may be able to help him simply by pointing it out when his pattern automatically goes into action. She may help him merely by not blaming him and by being patient and willing to communicate with him about the matter.

This kind of implementation gives Stan the opportunity to have a variety of experiences: he gets the feel of the alternatives; he consciously considers his style in action; he feels his style in action; he relives old thinking and feeling positions; he communicates with himself and others (his wife in this instance.) By doing these, Stan allows himself to experience, to feel, the differences (no matter how small) between his old ways and these other, newer ways. In effect, he gives his Adult a chance to stretch and to grow. Whatever Stan chooses to do from here on, he at least has given himself alternatives from which he can choose.

The differences between the ways the closed and the open person engage in this process of human interaction should be more apparent now. The closed person goes through the process again and again but tends primarily to reinforce his sameness. The open person goes through the process again and again but tends to widen his personal and interpersonal horizons, to experiment with and experience difference and newness, to change, and to grow.

Thus implementation does not become exciting until you consider the open (or partially open) person. When the open person implements his insights, that is where the real action is. It is fine (and useful) to talk and to learn about PFLs, patterns, self-concept, Child/Parent/Adult balance, communication, and interaction. It is like learning the words and music of the song. But only when the human being gives voice to the words and music—only when he implements what he learns about his self-system and his life-style—only then does he sing his song of life; only then does he combine what he has learned into a synchronized, harmonious, compatible movement toward autonomy and true freedom and joy.

When you start implementing, no longer is The System only something to be studied, learned, and appreciated; now it is something to be built in, taught, and lived, with awareness, fullness, vitality, humanness. It is no longer an intellectual matter. In implementing The System, you consciously and deliberately use all its steps and apply them to everything in your life: your thoughts, feelings, actions; your decisions; your sensory responses; and your past, your present, and your vision of the future. You test life and the alternatives it offers with your whole being.

By implementing the Interactional Therapeutic System, you put insights and skills together; you put them into practice; you are able to feel the richness, the wholeness, the consistency, and the healthiness of your being as you experience your movement away from former positions that have bound and limited you. As you experience and reexperience success in implementing your "you-ness," the joy and the thrill of feeling who you are and who you are becoming sweeps through you. These are the moments that cause significant long-term growth, since to implement The System is to grow.

Chapter 11 is devoted to explaining how to make The System work for you. Specifically it teaches how to use The System to change PFLs and patterns. In effect, Chapter 11 draws on and puts together the information presented in all the chapters of Part II and explains how to apply this information to your life.

Interaction experience

1. Using The System—and growing (p. 164)

Make a conscious effort to use The System for a week and keep a diary or daily log of your experiences. Try to be aware of how and when you use the various steps of the process of interaction (e.g., gathering information, decision-making). Try also to get in touch with the part your PFLs and patterns play in your efforts.

EVALUATION: Did deliberately trying to use The System make a difference in your usual ways of living? Did you gain more awareness and experience greater openness as a result of your conscious effort? What and how did you feel as you experienced using The System?

FOLLOW-UP: Continue to try to consciously use The System—working to achieve progress, not perfection. Try to become aware of how you use The System and try to get in touch with whether you use it in an open manner.

REFERENCES

1. Mullahy, Patrick: Psychoanalysis and interpersonal psychiatry: the contributions of Harry Stack Sullivan, New York, 1970, Science House, Inc., p. 246.
2. Ibid., pp. 245-246.
3. Howells, John G.: Theory and practice of family psychiatry, New York, 1971, Brunner/Mazel, Inc., pp. 25-26.
4. Coleman, James C.: Types of adjustive reactions. In Hamachek, Don E., editor: Human dynamics in psychology and education, Boston, 1970, Allyn & Bacon, Inc., p. 639.
5. Wolberg, Lewis R.: The technique of psychotherapy, vol. 1, ed. 2, New York, 1972, Grune & Stratton, Inc., pp. 181 and 469-472.
6. Ruesch, Jurgen: Synopsis of the theory of human communication. In Howells, John G., editor: Theory and practice of family psychiatry, New York, 1971, Brunner/Mazel, Inc., pp. 243-247.
7. Rogers, Carl R.: On becoming a person, Boston, 1961, Houghton Mifflin Co., pp. 111-113.
8. Nierenberg, Gerald I.: The art of negotiating, New York, 1968, Hawthorn Books, Inc.
9. Satir, Virginia: Conjoint family therapy, Palo Alto, Calif., 1964, Science & Behavior Books, Inc., pp. 13-18.
10. Ibid., p. 13.
11. Maslow, A. H.: Self-actualization and beyond. In Hamachek, Don E., editor: Human dynamics in psychology and education, Boston, 1970, Allyn & Bacon, Inc., p. 177.
12. McGinnis, Thomas C.: Your first year of marriage, Garden City, N.Y., 1967, Doubleday & Co., Inc., pp. 55-65.
13. Rogers, op. cit., p. 115.

chapter 11

MAKING THE SYSTEM WORK FOR YOU

This chapter is perhaps the single most exciting part of this book. Your use of the information and the instructions in this section can help you open yourself and your life to the limitless possibilities of personal and interpersonal growth. If you choose to embark on this adventure, you will have started on a journey of a lifetime because this is *a journey into self*—past, present, and future. It will take you into those rarely explored countries of your own and other people's minds and hearts. This journey can be one of continual discovery and fascination as you travel through life. The *Interactional Therapeutic System* will provide you with the map, the routes, and the vehicles. Your passport is your humanness.

The material in this chapter is intended to teach you how to apply The System consciously, constructively, and directly to your own life. If you do this, you can increase your awareness of your identity—who you are now, how you got to be who you are now, and who you might become. If you choose to implement your awareness, then you can discover alternative ways of thinking, feeling, and acting; you will most likely encounter difference and newness. As a result of these experiences, you give yourself opportunities to change and to grow, and this growth can enable you to develop greater personal and interpersonal competence and to become more open and more autonomous.

In effect, this is material you can use for a lifetime. If you learn to use The System and develop expertise in using it, you will be building in the tools for experiencing your own and others' humanness and for being more human with others.

SOME HELPFUL GUIDELINES

Some guidelines follow that will help you as you use The System. Although they are presented here in a particular sequence, you will find that you will cross and recross your own path and that you will probably be doing a number of different things at the same time. For example, you may be working with your defenses at the same time that you are implementing and building in an insight.

1. Try to get and to stay in touch with your insides. As you do so, you will be gathering valuable information and learning about who you are now and how you got to be that way.

2. To the best of your ability, try to accept yourself as you are now. For example, try not to kick yourself for what you may consider weaknesses or stupidity or flaws in you. Try to remember that you are human, and therefore you have psychological strengths and scars.

3. Any invitation to change—no matter how gentle, no matter how positive, and no matter how exciting—offers some degree of threat to your established ways of thinking, feeling, and acting. Since you have spent a lifetime building your self-system and life-style, you cannot expect to be strongly motivated to change it. Because this is so, you will need to encourage your-

self to try learning about yourself and letting some differences into your life. You can enter into and engage in changing *if and when you choose.* But keep in touch with your motivation, check it out frequently, and work on motivating yourself to keep on trying.

4. A knowledge of the past can be an effective tool in aiding you in the here and now and in the future. Who you are and what you do now and in the future are inextricably linked with influences exerted on you in the past. Thus if you gain some awareness of and feel for what happened as you were growing up, you will be able to identify many of the sources of your identity in the present, an ability that is necessary to bring about change and qualitative growth.

In addition, an awareness of how you have functioned in the past can help you in the present. For example, suppose you start feeling terribly "down." If you have been able to cope with feeling down in the past, then you have some assurance that you can probably do so again. Furthermore, you probably learned some techniques during your earlier experience that can help you in your present situation. Thus although it may be a source of some of your current problems or difficulties, the past can also be a source of important information and guidance. In this sense then it is your friend and ally.

5. As you gather information and acquire insights, try to relate what you learn to all three areas of human functioning—thinking, feeling, and acting. In other words, do not be satisfied with just acquiring intellectual insight; try to gain emotional and behavioral insight also.

6. Try to implement your insights in all three areas, also.

7. Anxiety and defensiveness are natural responses to newness and change. Just knowing this helps to attenuate their negative influence. Furthermore, once you are aware that anxiety arouses defenses, you are in a position to work thoughtfully, carefully, and sensitively with them, and by doing so, you can ordinarily work them through. If necessary, you can get another person to help and support you, or you can back off.

8. **Difference** does *not* mean antithesis. Rather it means something that is just not exactly the same as your usual way. In fact, difference can be so minute that it feels almost the same, but it is not because it *is* dissimilar. **Newness**, however, means a big or noticeable difference.

Do not be fooled into thinking that difference and newness mean taking the extreme opposite position (e.g., moving from cold rationality to impulsive emotionality). To swing so radically from one extreme to the other is indeed to change. However, for most people this kind of change is not constructive and does not mean growth. A few people are able to benefit by such big shifts, but most people merely get themselves into emotional hot water. Thus the following is the best guideline: take it easy—one small step at a time.

YOUR USE OF THE SYSTEM

The remainder of this chapter is devoted to teaching you how to apply The System to your own life. PFLs and patterns will receive primary consideration, since a complete discussion of self-concept and Child/Parent/Adult balance would make the chapter unwieldy.

We will deal with patterns first rather than PFLs (even though PFLs are smaller than patterns and are the foundation for them) because a pattern is an observable phenomenon. Thus it is easier to spot your patterns when you are first using The System because they have public, interpersonal dimensions, which can be helpful to you. You can watch for, see, and feel a pattern in operation; so can other people, and therefore they can help you identify them. In addition, the repetitious nature of patterns makes them more noticeable.

However, since patterns are the implementation of PFLs you cannot get far in an investigation of yourself without looking for PFLs. Thus the next step will be to help you identify and work with the PFLs that underpin your patterns. Once you get used to working with these two interlocking components, there is no reason why you cannot start with PFLs and move to patterns or vice versa.

Because PFLs and patterns require you to work with fewer psychological positions, the primary focus here is on teaching you how to work with them. Also they are the specifics of your self-system and life-style; when you figure them out and add them up, you get explanations about the workings of the broader, more general, and complex components like self-concept. Furthermore, if you start dealing with self-concept or Child/Parent/Adult balance, you must finally break them down into their specific parts (patterns and PFLs) to understand them fully and to work effectively with them.

Since, as we explained, there is a great deal of criss-crossing among the various steps as you employ them, we have used italics to identify the particular step(s) involved at significant points.

Applying The System to your patterns

To apply The System to your patterns, obviously you first have to determine what your patterns *are*. Depending on how much you already know about yourself, you can utilize one of two basic methods to identify your patterns. One method is to start from scratch; the other is to start with some prior knowledge. Each of these methods focuses on investigating one pattern at a time; to try to work with more than one at once is usually confusing. In addition, you will note that these two methods tend to overlap.

STARTING FROM SCRATCH

If you are setting out with little or no prior knowledge of your patterns, you can start looking by yourself or with another person. If you are at a loss about where to begin, try asking a good friend (or relative) whether any of your actions or responses strike him as repetitive. Since most of us are predictable to some degree, your friend may be able to give you some leads about your consistent ways of responding. If he can give you a lead, try to *gather* as much *information* from him as possible. For example, when has he observed your particular response? In what situations? Who was around at the time? How often has he seen you respond this way?

If you begin your search without a lead from a friend, then the way to initiate it is to become an observer of yourself. Try to observe and evaluate the ways you think, feel, and act. In effect—*watch yourself in action and apply the techniques of intrapersonal communication to what you observe.* Check yourself out. Ask yourself: What am I thinking? What am I feeling? What am I doing? As you do this over and over again, you may begin to notice a certain amount of repetition in some of your ways of responding.

Whether you get to this point as a result of a lead from a friend or your own efforts, you need to check out further. Ask yourself: Do I think or feel or act in the same particular ways over and over again? Do I think or feel or act these ways in similar (or similar-seeming) situations? If you answer "yes," then you can begin to suspect that some kind of pattern exists.

For example, suppose your friend tells you that sometimes you remind her a little of Lucy of *Peanuts* fame. Or suppose you observe yourself in action and catch yourself making nasty comments to a pleasant, unprepossessing Charlie Brown who lives down the street from you. Your sudden awareness may startle you. (Or your friend's comment may have startled you.) Hopefully, the shock of your discovery does not turn you off but rather makes you more alert and observant. **Pattern watching**—searching and being on the lookout for your consistent ways of responding—and **pattern discovering**—finding out what your patterns are—demand that you be attentive and sensitive to your actions and reactions.

Suppose you watch and wait. The next time Charlie Brown (or someone like him) ambles up to you, do you give him another sample of your sharp-tongued wit? Or are you pleasant to him? If you do not make any more nasty remarks to him for a week or longer, you may have to look elsewhere for a pattern. If, however, you check and find that almost every time you run into good old Charlie your tongue drips acid or you boss him around (or both), you have latched onto something that looks and acts suspiciously like a pattern. Watch it closely from now on.

In addition to getting help from a friend or observing your responses in the here and now, there is another way to initiate pattern watching that is sometimes easier and more productive because it allows you to maintain a certain emotional distance and objectivity. Look long and closely at your parents and other Significant Persons in your life and ask: How do they think, feel, and act? What repetitions do I see in their ways of dealing with life? What ways of thinking, feeling, and acting seem automatic, repetitive, and persistent? If you spot consistency in some of these people's responses, then check out your own responses in terms of theirs. Do you share any of their consistent ways of thinking, feeling, and acting? Have you learned from or copied any of these predictable ways? Or do you possibly act in ways that are opposite?

Suppose, for example, you discover that your father is rather passive; he takes all kinds of guff from other people and rarely says anything back to defend himself. Although it is perfectly clear to you that *you* are not passive, do you act in the opposite way? Do you refuse to take anything from anybody? Do you instead attack verbally almost before the other person has a chance to say much to you? Do you flare up and make sarcastic comments if someone does something you do not like?

If you answer "yes" to all or some of these questions, then you might profit from looking at other Significant Persons to see if your responses are modeled after those of one of these people. You would do well to ask: Have I seen or experienced this within my family or with others who have played important roles in my life? Who have I seen act the way I'm acting—or in a way that is similar to mine? Suppose you observe that your mother tends to be sharp-tongued, bossy, and sarcastic—especially to your father. If her responses tend to be repetitive and seem to be rather automatic, then you have probably identified a pattern (or a part of one) of hers. If at times you act the way she does, then you may have found a pattern of your own too. At least, it would be wise to check it out further.

Another helpful aspect of this approach is that once you identify another person's consistent way of responding, you can observe when it occurs and what person(s) and conditions seem to evoke these responses. If you begin to figure out these stimuli, then you can check to see if the same kinds of stimuli set you in motion. For example, suppose you determine that your mother is most sarcastic toward your father, and she tends to guard her tongue more when she is around you and your older brother. But she tends to be sarcastic to your younger brother, who is most like your father. You may infer that your mother's sarcasm occurs especially in response to passivity. If you continue to observe, you may discover that her sarcasm seems to increase in proportion to the passivity she encounters. Thus if your father finally stands up for himself, her sharp tongue either falls silent or softens considerably.

Drawing on these observations, you can check out what and who seems to evoke your sharp tongue. Do you act the same way your mother does or differently? Whatever answers you may garner, this whole approach can help you not only identify a possible pattern but also learn about how it specifically operates when you use it. Does *any* passive person—male or female—

arouse your ire? Or is it just the good old Charlie Browns of this world who call forth your serpent's tongue?

All these approaches, which are designed to help you pattern watch and pattern discover when you are starting from scratch, tend to require primarily intrapersonal effort. However, if you want to get help and support from another person and thereby use both an intrapersonal and interpersonal approach, by all means do so. Frequently, another person can see what we may have trouble seeing or may not want to see.

STARTING WITH SOME PRIOR KNOWLEDGE

The following example illustrates the second method you can use to identify a pattern. In addition, it explains how you can apply The System to a pattern to modify or change it.

Suppose you already know you are somewhat like Lucy—that you have a tendency to be sharp-tongued, bossy, and sarcastic. Even to recognize that much about yourself puts you farther down the road than many people. But where does your knowing this much really get you? Do you stop being this way once you realize it? Probably not. Even though you know that your tendency turns people off, you do not seem to be able to refrain from being that way. So now what? Instead of just sweeping through life, turning the Charlie Browns of the world upside down and inside out with your acid wit and aggressive putdowns, you start trying to *gather information* about your tendency. You may ask a friend to help you, or you may do it alone.

Using the intrapersonal communication process, you can check what you are thinking when you get sarcastic. You will also want to find out the specifics of when you get sarcastic, to whom, and under what particular conditions. In effect you are looking for the **situational triggers** for your tendency. For example, suppose you start closely observing your behavior when you are with females. Are you sarcastic and bossy with them? Or are you this way only toward males? Are you sarcastic around some people of either sex and not sarcastic around other people of either sex? If you can figure who specifically triggers your tendency, then you can concentrate on these particular people.

At the same time you are *gathering information,* you can also be trying to *identify* your *feelings* when you are sarcastic and bossy to someone. Suppose you run into your friend Charlie, who is being his usual, pleasant, vulnerable self. As usual, you are sarcastic and sharp-tongued. However, instead of going on your merry and uncaring way, you stop dead in your tracks and start identifying your feeings. What are you feeling? If you have trouble determining exactly what you are feeling, remember to offer yourself alternatives. Do you feel angry, annoyed, and irritated; smug, superior, and pleased with yourself; or mean, petty, nasty, and ugly? Are you ashamed of yourself and amazed at your own cruelty?

Suppose you are able to *identify,* to hold onto, and to vividly feel your *feelings.* You are extremely irritated, you feel superior, and you feel ugly and ashamed of what you have just done. Now you begin to evaluate each feeling. What exactly irritates you? As you begin to answer this (and other questions), you may be *acquiring insight.* Perhaps you determine that Charlie's vulnerability and his pleasant manner irritate you. It is as though his being nice challenges you to be mean; it is almost as if you cannot stand his being so pleasant and happy, so you "have" to ruin it for him. But what do you gain from ruining his pleasant moment? You begin to realize that ruining his pleasure allows you to feel superior to him because you can belittle him and make him feel bad, whereas you (apparently) come out of the incident unscathed. You *know* better than to wander around being happy; now you have taught him a lesson!

What about your feeling ugly and ashamed of yourself? Although it may seem paradoxical, a mixture of conflicting feelings is perfectly natural. That is, you like

Charlie, but you cannot stand his being so vulnerable and so nice. Now if you examine your mixed feelings and the order in which they occur, you may *acquire* further *insight.* You begin to realize that first you get irritated; next you act on your irritation, and your actions (sarcasm, acid wit, put-downs) evoke feelings of superiority over him. Then you feel ashamed of yourself because you have been so mean *(acquiring insight).*

When you examine and evaluate your feelings, you conclude that to become irritated with Charlie simply because he is pleasant, friendly, and vulnerable is not an appropriate response *(negotiation).* Feeling superior because you have put him down, that is, because you have bested Charlie, is appropriate in the sense that you *did* "win." But is your feeling of superiority appropriate if you measure your "win" against accomplishments that legitimately and realistically signify that a person is, in fact, superior.

The most appropriate feeling in your mixture is being ashamed of what you have done. It is not likely you would feel proud of yourself (although some people would). When you add everything up, the only appropriate feeling you have is the result of two other inappropriate feelings and your actions toward Charlie.

Everyone is entitled to a few inappropriate feelings and actions once in a while. The difference here is that with the insight you have acquired, you know that what just occurred between you and Charlie cannot be chalked up simply as one of those random moments. So you begin *negotiating* with yourself. You assemble, identify, and examine everything that you have learned so far. Your evaluation is that your actions with Charlie are too complex and that the feelings your behavior arouses in you are too important to ignore.

Since you have *decided* this much, you start trying to *develop alternatives.* You can try to be nicer to Charlie from now on. You can try to avoid him. You can try to ignore your behavior. You can try to blame it all on Charlie. Or you can keep working with your tendency and with this incident and try to learn more.

Suppose you *decide* to work with yourself to try to learn more. Your first *implementation* of this decision may be to try to find out if there is any discernible pattern to your tendency. To determine this, you need to *gather information* about your feelings and your behavior and evaluate them according to two criteria: First, are they repetitive? (Do you keep feeling and acting the same way each time you get into this situation?) Second, are they automatic? (Do you feel these feelings and act this way without even being aware of it or without thinking ahead what you will say, do, or feel)?

As you implement your decision to learn more, you will be gathering more information, identifying feelings, and negotiating by means of the process of intrapersonal (and perhaps also interpersonal) communication. Taking each part of the incident and your behavior at a time, you evaluate what is going on with you. Are your feelings of irritation, superiority, and shame repetitive? Is your sarcastic put-down technique repetitive? Do you consistently feel and act this way in response to this type of person or situation? That is, do you merely feel and act these ways once in a while, or do you feel and act these same ways every time you meet one of the Charlie Browns of the world?

Do you automatically feel and act these ways? Do you react to the sight of Charlie's smiling face like a bull to a red flag? Are you aware of what you are about to do before you do it? Or do you just move right in and cut Charlie to shreds before you or he even knows what has happened? If you answer "yes" to these questions, then you have a pattern.

To work more constructively with your pattern, it would help to know even more. How did you get this pattern? Where does it come from? You could start by asking yourself simply, "Where have I seen behavior like this before?" A faster way is to ask yourself if either of your parents acts this way. When you do, do not let difference in sex block your thinking: that is, if you are a female, do not discount your father as a possible influence; if you are a male, the same is true for your mother. In this instance, suppose you realize that you have seen your mother be sarcastic and sharp-tongued to your father, not just once but over and over again. In fact, you cannot remember a time when you have not seen your mother act this way toward your father. Now take a good, long, close thoughtful look at your father. Is he a Charlie Brown type? Or at least did he act like a Charlie around your mother?

It is at moments like this—when you are acquiring insight and when you are beginning to discover some of the less than pleasant facts about your parents and about yourself—that the going can get rough. In this instance you are having to face certain truths that you may have blurred or blocked out before. One is that although your father is a nice, easy-going sort of guy, he is overly passive, vulnerable, and not very self-assertive. You realize that you feel anger and contempt toward him because he never seems to stand up for his rights. Another truth is that your mother has pretty consistently put your father down for as long as you can remember and that you consider her to be unpleasantly aggressive and shrewish. Perhaps the truth that is hardest to take is this: you have long cherished the belief that you are different from your mother. Now you discover that you are not so different after all; in fact, you have built in a part of her that you dislike and disapprove of.

CHANGING YOUR PATTERN

So what happens now? If you do not like this pattern or if you do not like its automatic, repetitive nature, you can decide to work on modifying or altering or getting rid of it. Since we build patterns in, there is no reason we cannot build them out. But how? The "how" takes a lot of vigilance, a lot of work, and a lot of time. After all, you did not build the patterns overnight. So watch for the pattern and be prepared to *implement* alternative ways of acting.

The next time a Charlie Brown ambles up to you, be alert for the first stirrings of the pattern. Feel as sharply as you can the feelings that just his presence and behavior arouse in you. And then in any way you can (short of murder or other illegal acts), break in to your pattern. *Act differently from the way you have always acted.* Act as if you do not have this particular pattern. Do not worry if Charlie irritates you beyond reason—you do not *have* to be sarcastic to him. If you cannot stand it after a few moments, then cut and run. But do it differently. Let yourself *feel* the differences. Never mind what Charlie may think. At this point, you are not doing this for his benefit; you are doing it for *you.*

Suppose you are sarcastic to Charlie before you even realize what you are doing. Then break into the pattern at the next point: instead of glorying in your superiority, apologize to Charlie. Or, better yet, apologize to him and explain what is going on. You might be surprised at his response.

Incidentally, if you zoom through the pattern before you even know you have done it, try to break into it afterward. Instead of hanging your head in shame (which is a part of the pattern), try not to feel so bad about it and resolve to try again. Part of interrupting this pattern is a matter of accepting yourself as being something less than perfect.

Whatever measures you take and however you decide to deal with your patterns, you are likely to encounter certain demands and feelings. Pattern watching and pattern discovering take time, patience, and sharp observation. They also take a willingness to try to be honest about what you think and feel and do. Often these processes are plain hard work. When you do begin to understand your patterns and start trying to break into them, that takes more hard work. Furthermore, you will probably experience some feelings of discomfort—anxiety, annoyance, and phoniness.

This is natural, since change means giving up to some degree that which is familiar to you and that which tends to help you stay comfortable.

In addition, you may experience times of inertia and other times of backsliding. These also are natural. You do not change a pattern of fifteen or twenty years' standing without needing to rest occasionally or without wanting at times to go back to your old, familiar ways. Finally, try not to be too impatient with yourself or with circumstances when you find that your patterns are persistent and cannot be changed overnight. You may have taken from ten to fifteen to twenty years to build them in, so it is hardly reasonable to expect that you can build them out of your self-system and life-style in ten or twenty tries. Give yourself time and keep at it.

When you manage to break into a pattern—when you manage to do it differently—pat yourself on the back and allow yourself to feel a sense of triumph. It is these moments of delight and excitement at having accomplished something different and constructive that will help to motivate you to try again. And as you try and keep on trying, you will begin to experience the joy of having more control over who you are and the pleasure of becoming more autonomous and less of an automaton.

Applying The System to your PFLs

The other primary procedure for facilitating change and growth consists of working with your PFLs. Since PFLs inform, energize, and provide the shape and content of patterns, often it pays to deal directly with them rather than a pattern, especially if you are having trouble spotting or working with your patterns. Sometimes PFLs are easier to manage because they are the smallest units of the self-system and therefore may be less overwhelming than the larger units, patterns. Because they are the smallest units, PFLs are the basic building blocks of change and growth. If you alter PFLs, you are of necessity affecting your patterns because they are interrelated.

HOW TO BEGIN WITH YOUR PFLs

The key way for you to get in touch with your PFLs is to use the intrapersonal communication process in conjunction with your memory. Ask yourself: What rules have I heard and/or been taught to follow all my life? What rules do I live by now? What expectations? What values? What do I think now about such things as money, sex, education, trust, friendship, politics, and happiness? What do I feel? How do I act? What are the instructions or orders or guidelines that I "hear" in my head, feel in my heart, and respond to with my body? Who and what are *my* drummers?

Drawing on your memory, try to recapture what you were taught as you were growing up. But try to keep in mind that PFLs are conveyed in various ways. Perhaps the easiest ones to spot are those that were taught by direct verbal communication. Even so, remember that some or many of these may have been passed on to you as "famous family sayings" (e.g., "time is money," "the early bird gets the worm"). Frequently, these are more difficult to identify because they have become so familiar, so ingrained in you that you no longer "hear" them on a conscious level.

Remember, too, that many PFLs are taught nonverbally. To get at these, try recreating scenes from your childhood; imagine as vividly as you can how Significant Persons acted. Did your parents touch each other affectionately? Did they ever hit each other? How did they look at each other—with hatred, with pity, with concern, or with love? How did they look at you? What tones of voice did people habitually use? How often were your parents silent? When and under what circumstances were they silent? Were they noisy? Suppose your father habitually slammed doors—not in anger, but just as a matter of course. Did this give you a PFL that "fathers (or all adults) don't have to be careful about making a racket"? Did it teach you disregard for other people's noise rights? Or did it teach you to respect other people's noise rights?

Keep in mind also that PFLs can be taught by omission. These are perhaps the most difficult to get at because you have to think back and try to recall what things were *not* talked about or mentioned. For example, suppose you are deathly afraid of thunderstorms, yet you cannot remember anybody ever saying anything about them. At this point, you may be tempted to chalk off your fear as a stupid, irrational one with a totally mysterious origin. *Do not.* Think back. Feel back. What do you remember about thunderstorms when you were growing up? When a storm occurred, where were you? What did you do? What did you feel? Who else was around? What were they doing? What did they seem to be feeling? If you remember that the dog hid under the bed and whimpered while your mother talked a blue streak about anything but the storm the whole time it was occurring, then you may have tracked down the PFL source. What PFL did you learn? Depending on how you interpreted what you experienced, it might be "be terrified of thunderstorms." Or "thunderstorms could kill you." Or "there is no security anywhere during an electrical storm." Or "pretend the storm isn't happening and maybe you won't be so frightened." Thus the origin of these PFLs—taught by omission and avoidance—is not really such a mystery after all. In addition, you might do well to check out other possible "fear" or "unpleasantness" PFLs to see if you have developed a composite PFL that says, "when you're frightened of something pretend it doesn't exist (and maybe it will go away)."

In the process of *gathering information* about your PFLs, if you are able to discover one or more, it is important that you not stop there. PFLs come in packets, and it is from these packets that you will have your best chance to identify your composite PFLs. If you have a PFL about a particular subject, you can be sure it belongs to a packet that contains related PFLs about the same subject. For example, suppose you find that you have the PFL: "You should respect and obey people in authority." If you think and feel some more about this one, you can probably discover others that belong to the same packet, including some of the following: "Respect and obey your parents, teachers, policemen, clergymen, and the government"; "Respect and obey the laws they represent"; "It is wrong to go against authority"; "Those in authority are almost always right"; "You will be punished if you go against authority"; or "Feel bad (guilty, awful, wicked, sinful) if you challenge authority." You might derive the following composite PFL from this packet: "Always obey those in authority. If you go against authority, then you can expect (and you ought) to be punished."

Approaching PFLs as members of packets rather than an isolated entities has three important benefits.

1. If you discover and spread your PFLs out before you, you will be able to see and feel the impressive role they play in your life. If your PFLs are mostly negative, you will have collected irrefutable evidence of how limiting and closed your self-system and life-style tend to be. There are few things more convincing than seeing a long list of PFLs that belong to you and that in effect control you.

2. If you discover a large number of PFLs in many different areas of your life, you can begin to make accurate deductions about what attitudes, what feelings, and what actions are forbidden or encouraged. Information of this sort can help you develop a fairly clear notion of the basic "flavor" of your style. For example, good old Charlie Brown's list of PFLs about relating to other people might include the following: "Don't show (or feel) anger." "Don't talk back." "Don't pick fights." "Avoid arguments." "Always try to be pleasant." "Turn the other cheek." "Be friendly." "Nobody likes a loud-mouth."

"It's not right to impose your will on others." "Always obey the rules and laws." "If anybody's going to be wrong, it'll be you." "Who are you to demand so much attention?" "A soft answer turneth away wrath." "Don't be competitive, pushy, aggressive, boisterous, or forward." "The meek shall inherit the earth." "Silence is golden." "Don't stick your neck out; you'll only get your head chopped off." "Be careful." "Don't make waves." "Smile." "Grin and bear it." "People will like you better if you don't hassle them."

This is a powerful packet of PFLs that yields the following powerful and dominating composite PFL: "Don't be aggressive; *be passive!*" If Charlie compiles such a list and figures out the composite PFL, which synthesizes the instructions given by this packet, he will become painfully aware of having discovered a potent pattern and its roots. To make sure, however, he needs to check out his discoveries by watching to see if he consistently acts on these PFLs and others like them. If he finds notable consistency, he has found a pattern—and an important pattern, at that.

3. This approach can help lead you to other, related composite PFLs and their packets. In other words, if you have a central *don't* PFL, look for another major directive that is negative, for example, "Beware of . . . ." If you have packets of *beware* PFLs, your composite PFL might instruct you to be passive and mistrustful. If this were so, your packets would probably include messages such as "beware of getting involved," and "beware of others; they'll try to cheat you if you give them half a chance." Or your composite PFL might be less concerned with distrust than with fear. Then your packets would tend to include messages such as "beware of your emotions—they'll make you vulnerable and you'll get hurt." Suppose you look at another directive such as "*you aren't*" and find the following PFLs: "You aren't strong enough to face problems alone"; "You aren't smart enough to protect yourself against the dangers of life"; and "You aren't very good at figuring things out for yourself, are you?" This packet has the flavor of fear mixed with the need for someone stronger to help you, that is, dependency.* The composite PFL then might be one instructing you to rely on others for strength and help.

In your attempts to discover packets and to determine your composite PFLs, keep in mind that a composite PFL may never have been communicated verbally to you. It is possible, for example, that no one ever came right out and said to Charlie Brown, "Don't be aggressive; be passive." However, that is the loud and clear message that his packet of PFLs sends him, and, no doubt, Significant Persons sent loud and clear nonverbal messages to Charlie to be passive.

HOW TO CONTINUE WITH YOUR PFLs

Gathering as much *information* as possible about your PFLs is extremely important, but since the process of gathering information is primarily an intellectual one, it is not enough. To acquire insights, which can aid you in making significant changes, it is necessary that you *identify* and get in touch with your *feelings* about your PFLs and the feelings you experience when you act on them. In this way, you can *acquire insights* that are a blend of thinking, feeling, and acting.

Thus it is necessary for you to answer as many of these questions as possible: What do you think about your PFLs? What do they mean? How do they affect your thinking? What do you feel about them? What do they mean emotionally to you? How do they affect your feelings? What do you

*Incidentally, we do not mean to imply by this discussion that a central PFL such as "don't!" necessarily means that you will be passive. *Don't* PFLs can just as well teach someone to be aggressive ("Don't let anyone tell you what to do.") or impulsive ("Don't think so much—just do it.") You must know the *content* and *application* of the PFLs before you can determine what kind of style will evolve from them.

feel when you obey or rebel against them? What do you do with them? What do they mean in terms of action? How do they affect your action? Only when you have this kind of tridimensional grasp of your PFLs (or any other component of your self-system) can you deal most fully and effectively with them. If your PFLs—your reactions to them and your understanding of them—are limited to one or two areas of functioning, then your whole self-system is limited in the same way. Acting on one or two of the areas (thinking, feeling, and acting) and accepting or rejecting PFLs without careful thought about or considerable attention to the other area(s) of functioning is to put on blinders and to limit your functioning. To work in a constructive way with your self-system and life-style (in this case, your PFLs) you need to gain insights that take into account all three areas of functioning.

Another part of acquiring tridimensional insight is determining your feelings in regard to your PFLs. To do this you need to ask yourself various questions: When do I use a particular PFL? How often? Where? With whom? Under what circumstances? How do I feel when I use it? Essentially what you are trying to do is identify your feelings about your PFL and determine how it serves you. For example, assume that you have the following PFL: "If you don't have something nice to say, don't say anything at all." Suppose you figure out that you act on this PFL whenever you feel negative about yourself, others, situations, or anything. In fact, you have a reputation for being, calm, pleasant, and kind, a reputation for never saying a mean thing about anybody. As you investigate how you feel when you use this PFL, you begin to realize that your feelings follow a certain order. First, you feel negative, which calls the PFL into action. Then you feel guilty for feeling negative. But when you follow the PFL and determinedly shut your mouth on whatever negative statement you were ready to make, you feel thwarted and irritated. By the time you are through obeying this PFL, you feel thoroughly frustrated and annoyed because you have kept silent.

If these are the ways you feel when you obey your PFL, there must be some reason you use it in spite of your feelings. What purposes does it serve? People think you are nice because you never say anything mean about anyone. For the same reason, you also think you are okay. Moreover, using this PFL tends to keep you out of arguments, out of the limelight, and out of trouble. The other purposes it serves, however, are not so positive. It keeps you from getting more involved with yourself or with others. It can also make you look as though you do not have opinions or care about many things or know much. And although the PFL helps you in one way to think well of yourself, you may also have to deal with another, less pleasant feeling that you are hypocritical—that is, you feel negative, but you act pleasant and positive.

CHANGING YOUR PFLs

When you get to this point in the process of gathering information, identifying feelings, and acquiring insights about a PFL (or a packet of them), *you are ready to negotiate with yourself:* Do you want to keep your PFL as it is? Do you want to modify it? Do you want to try to get rid of it altogther? Do you want to substitute another PFL for this one? Do you have the motivation to try something different or something new?

As a part of your negotiating, you need to examine and evaluate the effects of your PFL(s). With the PFL against saying negative things, for example, you might decide that your dishonesty in the form of your silence affects the way others relate to you, that your feeling hypocritical undermines your ability to feel comfortable with yourself, and that suppressing negative thoughts and feelings means suppressing positive thoughts and feelings too—you simply do not express much of anything because you are so well trained to suppress.

You also need to *develop alternatives* to

your PFL and to evaluate those alternatives. For example, you might consider the following alternatives: You will simply say whatever comes into your head and heart; you will express your negative feelings only to your most trusted friends but not to the person who aroused the feeling; you will at least try to identify your negative feelings, hold them, feel them, and then try to determine what has evoked them; or you will try this last alternative but, in addition, will attempt to report your feelings to the person who evoked them if and when it is appropriate to do so.

You need to negotiate with yourself to decide what you want to do with the PFL. How appropriate is each alternative? How much risk is involved in each alternative? How much anxiety? What are you willing to do? Which alternative (or mixture of alternatives) will you try to implement?

You need to *implement* your decision. When you do put one of the alternatives into effect, remember that you will probably experience some discomfort because you are working with difference and newness. But remember also that unless you allow yourself to experience difference and newness, you cannot hope to change and grow.

CHARLIE BROWN CHANGES SOME PFLs

Let us now observe Charlie Brown as he uses The System to alter or change some of his PFLs. Suppose Charlie has *gathered information, identified* his *feelings,* and *acquired insight* about some of his "passive PFLs." He *negotiates* with himself and *decides* he wants to become less passive (not aggressive, just less passive). He especially wants to get rid of those worthless PFLs that direct him to "grin and bear it" and to "turn the other cheek." So good old Charlie *develops* some *alternatives* and *decides* that he will try to modify these two PFLs (knowing that if he alters one or two, his actions will affect other PFLs also).

How will Charlie go about altering his PFLs? What are his alternatives? Yelling at Lucy the next time she pounces on him or poking her in the nose? No. Those would be complete reversals for Charlie. He decides that he will *not* smile pleasantly the next time Lucy lets him have it, and he will *not* turn the other cheek. Instead, the next time Lucy comes along and delivers one of her devastating broadsides, Charlie *acts differently* from his usual way. He does not stand there wringing his cap or helplessly saying "Good grief!" while Lucy sails off in triumph, nor does he smile and say nothing.

What does he do? Charlie speaks up! "Wait a minute, Lucy. What you just said really hurt my feelings and I don't like that. So please don't do it again." Charlie looks Lucy straight in the eye. He does not look away. He does not say he is sorry. And *he does not smile.* In fact, if he has any strength left, he may muster up a slight growl or at least a frown.

Imagine Lucy's surprise. Interestingly enough, no matter what Lucy says or does—even though she may make another devastating remark—she cannot take Charlie's experience of difference away from him. It is true that Charlie may have to spend the rest of the day recovering from his surprise at his own boldness and from his worry about Lucy's hating him. But the point is that he has done it, and if he has done it once, *he can do it again* and again—until he makes significant alterations in his seemingly (to him) unchangeable PFLs.

As Charlie continues to work on significantly altering these and other PFLs, he will gradually be changing the nature of his PFLs. They will stop being ironclad *rules* ("You *must* grin and bear it") and become guidelines ("Grinning and bearing it is one way to handle a sticky situation, and I'm free to act this way if I think and feel it's appropriate. But I'm also free to object and refuse if I think and feel that that is not an appropriate way to act."). When Charlie moves away from rules to guidelines, he is on his way to greater openness and autonomy.

Self-concept and Child/Parent/Adult balance

In this chapter we have deliberately limited our considerations to PFLs and patterns. However, it is not really possible to ignore self-concept and the Child/Parent/Adult balance. Because the parts of the self-system and life-style are so interrelated, the treatment of any one part touches on (at least by extension) every other part. If we talk about PFLs, we are talking about the things that shape and direct patterns; patterns implement PFLs and are the ways we think, feel, and act in relation to our self-concept; self-concept is built on patterns and PFLs; and the Child/Parent/Adult balance is a particular way of viewing the relationships among PFLs, patterns, and self-concept. All these components, taken together, form the self-system and the life-style. Each smaller unit is a building block for the next larger unit, all the way up to the largest units, the self-system and life-style.

Since this interrelationship exists, it follows that what happens in one part of the self-system and life-style will affect all the other parts. That is one of the joyous aspects of The System. If, for example, you loosen the hold of one PFL, you loosen the rigidity of the packet to which it belongs. If you make the packet less rigid, you ease the tightness of the pattern which that packet directs. Gradually, as you modify and temper a number of packets of PFLs and a number of patterns, your self-concept begins to change. Because altering PFLs, patterns, and self-concept means becoming more open and more autonomous, you are of necessity affecting the Child/Parent/Adult balance by helping the Adult in you to gain strength and to grow.

Even if you cannot immediately see or feel much difference in yourself when you successfully break in to any part of your self-system and life-style, try to be patient. If you keep at it, change and growth will come—if not today, then tomorrow; if not tomorrow, then next week; if not next week, then next month. Remember that you have embarked on the journey of a lifetime, and each step—no matter how small—contributes to your progress. Whether it be challenging a PFL, breaking a pattern, looking at something in a new way, sensing an alternative, deciding to act differently, feeling a feeling, or tentatively trying to communicate with someone, each step places you in a slightly different position from the one you occupied before. By experiencing difference, you become slightly different from who you were before, and you start growing. The final goal is not so all important (and who knows exactly what anyone's final goal consists of), so do not miss the scenery along the way by straining your eyes to see the final goal. What is truly exciting is not so much the final goal but the process of growing more human, more autonomous, and more open. The joy is in the journey.

Where should you begin?

Having read the book to this point, you may feel that you are faced with a dilemma. If it is possible to work with any part of the self-system and life-style, which part is it *best* to start with? Other questions are relevant to this dilemma as well. What subject matter should you try to deal with first? Family relationships, friendships, education, sex, money, goals, expectations, social life, marriage, or jobs? Should you start with the past, present, or future? Which should you begin with—thoughts, feelings, or actions? Should you try to work first on an intrapersonal or on an interpersonal level? The answer to all these questions is that because of the interlocking nature of the self-system and life-style and of The System, it really does not matter where you start or what you work with. As long as you try to be honest with yourself and others, as long as you try to keep to specifics, and as long as you try to get and stay in touch with your insides, then you cannot go wrong.

You may also be wondering if there is any best or better order to follow once you start. No. The organization of the book presents you with one possible structured way to proceed, but once you understand The System, there is no reason you cannot develop and follow the order and procedure that suits you.

THREE GUIDELINES

As you use The System, we urge you to keep three particular guidelines in mind.

Balance. Try to keep some kind of balance in whatever you do, a balance among whatever parts you deal with—past, present, or future; subject matter; intrapersonal and interpersonal interaction; or thoughts, feelings, and actions. For example, try not to concentrate just on feelings to the exclusion or denial of thoughts and actions. If you try to maintain this kind of balance, over a period of time you will find that seemingly unrelated pieces fall into place so that a clear picture of self will emerge from the apparent jumble of pieces.

Building in. When you do something a significant number of times, it is inevitable that you will build it in and make it a part of your repetoire. It is perhaps disconcerting that a child inevitably builds in much of what is presented to him as he grows up, including a lot of negative material. But it is heartening to consider the other side of the coin: if you work at consciously and deliberately using The System again and again, you will inevitably build in your developing personal and interpersonal competence. That is what contributes to long-term growth. Perhaps what is most exciting is that as you build in what you learn from utilizing The System, you are building in the ways *you choose* to live your life. That is what we mean by growth toward openness and autonomy.

Teaching The System to others. Teaching what you have learned is the ultimate in implementation: it will help you clarify your knowledge, increase your understanding, sharpen your skills, gain greater expertise and competence, and feel yourself in action. To teach something well, you must *really* know it, feel it, and do it. And that is the essence of The System.

Teaching The System will benefit not only you but those you teach. Constricted by narrow and closed self-systems and life-styles that they have acquired they know not where or how, too many people live out their lives in a desert of boredom, quiet desperation, unfulfilled hopes, and deep loneliness. But life does not have to be like that. People *can* learn to become more open; they *can* learn how to tap their own wellsprings of strength, inner richness, and creative power. That is where you come in. If each of us who knows how to use The System teaches it to at least one other person, we can begin to make the desert flower.

> In the deserts of the heart,
> Let the healing fountain start. . . . *

Concluding remarks

As we close this part of the book and look ahead to Part III, which will apply The System to dating, living together, marriage, and the family, we wish to comment on two issues. First, real freedom comes not from denial or rebellion but from working through those matters in your life that you find narrowing and constricting, so that you become an independent, decision-making, autonomous adult.

Second, as you become more open, you will find that you have developed methods for maintaining your openness. What will happen is that if you use The System to become more open, you will incorporate it into your life-style as a set of *guidelines for living.* As we have often seen happen, eventually you will think of The System as

---

*From Auden, W. H.: In memory of W. B. Yeats. In Coffin, Charles M., and Roelofs, Gerrit H., editors: The major English poets: English and American, ed. 2, New York, 1969, Harcourt, Brace & World, Inc., p. 533.

something you thought of because it will have become yours.

The following chapters are designed to help you apply your knowledge of dating, marriage, and the family and your understanding of The System to any two-person (or more) relationships. These chapters focus on the dynamics of relationships, a subject requiring a fairly thorough grasp of The System. Thus we urge you to review the chapters in Part II before you read further so that your understanding will be enhanced.

The chapters that follow are designed to encourage and enable you to apply the understanding and skills you have learned about yourself and others to dating, going steady, being engaged, living together, marriage, and family and indeed to all your relationships. These chapters explain the dynamics of human relationships, that is, how they work and why. Once you understand these dynamics, you are in a position to make maximum use of your knowledge and your skill in applying The System in developing and maintaining more open relationships.

part three

THE DYNAMICS OF HUMAN RELATIONSHIPS

chapter 12

DEVELOPING MORE OPEN RELATIONSHIPS dating, going steady, being engaged, living together

Part I discussed changes in societal attitudes and values since 1900 and the impact of these changes on dating, marriage, the family, and the individual. In many cases the individual finds himself caught in double binds between rigid, authoritarian, closed PFLs of the past and more open, flexible, self-fulfilling PFLs and situations of the present. The results of this dilemma may take various forms: alienation, depression, confusion, anxiety, unquestioning conformity, denial, or outright (sometimes destructive) rebellion. The greatest hope for the individual who is caught in these binds lies in expanding his awareness and understanding of what has been and is happening to him, his institutions, and his society and in learning what to do about it.

Part II was designed to provide the individual with the knowledge, experience, and skills necessary to becoming more open and autonomous. Thus this part was intended to give encouragement and hope to the individual that there *is* a way to free himself from these double binds—from the chains of the often closed past and the tyranny of the often directionless open present. The Interactional Therapeutic System teaches the way to become more free through awareness and skills that can enable the individual to change and grow and become more open and autonomous.

Part III examines and explains the interpersonal realm in some detail to help the individual change and grow and develop more open relationships. Thus the focus is on the dynamics of relationships—especially dating (this chapter), marriage (Chapter 13), and the family (Chapter 14). This examination centers on learning how relationships function, why they do or do not work, and how they can be made more qualitative. Achieving greater quality means becoming aware of and learning to alter the masks, games, roles, stereotypes, distortions, and closed PFLs that get in the way of open communication and interaction. Achieving greater quality means learning to apply The System to self and to relationships—specifically those of dating, marriage, and the family but ultimately to all relationships.

This chapter is devoted to some of the basic principles that govern relationships. Specifically, the chapter explains the following: (1) how the interplay between outsides and insides affects the perceptions and responses of each person in a relationship and how these perceptions and responses both comprise and influence the dynamics of relationships; (2) how this interplay determines the balance, nature, course, and quality of relationships; and (3) how The System can be applied to the dynamics of relationships to make them more qualitative. Because this chapter is intended as both an introduction to the dynamics of relationships and as an examination of dating,* the dynamics of the

---

*In this chapter, we use the word "dating" to refer to dating, going steady, being engaged, and living together. In essence it refers to any nonmarital, two-person relationship.

dating relationship will be used as the focal point of the discussion. Ultimately the discussion is aimed at helping you understand the dynamics of *all* relationships so that you can apply your understanding and The System to your own relationships.

One specific aim of this chapter is to try to allay some of the anxiety that many people feel when they anticipate the prospect of dating, when they are involved in dating, or both. Often a certain amount of anxiety is natural; dating presents a new and different atmosphere and different expectations from those that people have been used to in their families and groups of friends. Much of the anxiety results from a person's being in a nongroup situation and feeling that his individual actions and decisions are spotlighted by the demands of a one-to-one relationship. Many a person feels stupid, incompetent, doubtful, or awkward. Many a person first experiences these feelings of anxiety in their early teens when dating frequently begins. However, many people experience these feelings (either for the first time or again) in their late teens or early twenties.[1]

But dating does not have to be like this. It does not have to be an agonizing experience of sweaty palms, nervous stammering, embarrassing flushes, or anguished guessing and wondering about what to say or what not to say, what to do or what not to do. Although some anxiety is natural when you are meeting new people or are getting to know someone in a new way or are establishing a new relationship, anxiety need not be the predominant feeling. Rather, we believe that excitement, fascination, wonder, delight, joy, and exhilaration can be the predominant feelings when you involve yourself in new experiences. These feelings are possible if you learn to (and do) communicate effectively and interact openly.[2]

Effective communication and open interaction are important not only because they enable you to experience these positive feelings but also because they can help you to develop healthy dating relationships. This latter ability is crucially important because as you date you are usually moving toward choosing a long-term partner. Thus if you communicate effectively and interact openly, you are taking the best measures possible to ensure that you will make a healthy choice and thereby enormously increase your chances for establishing a healthy long-term relationship, whether it be living together or marriage. This is the reason it is so important for you to learn about yourself and to learn to use The System.

RELATIONSHIPS: SOME BASIC CONCEPTS

The subject of the dynamics of relationships covers an enormous range of human experience. It includes such matters as the kinds of relationship (e.g., social, business, dating, marital); the depth and intensity of the relationship (e.g., casual, close, intimate, intense, passionate); the duration of the relationship (e.g., an hour, a day, a year, many years); the time devoted to the relationship (e.g., a couple of hours a day, a few hours once a week, several hours every day); the purpose of the relationship (e.g., work, companionship, reassurance, family, sex, love); and the quality of the relationship (e.g., hostile, shallow, intense, cooperative, punitive, loving, supportive). Whether a relationship comes into being and whether it will continue or die depend on complex interrelationships among many variables.[3] Part III is devoted to analyzing and explaining these variables and their interrelationships.

In the following analyses of the dynamics of relationships we give numerous examples to cover as many different combinations of variables as possible and to give numerous different perspectives on those dynamics. There is no attempt to cover all possible combinations; instead the ultimate aim is to help you understand the principles governing the dynamics of relationships.

Intrapersonal dynamic equilibrium

Every person brings his self-system and life-style to every relationship he engages in, and every person in every relationship is continuously involved in trying to achieve and maintain his own **intrapersonal dynamic equilibrium** as he takes part in the relationship. That is, he is incessantly trying to acquire or retain that vital balance by which a person keeps his sense of self and stability intact while at the same time allowing for and adjusting to newness, to difference, to change, and to the unfamiliar.* (Refer to the discussion of dynamic equilibrium on pp. 87 to 89.) The equipment the individual utilizes to do his balancing act consists of his self-system and his life-style.[4,5]

Interpersonal dynamic equilibrium

By definition, any relationship involves some kind of connection between at least two entities. As soon as two people "connect," that is, form any kind of relationship (e.g., business, social, casual, friendship, romantic, marital), they become involved in a balancing act between them. A relationship between two people is like being on a seesaw. Each person must try to keep his own balance (intrapersonal dynamic equilibrium). At the same time, he must take the other person into account and make allowances for the other's presence. By means of their mutual and concerted efforts, the two people may be able to keep the seesaw level. However, the weight or greater influence of one may tip the seesaw so that he has his feet on the ground while the other person is dangling in midair. Whatever the particularities, however, the essential fact of a relationship is that it means people are *in relation to* each other. This means that of necessity each must in some way adjust to and make accommodations for the other person. Thus each person must strive to achieve and maintain some kind of balance between him and the other person, which is what we mean by **interpersonal dynamic equilibrium.**

*Whenever we deem it necessary or helpful, we will repeat definitions or explanations that have appeared earlier in the text.

Definition of a relationship

A **relationship** may be defined as the outcome of the moment-to-moment ongoing interaction between at least two people (their self-systems and life-styles); this interaction involves achieving and maintaining some kind of intrapersonal and interpersonal dynamic equilibrium.

Functional and dysfunctional relationships

To carry out the process of establishing and maintaining interpersonal dynamic equilibrium and therefore the relationship, each person uses his self-system and life-style. Because life-style is the observable and/or inferable part of an individual's personality, most people in relationships tend to measure and respond to one another mainly in terms of life-style. This is particularly true when effective communication is limited or nonexistent; without effective communication, it is not possible to learn much about or become aware of what is happening to the other person's insides (his self-system). If such is the case, then the ways of finding and sustaining interpersonal dynamic equilibrium are limited by a lack of information about and a lack of awareness of the other person's thoughts and feelings. Nevertheless, many relationships do exist and do achieve a dynamic equilibrium based on minimal information and awareness and a great number of assumptions, stereotypes, and guesses. Obviously this kind of dynamic equilibrium is frequently a tenuous, fragile, discordant, conflictual, neurotic, or destructive kind of balance. When this is the case, the relationship itself tends to be **dysfunctional.** That is, the relationship works, but its functioning is limited, impaired, or both.[6] Its functioning is less qualitative, less healthy, and less constructive than it might be. Conversely, a **functional** relationship is one in which the functioning is qualitative, healthy, and constructive (e.g., communication is clear and undistorted; patterns of interaction are not automatic and repetitious but are under conscious control).[7]

DYNAMICS OF RELATIONSHIPS

To understand the **dynamics of relationships** (how and why relationships work in the ways they do), it is necessary to examine the interplay that exists between a person's self-system and life-style and that influences his perceptions of others and his responses to them. In addition, it is necessary to consider how this interplay between the self-system and life-style of each partner affects the relationship.

Function of the self-system and life-style in relationships

Every human being takes in, perceives, evaluates, and responds to the world outside him on the basis of his self-system. However, his responses, based on his perceptions and evaluations, are conveyed to the world outside him through his life-style; the patterns of his life-style translate a person's insides into external, observable actions and responses. In effect every person takes in stimuli from the world outside and perceives, interprets, and evaluates them in light of his self-system; his self-system determines his responses; and the interpersonal patterns of his life-style implement the responses determined by the self-system. For example, suppose Don is walking to work, slips on a patch of ice, and falls. A stranger helps him up, smiling as he does so. If Don has a PFL that says, "Cruel people laugh at others' misfortunes and should not be trusted," he may interpret the stranger's smile as a mark of cruel laughter and push the stranger away. If, however, Don has a PFL that says, "People who help others are good and should be appreciated," then he may read the smile as one of concern and relief and accept the stranger's help with thanks.

SELF-SYSTEM: DETERMINER OF INSIDE PERCEPTIONS AND OUTSIDE RESPONSES

How a person perceives, interprets, and reacts to the world outside him depends on his self-system. If a person is aware of and in touch with his self-system, then his self-system is operating primarily on the basis of conscious material. If the self-system is governed essentially by the conscious, if it is not plagued by unresolved conflicts, and if it is not rigid, distorted, and inflexible, then the directions from the self-system, which the life-style implements, are likely to be clearly attuned to the reality of the stimulus from the outside and are therefore appropriate. Thus if someone angrily yells at Sally, whose self-system is basically healthy and undistorted, she probably will not yell back in automatic response, which results from a rigid PFL or a frightened Child position. Instead she will perceive and evaluate the yell in terms of the realities of the situation, in terms of her thoughts and feelings at the moment, and in terms of what might constitute the appropriate response. Then she will implement that response. According to what is appropriate, she may yell back, she may calmly tell the person to stop it, or she may softly ask the person what is wrong and negotiate the matter with him.

Both intrapersonal and interpersonal problems occur when a person is *not* in touch with his insides and when he is *not* aware of the contents or operations of his self-system. Then his self-system operates primarily on the basis of unconscious material, and both his self-system and his life-style are largely controlled by unconscious material. If his self-system is largely governed by the unconscious, if it is plagued by unresolved conflicts, and if it is rigid, distorted, and inflexible, then the directions from the self-system, which the life-style implements, are likely to *not* be clearly attuned to the realities of the stimulus from the outside and are therefore probably inappropriate. For example, suppose someone yells angrily at Celeste, whose self-system is basically rigid and distorted. If Celeste has a rigid PFL that says, "You should never take any guff from anyone," she will automatically yell back. If she has a rigid PFL that says, "If someone yells at you, you shouldn't fly off the handle; if you keep your cool, you'll show the other person you're better than he is," then Celeste will automatically answer in a coldly contemptuous manner. Or if Celeste is burdened by a frightened Child, she may have a PFL directing her to apologize to someone who seems to be angry with her; thus she probably will automatically apologize to the person who yells at her.

The meaning and significance of these phenomena are that a person with a closed self-system will tend to perceive and evaluate stimuli from the world outside him in rigid, often distorted ways; his self-system will give directions to his life-style; and his patterns of response to the outside world will implement these directions automatically, repetitiously, and frequently inappropriately. The ultimate meaning and significance of all this are that what a person says and does (his outsides) can often be distorted, misleading, and inaccurate. When this is so, then his outsides will serve as insufficient (indeed sometimes deceptive) means by which the world can evaluate him.

EXAMPLES OF THE INTERPLAY BETWEEN INSIDES AND OUTSIDES

Since even the most open person has some psychological wrinkles and scars, any relationship that is formed and based primarily on outsides, on life-styles, risks being built on some degree of distortions, faulty perceptions, and misassumptions.

When two people first meet and begin to form a relationship, unless each person effectively communicates about his own and the other's insides and outsides, the relationship will be based primarily on appearances—each person's outsides. Appearances can be enormously appealing, or they can be repellent, and they frequently can be deceiving.

What happens under these circumstances is that Person 1 receives stimuli from Person 2 and perceives and interprets these stimuli according to his self-system. The self-system of Person 1 then directs him to respond in particular ways to these stimuli, and by means of the patterns of communication and interaction of his life-style, he implements the directives and conveys these responses to Person 2. In turn, Person 2 reacts by taking in these responses and perceiving and interpreting them according to *his* self-system, which then directs him to respond in particular ways to these stimuli (the other person's responses). Then through the patterns of communication and interaction of his life-style, he implements the directives and conveys his responses to Person 1. And so it goes, back and forth from moment to moment.

This paradigm of a relationship can be fleshed out in various basic ways.

Example 1. One possibility is that both people can communicate effectively, can interact with awareness and competence, and are basically open and autonomous. Their relationship is likely to be relatively free of distortion, marked by mutual respect, and based on honest communication and open interaction. This kind of relationship is unfortunately rather rare because most people have not been taught to be very open or aware.

Example 2. Another possibility is that two people form a relatively healthy, open relationship based almost totally on their life-styles. That is, neither of them is very aware of or in touch with his insides, and therefore they do not communicate much about their inner thoughts and feelings.

Nevertheless, because each has a self-system that tends not to distort or misinterpret, their relationship will probably be fairly open. Each person says what he means and responds in reasonably clear and direct ways to what the other person says and does.

For example, June and Ted have been living together for five months; prior to that, they dated for eight months, so they know one another's outsides well. Ted tends to be blunt and outspoken: if he does not like something or does not want to do something, he says so in no uncertain terms. Yet he is not a cruel person, and he can be sensitive to another's needs and wishes if he cares enough about the other person. June is rather quiet and shy, but she will speak up if she feels someone is pushing her or if she really wants or needs something. Thus if June casually asks Ted to do something that he does not want to do, he may flatly refuse, and she will tend to accept his refusal, chalking it up to "that's the way he is." If, however, she asks him in a serious and earnest tone or if she says she really needs him to do something with or for her, he will agree, although he may grumble a bit. This then is one of their life-style ways of maintaining their intrapersonal and interpersonal dynamic equilibrium.

Although June's and Ted's relationship tends to be fairly straight and open, it is also rather superficial, since they deal primarily with outsides. There tend to be some distortions simply because outsides per se can be misleading. Thus if Ted comes home feeling sick to his stomach and June asks him to go grocery shopping with her because she has to buy a lot of heavy groceries, he may snap at her and refuse. If Ted is the kind of person who does not say much about sickness and if he continues to feel sick for several days but plays down or says nothing about his nausea, he may snap at June several times during this period. She may then begin to assume on the basis of what is really happening that Ted is angry with her. If she asks him, he will say "no" because he is not angry with her. This situation is obviously a distorted one. Given enough distortions caused by outside circumstances or by a really stressful situation, problems will occur even for people with relationships based on well-matched life-styles.

Example 3. Another basic type of relationship is one in which one of the two people has a self-system that causes him to misperceive or misinterpret or distort the stimuli he is receiving (what the other person says, does, and implies). Thus he in turn sends out distorted stimuli to the other person. Just what this relationship is like depends greatly on the degree of distorting that Person 1 does and the degree of personal and interpersonal competence of Person 2. If Person 2 operates primarily on the life-style level (i.e., he does not communicate much about his own or the other person's insides), then although he may try to deal with the other person's distortions, he is bound to misperceive and misinterpret because he is receiving distorted inputs.

For example, Sarah has a low self-concept. Even though she is a good-looking blond who is intelligent, easygoing, and friendly, she feels woefully inadequate. She sees herself as fat and dumpy, ugly, and rather dull. (She bases this self-concept partly on experience; when she was in junior high, she *was* extremely overweight and not too attractive, and because she felt so bad about herself, she seemed rather dull. Another contributing influence was her parents' overconcern about her at that time.) Underpinning her low self-concept are PFLs that say, "Your true friends are those who like you no matter how you look," "People only give compliments when they're trying to make someone feel better," and "Always try to look your best." Sarah has turned down many dates with guys who are attractive because their compliments to her seemed condescending and because she could not really believe that they would want to date *her*. When she met Dave, who is fairly attractive, quiet, somewhat shy, rather soft spoken, sincere, warm, and gentle, she agreed to date him because he came across as nonthreatening.

Dave likes Sarah very much, and she feels the same toward him. They have been going steady for three months, but the relationship has become rocky and may not last much longer. The reason is that almost every time Dave compliments Sarah, either she says, "Oh, you're just saying that to be nice," or she gets annoyed and pouts. Yet if Dave shows the slightest sign of not liking something she is wearing or even if he says he prefers one of her outfits to another she gets annoyed and pouts or sulks. No matter how much Dave tries to deal with either of Sarah's reactions he cannot seem to get anywhere with her, and they often end up fighting with each other. Gradually Dave has begun to feel that either Sarah is interested in someone else or she just does not like him much. But when he asks her, she becomes upset, cries, and says she needs and loves only him—which is the truth. Unfortunately her distortions help create a situation in which Dave also misperceives her actions and feelings because he is dealing with Sarah on a life-style level. This relationship is dysfunctional; in addition, it is divisive. A **divisive relationship** is of the kind and quality that tends to drive people apart.[8] Even though only one person in a relationship (Sarah) has a self-system that causes her to misperceive, misinterpret, and distort, the other person (Dave) is presented with distorted stimuli, which he will more than likely misperceive or misinterpret *unless* he is an effective communicator.

If one person in a relationship distorts, then the other person is inevitably affected by those distortions; a relationship is a two-way street. In the relationship just described, Sarah's distortions tend finally to evoke distortions from Dave. However, the two-way street nature of a relationship can also work for rather than against a relationship. If one person tends to distort, but the other does not tend to do so, there may be hope for the relationship. If one person is in touch with his insides and is an effective communicator and interactor, then he may exert a healthy, corrective influence on the relationship and the person who distorts. Thus if Dave were an effective communicator and interactor, he would probably be dealing directly with Sarah's anger and pouting when complimented or criticized. He would try to check out her feelings, give her feedback about his, and teach her how to communicate and interact more openly. Unless Sarah is extremely closed, she can benefit from Dave's approach and learn how to communicate and interact more effectively and openly. Even if she and Dave were to break up at some later time, the breakup would be based on more realistic and appropriate factors.

Example 4. Another basic type of relationship is one in which both people distort. In this case, the result is far more than double trouble: it is multiple trouble. For example, suppose Person 1 is a Charlie Brown type—a "people pleaser." No matter how irritated he may get by what another person does or says, he tends to smile and act in an ingratiating manner. Suppose Person 2 is a Lucy type—sharp-tongued, sarcastic, short tempered, and impatient. One of her PFLs is "attack first so you keep the other person off balance"; another is "never let another person know that you're upset or he'll laugh at you." If Charlie and Lucy have a relationship, it is bound to be rather dysfunctional (distorted). Suppose Lucy is feeling upset because she just received some bad news. Charlie comes along, says "Hi!" in a cheery voice, and smiles pleasantly at Lucy. Lucy takes all this in but perceives and interprets Charley's pleasantness as his laughing at her. Angrily she thinks to herself, "Somehow he has found out I'm upset and he's laughing at me!" So she responds with a sarcastic comment. This angers him, but his self-system directs him to smile, to be a people-pleaser. So he smiles again. Lucy responds angrily again. Charlie smiles some more, but he is now feeling extremely angry yet at the same time guilty. He feels that surely he has done something wrong, since Lucy keeps pouncing on him. He is upset because, try as he may, he cannot seem to please her. If his feeling of upsetness finally overrides his PFL pattern of people-pleasing, he may switch to another pattern of withdrawing—becoming quiet and looking sad. When Lucy sees this, she may suddenly become nicer but condescending as she interprets Charlie's withdrawal as an apology.

This is a simple example of a single incident in a relationship, but it gives some notion of the complex interconnection between the self-system and life-style of each person and the interplay between each person's life-style and the other person's self-system. Furthermore, this example strongly underlines the need for each person to be in touch with his insides and outsides and the need for each person to *share* his insides with the other person. If this kind of communication and interaction is not present, the relationship will be hampered or crippled because it will be based primarily on outsides, which are far too susceptible to misperceptions and misinterpretations.

Relationships: the need for detailed analyses

The preceding discussion has presented a relatively brief, theoretical overview of self-system, life-style, and possible variations in the basic forms of relationships. Now, however, it is necessary to examine relationships, especially dating relationships, in more specific detail. It is important to provide you with a working knowledge and practical understanding of the actual processes that occur during the formation, development, establishment, and maintenance of dating relationships.

The reason it is important to gain this knowledge and understanding is that although most people date, many go steady, some live together, and many get engaged, most people have little notion and often less understanding of the processes they involve themselves in. Unfortunately when it comes to people's most important relationships—those which prepare them for and those which can provide them with intimacy—far too many people approach and work with these relationships on the basis of fuzzy intellectual and emotional positions. They tend to have little or no clear framework or methods for evaluating themselves, others, or relationships.

Too many people do not even ask themselves, "What do I want from my relationships? What do I expect to gain? To give?" Few people think to ask the following questions: "Is what I'm seeing in another person what I'm really getting?" or "Is what I know about another person what he is really like?" Instead most people tend to enter and maintain relationships on the basis of idealistic notions, romantic ideals, hopes, dreams, fantasies, and rationalizations, which evade or ignore or deny those realities that might clash with their hopes, dreams, needs, and wishes. Unfortunately these are views and feelings that society has long taught and encouraged and that parents, friends, and peers have also helped to perpetuate.

Thus far too many people enter and develop important relationships with the vague (and often naive) hope that matters will turn out for the best. Often their goal is some kind of instant happiness. If happiness does not occur immediately or if it seems to be just beyond reach or if it disappears like a puff of smoke, many people hang around and hope that someday happiness will somehow just happen. They tend to think and hope that "he'll change after we're married" or "she'll see the light" or "he'll come around" or "things will get better; we just need time." Sadly enough, as the divorce statistics suggest, many people feel cheated when "later" never comes and matters do not get better.

Interestingly it does not seem to occur to many people that happiness is only one offshoot of a far more appropriate goal—that of engaging in the exciting, lifelong process of working on, developing, and nurturing relationships. The remainder of this chapter is specifically geared to helping you acquire the understanding you need to work more consciously and constructively with your relationships. The analyses that follow are intended to help you identify any fuzziness obscuring your intellectual and emotional positions about relationships, to help you realize that there are identifiable processes which are a part of the development of a relationship, and to help you develop the skills that can enable you to make your relationships healthier, more open, and more growth producing. In effect these analyses are intended to help you understand what goes on in any relationship so that you can consciously and deliberately apply the principles and methods of The System to your own relationships and thereby work on making them more qualitative and satisfying.

The word "work" may suggest struggle, dullness, or obligation, but the **psychological work** we refer to is that which involves becoming more aware, bringing things to the conscious level, and using your skills and talents of communication and interaction. Thus we feel that working in this way is one of the most exciting lifelong experiences available.

Interestingly enough, *not* working on yourself and your insides means ultimately that you do far more work in the sense of struggling. To maintain closedness requires a lot of inside and outside psychological work: it means having to deal with guilt, blame, anxiety, and defenses; and it involves you in superficialities, distortions, emotional tangles, masking, and game playing. Thus in the long run the healthier and more open your relationships the less you have to work at or struggle with them (and yourself). ►IE-1, p. 218.

Dating relationships

Because of the social, moral, and religious conventions and MIFs regarding dating, certain disadvantages are almost inherent in dating relationships (which also include going steady, being engaged, and living together). Frequently, it is the nature of these relationships, particularly in their early stages, to be based primarily on impressions, on outsides. Societal and personal PFLs teach most people to respond and to evaluate mainly on these bases.

Thus too often people's initial choices of partners and their later continuing choices are based primarily on their perceptions of others' outsides. As was discussed earlier, these perceptions can all too easily be misperceptions or distortions. At the least, people's perceptions can be limited if they lack information and do not communicate about their own and others' insides. In addition, because personal and societal PFLs tend to emphasize outsides, many people often feel the need to manipulate or "fix" their outsides so that they are more desirable to others. For example, many girls/women act far more retiring, acquiescent, and passive than they really feel because they do not want to be seen as aggressive females, and many boys/men act far more positive, competent, and aggressive because they do not want to be regarded as "weak." These kinds of emphasis on outsides then tend to increase the possibilities for distortion in the dating situation and in dating relationships.

Dating is not, however, necessarily a negative experience. Many people find dating a delightful experience. Often it is dating relationships that give a person the opportunity to try new ways of communicating and interacting. Frequently, dating is a person's first experience with the intoxicating joys of intimacy. Many times dating brings out and helps a person develop his sense of play. Often a person comes into his own as an individual: in a dating relationship, he is not somebody's brother or somebody's son—he is himself on his own, with the chance to be an autonomous individual.[9]

With all these factors and considerations in mind, it is time to look at the various processes involved in entering, developing, and maintaining dating relationships.

INITIAL PREVERBAL SCREENING PROCESS

It is important to look at the dynamics of the initial preverbal screening process first because it is a process that every person employs every time he imagines or sees a person unfamiliar to him. Until there has been some time and opportunity for verbal communication between people, the initial screening process is of necessity based entirely on each person's perceptions of the other person's outsides.[10] Thus if you are operating on the basis of a closed and/or distorted self-system, you may perceive the other person not as he really is but in terms of the way he matches up with the directives of your self-system. This can lead to various occurrences. You may perceive and evaluate the other person favorably but unrealistically, or you may perceive and evaluate him unfavorably and unrealistically. Thus you may move toward him or you may block him out completely. Or your perception may by chance match up with the way he really is. But whichever of these circumstances occurs, the problem is that if you perceive and evaluate on the basis of a closed and/or distorting self-system, you run risks of thinking and feeling that someone is what he really is not and risks of aborting a relationship that might turn out well if you were to share your insides with the other person and vice versa.

It is important therefore to consider what happens as you screen people; it is through this process that you make your initial choices about whom you will and will not relate to. In addition, so much happens when you first see a person that you need to gain some awareness of what can occur during this process. With this awareness, you can learn from your first encounters and can practice becoming more aware of what goes on inside you when you see a new person. In this way, you can learn a good deal about how your self-system operates, and you can begin to modify or change those aspects that may limit or restrict you in new encounters. In addition, the initial screening process is a good place to do your learning and practicing. One reason is that you can briefly (or indefinitely) delay meeting someone you see and thereby gain time to concentrate on and analyze your inside responses to others' outsides. Another is that this process has the advantage of "purity"; that is, there is no possible influence from the other person's insides. Therefore you know that your responses are definitely based on your insides and his outsides. Thus the operation of your self-system may be clearer to you under these conditions, and therefore you have a good chance of learning a great deal about how you screen other people.

A person starts to respond to another person as soon as that other person even *potentially* exists. For example, Lily tells Scott that she can get him a date with her friend Judy who is good-looking, outgoing, enthusiastic, and friendly. Even though Scott has never seen or met Judy, she potentially exists for him now, and he begins to react. His responses, of course, will be generated and directed by his insides. For example, how does he feel about Lily? Does he trust her? Does he feel that he would like someone who is a friend of hers? Does he have a PFL against blind dating? Does he feel good enough about himself to believe that he might be attractive to a good-looking girl? Scott's responses to Lily's offer will also be affected by MIFs. (Is Lily a significant other whose opinions and feelings have meaning for Scott? Does he have time? Is he motivated to meet Judy at this point, or is he content with the girls that he is already dating?) What Scott does will be directed by his self-system and implemented by way of his life-style. (If he is a passive person, will he allow Lily to decide for him? If he is an impulsive type, will he immediately ask Lily for Judy's number and then go call Judy and ask her for a date?)

Thus even before he has met Judy, Scott has gone through a complex screening process. However, if Scott is not in close touch with his insides, much of this screening process will have occurred without his being aware of it, and it will have happened so fast that (if he even thinks about it at all) he probably will think he made a simple decision.

Suppose Scott likes Lily as a friend, but he feels that she is overly positive and assertive for a female. Although he may be aware of this feeling, suppose (because he is not very in touch with his insides) he tends to automatically assume that any girlfriend of Lily's is also too positive and assertive. Suppose also that he has a PFL that tells him to avoid assertive women because they are domineering. On the basis of these factors, he decides not to date Judy. Although he may be unaware of these reasons for his decision, they nevertheless have limited his actions, and he has rejected Judy before he has even met her. If he were more aware of his insides, he might decide differently; he might at least decide to meet Judy to see what she is like. The point is that the greater a person's awareness is the wider his choices tend to be.

The screening process also occurs when people just see each other across a crowded room before they have even met. For example, Cindy, a nice-looking redhead, goes to a party given by friends. She gazes across the room and sees Saburo, a handsome Japanese boy who looks straight at her and smiles in an engaging way. Perhaps she is turned on by his good looks and by his signal, but if she has a PFL that says, "Don't get involved with guys of other races (or nationalities)," then she may look away, refusing to return his smile. In effect she has screened him out on the basis of a PFL regarding a core characteristic (race). She may or may not be aware of her PFL and her response—all of which is processed in a flash.

Suppose, however, Cindy is feeling rebellious. She may then go against her PFL and at least make Saburo's acquaintance. If she does so, she may feel rather uncomfortable, and she may act in an exaggerated manner—perhaps extremely reserved or perhaps wildly impulsive. Her exaggerated manner would be a distortion and would contaminate the interaction between Saburo and her.

Suppose, however, that Cindy is aware of the PFL and has been working with herself to become more open. Then she may deliberately seek Saburo out, meet him, and talk with him; see what happens and how she feels as she goes along; and work with her insides. (Obviously what happens also depends on Saburo's reactions.) Whatever happens, the important factor is that she is not simply closing off a relationship before it even has a chance to get going, and presumably if Cindy is working with her insides, the decision she reaches about continuing a relationship with Saburo will be based on more realistic appraisals.

The preceding examples concern Cindy's inside responses and outside reactions to another person's outsides (in this case, Saburo's core characteristic of race). Another aspect of the screening process relates to the preformed images of "acceptable others" that a person with a somewhat closed self-system carries around. For example, Cindy is 5 feet 11 inches tall. She is well proportioned but has a large build and weighs a good deal, although she is not fat. Depending on many things, she may feel good or bad about her size. If she feels self-conscious about her size, then her image of acceptable others likely includes men who are taller and larger than she. Those who are her height or shorter and who have slighter builds are unacceptable to her. When she sees a man who is shorter or slighter, she automatically screens him out without ever having said one word to him. The function of her preformed image is to protect her against possible embarrassment and against her feeling bad about her size. But the image also functions to cut her off from meeting men who do not match up, from getting to know them and perhaps liking them, and from dating them.

Suppose, however, Cindy feels good about herself in general and okay about her size. Although she may feel that she would prefer to date a man who is taller and larger, she does not necessarily screen out all men who are not. In effect she remains open to new and different possibilities because she does not operate according to a strict, preconceived image of acceptable others.

All these examples of the initial screening process indicate that if a person is functioning in terms of a closed, inflexible, restricting self-system, he may cut himself off from all kinds of opportunities for relationships before he has even made contact. As he progresses, he will—if he keeps functioning in a closed manner— probably continue to narrow his field and range of experience. If, however, a person operates with a certain degree of openness, although he risks feeling anxious at times, he also widens his range of experience and increases his chances of meeting and knowing all kinds of interesting people.

This whole process of initial screening is, like all the subsequent interactions that occur, aimed at establishing personal (and interpersonal) dynamic equilibrium. For example, when Cindy screens out Saburo because she has a strong PFL against involvement with men of a different race, she is maintaining her dynamic equilibrium: she is staying the same in face of newness. Or as we described, Cindy may try to become more open and therefore decides to try a new experience and work with herself as she goes along. Although she is deliberately altering her old balance (based on the PFL) and is therefore exposing herself to some anxiety because newness changes the old balance, she is nevertheless working with herself and thereby gaining a new and more constructive balance.

The initial screening process does not, of course, always occur across a crowded room. We have presented it this way to isolate the process so that we could analyze it, since this process ordinarily occurs so rapidly that most people are hardly (if at all) aware that it is happening. Often (perhaps the majority of times) this screening process occurs in those few seconds before people speak to one another the first time. Once they speak, the screening process continues but it takes on added dimensions.

INITIAL VERBAL ENCOUNTER

In any social meeting between people, each person is attempting to establish some kind of comfortable match-up with the other person; each is trying to establish intrapersonal and interpersonal dynamic equilibrium that is satisfying. Thus each person is seeking responses from the other person that will help him feel comfortable and that will in some way meet and fulfill his inner needs, desires, and wishes.

This means that each person is doing a lot of rapid evaluating of the other, and if a person is the least bit interested in getting to know and perhaps form a relationship with the other person, then he is involved in certain maneuvers aimed at buying time. Each person is trying to hold the other in the interaction so that he can evaluate the other person; at the same time, each person is trying to appear attractive and to put his best foot forward. It can frequently be a complex balancing act.

In the course of this process, many (perhaps most) people tend to avoid communicating about or sharing inside material. They may not know how, they may feel that to do so would be rude, or they may be afraid that doing so would offend or scare off the other person. Moreover, because in early meetings each person is dealing with a relatively "unknown entity" (the other person) and because there has not been enough time or opportunity to build up trust, most people back away from the risks involved in being open and communicating about insides. Obviously if there is little or no communication about insides, each person must of necessity evaluate the other on the basis of the other person's outsides.

Let us look now at an example of what can occur during an initial verbal encounter, using Harry and Janice Johnson's first meeting. They already initially screened each other when they saw each other talking to other people a little earlier. Now a friend has introduced them, and they start to talk. As most people do when they first talk in a social situation, Harry and Janice trade information such as their ages, occupations, backgrounds (social and perhaps religious), experiences, interests, goals, likes and dislikes, and maybe families. On the face of it, Janice and Harry are simply carrying on a conversation, sharing information (and perhaps some feelings) and chatting about casual matters. But much more is going on: each of them is both consciously and unconsciously evaluating the other.

More specifically, two extremely important operations are occurring. First, each of them is processing whatever information he or she receives about the other in terms of self-system, especially PFLs (expectations, rules, and values). For example, Harry tells Janice that he is studying chemical engineering so that one day he can get a top position with one of the big chemical companies. This piece of information indicates to Janice that Harry fulfills several of her expectations concerning the kind of man she wants to date: (1) a man who cares about his future (and possibly hers, by extension); (2) a man who is studying something "solid" (practical, useful); and (3) a man who is going to get a college education. The rules that Harry measures up to are as follows: date (marry) a college-educated person (do not date or marry beneath your class and status) and date a practical, ambitious man (watch out for lazy, uncertain, indecisive men). Not only Janice, of course, but also Harry is doing this kind of evaluative processing of each significant piece of information they share with each other.

Another extremely important operation that is occurring during Janice's and Harry's interaction is that consciously and unconsciously each is sending, receiving, evaluating, and responding to all kinds of signals and messages. As they do this repeatedly, each of them begins to get some feel for the other's outsides, especially of the other's interpersonal patterns.

For example, Janice responds to something Harry says by reaching over and touching his arm for a moment, smiling at him, and saying in an admiring tone, "Gee, Harry, I think if anybody could qualify for that job, you could." She is sending various signals and messages—all of them positive ones. Her touch, her smile, and her tone signal that she admires Harry, that she wants to underscore her admiration by some physical contact with him, and that she is impressed by him. The verbal message is clear and complimentary. The metamessage is "Wow! I really think you're great! I like you. I hope you like me."

Now suppose Harry's heart lurches slightly when Janice reacts this way; he feels a sudden burst of delight and a certain amount of sexual arousal. If Harry's style were an open one, he might identify and report at least some of his feelings to Janice. However, Harry's self-system and life-style are closed: one of his patterns is to deny feelings.

Another is to be intellectual. So although Harry's response to Janice's input is a positive one, his self-system through his interpersonal patterns censors and shapes the content and intensity of signals and messages he sends back to her. He may look somewhat gratified but also uncomfortable. He may look down at his feet and shift his weight from foot to foot. He may say to Janice in a stiff but pleased way, "That's nice of you to say so." Then he probably will launch into a logical, intellectual analysis of the job's possibilities or an explanation of how the experience could be extremely useful to his career.

The signals and messages Harry sends to Janice therefore are shaped and censored and muted by his patterns of denial and intellectualizing. His signals are that he is pleased but does not want to talk too much about it and that he is not comfortable. His verbal message is a muted response to

Janice's rather emotionally charged input. His metamessage is as follows: "Don't stop saying (and doing) nice things like that, but don't expect me to respond in an emotional way. I'm a no-nonsense, logical man who thinks straight and who looks at life clearly and unemotionally. I'm in command of myself and what I do."

As Harry and Janice communicate and interact in this fashion, they are continuously processing their experiences of one another to see if they are comfortable with each other and if each meets the requirements established by the other's self-system. According to the results of this process, each is deciding whether he or she is interested in continuing the relationship.

A DEVELOPING RELATIONSHIP

As people date each other over a period of time, they begin to develop a relationship. They slowly become familiar with one another's ways, familiar enough to be aware of and to discern a certain consistency in the ways the other person thinks, feels, and acts. (These consistent ways of thinking, feeling, and acting are what we term "interpersonal patterns.") If these patterns—as each person interprets the other's patterns—help each of them to feel comfortable with one another and to establish and maintain intrapersonal and interpersonal dynamic equilibrium, then each will probably try to nurture and develop the relationship. Moreover, if both feel that there is a comfortable match-up between them and if nothing much challenges the balance (e.g., outside influences, stresses, the growth of one or both of the partners, crises), then they probably will continue the relationship; it will likely be satisfying to them.[11,12]

Using Janice and Harry as an example, let us look at what occurs in a developing relationship that is based primarily on each person's inside reactions to the other's outsides. This example highlights two specific phenomena that occur in a developing relationship: (1) each person gradually becomes aware of the other's patterns and interprets them in terms of his self-system, and (2) each person's interpretations encourage him to feel that their personalities interlock in meaningful and satisfying ways.

As Janice and Harry interact with each other in a number of different situations over a period of time, each begins to become aware of the other's patterns, to feel the interlock between their patterns and self-systems, and to sense the comfortable match-up between them.

Interlock 1. Harry's logical, intellectual ways attract Janice. They offer her a kind of security, since she tends to feel and act confused and vague. Furthermore, she admires these qualities because she lacks them, because they are useful qualities to have, and because they signify strength to her. Janice's pattern of confusion, vagueness, and self-belittlement tends to evoke feelings of protectiveness and superiority in Harry. In effect, he feels needed and adequate in the face of Janice's "weakness." In addition, naivete and confusion are a welcome and charming change from his inner and outer world of logic, reason, and order.

Interlock 2. Janice interprets Harry's tendency to deny emotion primarily as denoting traits of calmness, coolness, and self-assurance. (Also she is so busy being emotional that she tends not to see just how unemotional Harry is. She tends to project some of her own overemotionalism onto him and to think it is really his.) Janice regards Harry as a calm port in her emotional storm, and she reads his traits as indications of strength. Also his quietness and lack of spontaneity come across to her as an air of mystery and loneliness, something which she responds to emotionally and impulsively. In addition, his quietness complements her tendency to talk all the time.

Harry responds positively to Janice's overemotionality, her impulsivness, and her spontaneous entertainment. She fills a large gap in his life of little emotionality. Her overemotionality also makes him feel superior and protective because he *knows* the facts and logic about matters and is not swept along by fits of emotion. Her impulsiveness and spontaneity delight him because they are refreshing changes from his own rather plodding, highly ordered, and rigid ways of experiencing life. Furthermore, her constant entertaining chatter is a welcome diversion from his slow and methodical approach to social situations. In effect Janice relieves him of much of his social burden because she carries the conversational ball.

Interlock 3. Harry's aggressiveness and sureness about himself tend to awe Janice somewhat. But his sureness impresses her and attracts her because she feels as though she can draw on his strength. Mainly she sees him as strong and competent, as someone she can depend on and get support from.

Janice's unsureness, her childish, little girl anxiety, and her dependence attract Harry. He feels superior, needed, strong, and desirable. He feels protective toward her (which contributes to his feeling more sure of himself).

Interlock 4. If Harry's hostility comes across at any point, Janice distorts it by interpreting it as his "positiveness," his strength, and his assertiveness. If he is too sharp with her (to the point where even she cannot ignore or distort the signals and messages), her feelings get hurt, and she acts terribly insulted and injured. Usually, however, she distorts, filters out, or denies any hostility he may show. Also she tends to try to smooth matters over.

Because Harry operates from a hostile base, Janice's tendency to smooth matters over (or to distort or deny hostility) offers him a kind of refuge from his own hostility. Her pattern has the effect of a mother soothing a child by saying, "There, there, Mother knows you don't really mean to be angry. You're really a nice, lovable boy." Janice's pattern of denying negative emotions also fits another of Harry's patterns, which is to deny his emotions.

Interlock 5. Harry's rigidity and authoritarianism come across to Janice (who romanticizes and distorts) as Harry's having the courage of his convictions and knowing his own mind. Furthermore, because other things about Harry turn her on, Janice blocks out what is negative by interpreting it positively. In effect she idealizes Harry.

Harry's response to Janice's romanticizing and idealizing of him is pleasure, since it helps reinforce the way he *sees* himself—as intelligent, superior, and competent. Her response also helps him to feel likeable and valuable. She is critical of others but not of him, and the difference between her two reactions makes him feel "special."

• • •

We have discussed the interlocks between Harry's and Janice's interpersonal patterns and insides in a one-to-one order. Obviously, however, their patterns crisscross. That is, there is much more interweaving of patterns than our straight-line account would indicate. For example, Janice romanticizes or idealizes Harry's intellectualizing tendencies and she tends to overdramatize his achievements; in response, his sense of sureness increases. Also the more vague, confused, and naive Janice becomes the more assertive, directive, and controlling Harry becomes.

Another important facet to note about patterns is that different ones operate more strongly than others at different times. Sometimes a pattern does not get called into action at all. In large part, whether this occurs depends on what MIFs are operating. For example, as long as Harry is in a good *mood,* he is not too likely to turn his hostility on Janice. But if he wants to discuss something important with her and they have had little *time* and *opportunity* to get together or if Janice acts flighty and silly when Harry is trying to be serious, then he might become impatient and exhibit some hostility toward her. The particular MIFs that are operating at any given moment can strongly affect any interaction. This is especially true if people are interacting primarily on the basis of their outsides because many MIFs exert pressures or provide influences that encourage staying away from inside material (e.g., having insufficient *time*). Thus many times the MIFs that are present in a developing relationship tend to foster a certain amount of masking or distortion.

MIFs AND DATING

The interplay between the nature of particular social situations and their governing PFLs and MIFs can frequently foster masking, distorting, or game playing. All too often dating and the MIFs that occur within this social situation work together against openness and, instead, tend to encourage masking and distorting. (For the sake of clarity in the following discussion, MIFs are identified by italics.)

In a dating situation, a person may disregard the fact that his date does not really live up to his expectations. For example, he may expect his girlfriend to be attentive to him and not to flirt with other men when they go out. If his *psychological desire* is to impress his date that he is open minded, he may not make his expectations known to her. Or he may not reveal his expectations to her because his *intent* is merely to have a good time and not get into any close kind of relationship.

Frequently, when people date, they conform at least outwardly to the traditional male/female role stereotypes because their *intent* is to show others, by the shorthand of role playing, their acceptability and desirability as dates. For example, a fairly aggressive woman who knows that she has only one initial opportunity to impress a man with her desirability may temper her aggressiveness considerably by assuming the more conventional role of a quiet, unaggressive female. Many women, if their *goal* is marriage, tend to fit as best they can their own particular styles into the traditional female role. These women are frequently encouraged to do just this by *societal pressures.*

In a dating situation, people's actual patterns of communication are not always easily recognizable. For example, if the *intent* is to get to know something about one another to see if they want to continue dating, people will tend to trade a good deal of information. Thus if a person has a pattern of not communicating much about feelings, this fact would be covered over by the information trading. Furthermore, there may not be much (or people may not take) the *time* or *opportunity* to communicate on more personal levels. Another factor that can mask the nature of people's patterns of communication is their *motivation.* For example, a person who is highly motivated to have many dates so that he is not lonely may avoid making any critical comments or revealing negative feelings.

People's patterns of interaction do not always come across sharply in dating (especially casual dating). One reason is that the *social situation*—that is, the often rather public aspect of dating—can encourage people not to act on significant feelings but to keep matters on a somewhat lighter or more superficial level. Thus if a person tends to demand perfection and be critical of other people's performances, he may keep that tendency in check when he is in public. Another problem in dating is that people often do not have the *time* or *opportunity* to feel the weight of the repetition of patterns. Usually there is not enough time or opportunity to get some feeling for a person's *intrapersonal* patterns. One other problem is that people are often not *motivated* to deal with the really difficult matters of life, such as serious disagreements about basic matters such as roles. In addition, in casual dating, people simply do not get the same range of experience in living as do those who work and live together; therefore patterns may not show up clearly.

Although people have to make decisions all the time no matter what they may be doing, in casual dating many major decisions can simply be ignored or avoided. Furthermore, the *opportunity* to make major decisions may not arise, or people may avoid important decisions because their *intent* is to keep the relationship casual. Or a power-player may act like a compromiser if his *goal* is to convince his partner to continue dating him.

In effect, many social circumstances (such as dating) tend *not* to encourage a great amount of openness. In fact, in situations like dating, in which a person may want to impress others and to see and hear what he wants to, there is sometimes a tendency to present one's own and to perceive others' life-styles in a romanticized, limited, or distorted light. Such romanticizing or restricting of perceptions can occur partly because people are interacting within a limited number of situations and within a certain type of situation. Also usually less stress is involved in these situations and thus less opportunity exists for revealing at least a part of one's true nature as a result of stress.

DATING GAMES

Since the dating situation has traditionally been the arena in which people look (whether consciously or not) for potential long-term partners, there is often a good deal of pressure to work primarily on attracting and developing (as rapidly as possible) some degree of holding power with others. This means making one's outsides as attractive as possible and attempting to develop quickly an agreeable dynamic equilibrium. These pressures tend unfortunately to encourage people to play **dating games**—stereotyped, highly visible, and rather exaggerated ways of acting and reacting, which evoke equally stereotyped and exaggerated actions and reactions. Thus dating games consist of predetermined, automatic, and repetitious sets of actions and reactions (much like an intricate dance), which help the partners achieve certain psychological ends: the establishment and maintenance of intrapersonal and interpersonal dynamic equilibrium. Each person's vehicle for playing or carrying out the moves in these games is his life-style, but the psychological reasons that he plays and the choice of the particular games he plays are determined by his self-system.[13]

The following is only a partial list of dating games that people engage in. Presumably you have seen (or played) others and can add them to the list. Some dating games are geared primarily to *attracting others,* at least originally. Among these are games like "I Am Desirable" (pretty, handsome, popular, sophisticated, sexy, mysterious, hard-to-get, interesting, sensitive, thoughtful, warm, outgoing), "The Attentive Listener" (which signals that "I am easy to talk to" or "I am interested in you" or "I really care who you are"), and "The Last of the Big Spenders" (designed to impress and awe the beneficiary).

Other dating games, although they also serve to attract, are used more in *holding on to* others and tend to stress the player's agreeable nature. These include games like "Whatever You'd Like to Do Is Fine with Me," "Mona Lisa," (whatever happens—bad or good—the player always smiles), and "There's No One Else Like You."

In addition to these games, there are others that may come into play early, but are more likely to turn up if things begin to get a little rocky. These games can be highly manipulative, geared to *getting the other person to stay (or get back into) line.* They often achieve their purpose by arousing guilt, fear or both or by evoking anxiety. These include the following: the "Sulking" game ("you'll be sorry you crossed me") the "If You Really Cared About Our Relationship, You Would—" game, the male game "You Must Be Frigid" ("or you'd be sexually turned on and wouldn't fend me off like this"), the female game "You're Just an Animal" ("you demand too much sexual activity too fast; it's unnatural"), and the "There Are Other Fish in the Ocean" game ("if you don't treat me better, I may just leave you and go fishing").

Although dating games can yield a certain amount of fun if they are not played seriously, too often they are generated by feelings of anxiety, inadequacy, and insecurity. Actually they tend to be basically dishonest and distorting because they manipulate and maximize appearances—outsides. Therefore they can be essentially destructive. Dating games too frequently make possible and foster interaction and the development of relationships that are based on minimal communication and minimal honesty or openness. Furthermore, they make possible the development of pseudodynamic equilibriums, which often buckle later under the onslaught of change, challenge, or stress. All in all, dating games provide poor training and preparation for the more serious, long-term commitments of living together, marriage, and family life.

KINDS OF DYNAMIC EQUILIBRIUM IN RELATIONSHIPS

As two people form and develop a relationship over a period of time, they have the opportunity to interact in a greater number of situations and, whether consciously or unconsciously, to evalaute one another according to a much greater number and range of manifestations of their life-styles (and partially their self-systems also). As people interact, they begin to reveal more about themselves such as personality traits, patterns of communication, and patterns of interaction. Obviously no one reveals the full range of his interpersonal patterns during one or even a hundred interactions, but over a period of time, it is possible to get some understanding of and feel for the other person's life-style.

Gradually each person also gets an understanding of and a feel for the interlock between his self-system and life-style and the other person's self-system and life-style. This interlock constitutes the dynamic equilibrium of their relationship. These interlocks can be described and viewed in an organized way, that is, according to whether they are "complementary," "alternating," "supplementary," or "mixed." The terms that describe the quality of a relationship's dynamic equilibrium are "functional" and "dysfunctional." The terms that indicate whether the kind and quality of the relationship's dynamic equilibrium will tend to keep the people together or drive them apart are "cohesive" and "divisive."[14]

Complementarity. In a **complementary relationship** between two people, each person's life-style fills in or supplies much of what is or seems to be lacking in the other's life-style. Examples of complementary relationships are a passive person and an aggressive one; introvert/extrovert; sadist/masochist; dependent/independent; obsessive-compulsive/hysteric; impulsive/deliberate; sociopathic (con man type)/naive idealist; and paranoid (intensely mistrustful type)/passive dependent. (Obviously most of these examples draw on what are usually rather closed styles. These are used because their characteristics are sharp and vivid and therefore easy to describe and to observe.)

Following is a detailed example of a complementary relationship:

Introvert (Jerry)	***Extrovert (Sylvia)***
Shy	Bold
Withdrawn, aloof, loner	Outgoing, gregarious
Moody	Cheerful
Low-keyed, sometimes depressed	High-spirited
Intellect oriented	Emotion oriented
More interested in own inner world	More interested in outer world
Unemotional on surface	Emotional on surface
Slow to anger	Quick to anger
Friendly but distant and reserved	Friendly, warm, moves in fast
Thinks first, then acts	Feels first, acts, then thinks later
Careful, cautious	Impulsive
Follower	Leader
Quiet	Boisterous
Articulate but not talkative	Articulate and talkative

This relationship has a high degree of complementarity. Jerry (the introvert) is moody and at times depressed, but he finds that when he is with Sylvia (the extrovert), who is generally cheerful and high-spirited, he tends to get caught up in her joyfulness and usually feels happier. She enjoys being able to cheer Jerry up because she likes him and because she likes being helpful to and needed by others. Furthermore, Sylvia has found that her quick impulsive emotionality can get her into trouble; sometimes without thinking she will say or do things that hurt or annoy others. To her delight, Sylvia finds that when she is with Jerry, she tends to pick up or copy some of his more intellectual, quiet calmness and thoughtfulness. For his part, Jerry finds that Sylvia's impulsiveness and spontancity encourage him to be a little less cautious and a little more spontaneous and outgoing—qualities that he admires and that he realizes are social assets.

In this description, Jerry's and Sylvia's styles match up and complement each other in a **cohesive** way. That is, the complementarity tends to draw them together, to attract them to one another.

Suppose, however, that their high degree of complementarity is divisive rather than cohesive. Perhaps Jerry's moodiness and depressiveness irritate Sylvia because when she gets around Jerry she tends to get moody and depressed too. And Sylvia's cheerfulness and high spirits get on Jerry's nerves because when he is down he wants to be quiet and alone. When he feels down, cheer and high spirits irritate him. Jerry also likes to think problems out for himeslf and to plan with care what he will do; he does *not* like to be rushed into matters. Thus Sylvia's impulsive, emotional approach to life and her "let's try it now and talk about it later" approach rub Jerry the wrong way. Conversely, Jerry's cautious, careful, intellectual approach to life turns Sylvia off because she feels his way takes all the joy and surprise and spontaneity out of life. If these were typical of the ways Jerry's style affected Sylvia and vice versa, then the complementarity of their styles would be divisive.

Depending on what Jerry's and Sylvia's relationship is (e.g., friends, dating, going steady, living together, married), how long it has existed, and how much interest each has in it (plus other factors), the divisiveness may or may not break up the relationship. If they do stay together in spite of the divisive nature of the complementarity, then the relationship is almost sure to be dysfunctional; their staying together indicates the presence of strong but probably unidentified needs for one another or even needs for a divisive kind of relationship.

If their relationship is complementary in a cohesive way, whether it is functional or dysfunctional depends on many factors also. One important factor is whether the relationship is an open or closed one. If it is closed, it will likely be dysfunctional. The example that now follows is intended to illustrate how a complementary relationship can be cohesive and dysfunctional and has the potential to become divisive and dysfunctional.

On the life-style level Jerry (distant, aloof, reserved, a loner) and Sylvia (gregarious, outgoing) seem well matched: their patterns are complementary and, let us assume, cohesive. But if they interact primarily on this level without dealing with their insides, then the relationship is by definition **dysfunctional**—it is marked by functioning that is limited, impaired, or both; and that is less qualitative, less healthy, and less constructive than it might be. For example there is no provision at this level for times when Sylvia may feel unfriendly, withdrawn, or depressed or when Jerry may feel angry, hostile, or aggressive. In the event that one (or both) should enter into one of these nontypical emotional states, the dynamic balance of the relationship could be upset. Even so, occasional forays into these kinds of nontypical emotional states would not necessarily be divisive.

The potential for divisiveness lies in each persons' self-system. If you look at the PFLs governing Jerry's perceptions of signs of independence in another (gregarious outgoing people are "safe"—they are not the dependent type) and the PFLs governing his feelings about others' dependency (avoid dependent people; dependency makes me feel trapped), you can see that his pattern acts as a defense against his fears of others' dependency. If you look at Sylvia's PFLs about what she perceives in another as indications of strength (distant, aloof, reserved loners are strong and self-assured; they don't mind if others are dependent on them) and her PFLs about her own dependency needs (I need a strong person I can be dependent on because I'm afraid of being alone), you can see that her pattern is a way of compensating for her fears and need for someone to lean on. Each of them chooses the other because of a distorted inner perception of and response to the other's pattern, but the inner needs and feelings of each clashes with the other's. That is, Sylvia wants someone to lean on; therefore she picked Jerry because he is a loner who is distant, aloof, and reserved, which signifies strength to her. Jerry wants someone who is strong and independent and picked Sylvia because her being outgoing, and gregarious signifies strength and independence to him.

What do these interlocks mean in terms of their relationship and their interactions? They have various meanings, depending on what MIFs are operating at any given time.

1. If nothing challenges the complementary balance between Jerry and Sylvia and if they feel reasonably happy and secure, then each will probably act on his or her overt patterns. When both are operating primarily on the life-style level, then their complementarity tends to be cohesive.

2. If, however, Jerry were to become depressed because he loses his job and is having difficulty finding another, he may withdraw, become extremely aloof, reserved, and distant. He may emotionally shut out Sylvia—not talk to her much, avoid being with her, and treat her coldly when they are together. As a result, Sylvia may feel alone because what had seemed like strength that she could lean on now comes across as a weapon for shutting her out. In response Sylvia feels isolated, lonely, and rejected, and these feelings trigger strong feelings of dependency. Thus she may intensify her gregarious and outgoing pattern to try to push herself on Jerry and to be constantly with him because she feels alone and dependent. He may in turn withdraw even more. If this vicious circle continues, Sylvia may begin to berate herself or Jerry or both for the false interpretation of his pattern. In other words, she may come to feel that his withdrawal, his loner quality, and his reserve do not mean that he is strong, self-assured, and accepting of dependency but rather that he is cold, uncaring, and self-centered. If this occurs, she is likely to feel cheated and duped. All of this is what we mean by divisiveness.

However, if either Jerry or Sylvia is at least moderately open (or, better yet, if both of them are), they have a good chance of working constructively with their complementary life-styles and forming a solid, functional relationship. If they work (through intrapersonal and interpersonal communication) on their individual growth and the growth of their relationship, they may be able to fashion themselves a healthy, open relationship. (The approach and methods leading to a healthy, open relationship will be discussed in detail later in the chapter.)

Alternating. The second kind of dynamic equilibrium is that of **alternating**—an essentially complementary relationship in which the two people alternate between the two dominant styles of the relationship. Such alternating is possible in any of the complementary relationships we have mentioned previously (e.g., passive/aggressive, sadist/masochistic, introvert/extrovert, obsessive-compulsive/hysterical).[15]

The meaning of alternating can be illustrated by the following example of a passive/aggressive relationship between two people who are living together.

Passive (Denise)	*Aggressive (Steve)*
Introverted, mostly listens	Outgoing, talkative
Shy, hangs back	Socially a mixer, a mover
Aware of the emotional atmosphere, in touch with own and others' emotions	Operates primarily on the surface, not very in touch with own emotions
Friendly in a quiet way	Sociable, friendly
Insecure, unsure of self	Self-assured, self-confident

Passive (Denise)	*Aggressive (Steve)*
Agreeable, peacemaker	Quick to anger, argumentative
Dependent, tends to rely on others	Independent
Follower, will yield to a dominator	Leader, sometimes a dominator
Hesitant, cautious	Decisive, acts fast
Timid, just lets things happen	Forceful, strong
Does not fight, seeks agreement	Stands up for own beliefs and rights
Noncompetitive, avoids limelight	Competitive, seeks recognition
Easygoing, placid, slow mover	Energetic, takes initiative, active

There is a high degree of complementarity in this relationship. With this basic pattern of complementarity (i.e., Denise is passive; Steve is aggressive), let us assume that the relationship is somewhat dysfunctional but strongly cohesive. Ordinarily, Denise's style is passive and Steve's is aggressive, but at times they alternate or switch styles. This is not to say that each takes on every characteristic of the opposite style. Rather, in response to particular circumstances and to each other, Denise will become aggressive in specific ways and Steve will become passive in specific ways. For example, suppose Steve gets a serious case of the flu. The worse he feels the more insecure and dependent he becomes. In response, Denise, who is usually the insecure, dependent one, becomes assertive, competent, and decisive. She takes care of Steve, and during this whole time it is as though she has never been a passive person. This kind of switch is functional and cohesive. (If, however, only Steve switched and Denise remained dependent, passive, hesitant, and unsure, then the relationship might become at least temporarily dysfunctional and divisive.)

The outcomes of this alternating style, like those of the other styles of relationships, depend primarily on whether Denise's and Steve's relationship is open or closed. The more closed it is the greater the chances that it has been dysfunctional to begin with and the greater the chance that the switch may be divisive.

Supplementarity. Whereas the complementary relationship bears out the old adage that "opposites attract," the supplementary relationship bears out another old adage: "Birds of a feather flock together." In a **supplementary relationship,** each person's life-style or parts of it adds to, completes, and enhances the other person's life-style (or parts thereof). Essentially the two people in a supplementary relationship have significantly similar styles. Thus examples of this kind of relationship are ones in which there are two extroverts, two introverts, two passive people, two aggressive people, or two obsessive-compulsives. (This is not to say that these people's styles are exactly the same but merely that the similarities significantly outweigh the dissimilarities. In fact, it would be startling, if not impossible, to find two people who did not differ in any significant way.)

An example of a supplementary relationship follows. This particular relationship is between two people who have (to varying degrees of intensity) the specific characteristics of what we call the "independent-intellectual style."

Independent-intellectual

Decisive, determined, sometimes stubborn
Has strong likes and dislikes
Individualistic—strong ego, inner directed
Has courage of own convictions
Rational, intellectual, fact oriented
Backs away from emotionality, sensationalism, sentimentality
Intelligent
Well read, well educated
Bright, articulate
Idealistic
Stands up for and is fiercely loyal to own beliefs
Politically minded, politically concerned
Supports and works hard for causes he or she believes in
Intellectually passionate
Deeply concerned about mankind but not close to many individuals
Personally somewhat cool and detached although not necessarily cold
Puts up barriers to intimacy
Intensely private

The relationship between Kurt and Nina, each of whom these characteristics (or most of them) describe accurately, has a high degree of supplementarity. Both attend graduate school: he is studying economics, and she is studying international law. They first met in a seminar on American foreign policy since World War II, a course that each of them took because of interest rather than requirement. Since the course was conducted primarily by means of discussion and report, Kurt and Nina got a chance to evaluate one another's intelligence, views, and ways of thinking and of presenting ideas and beliefs before they even began to date. The content of the course naturally elicited people's social and political beliefs, and frequently, both Kurt and Nina were right in the middle of heated discussions and arguments, arguing passionately and often brilliantly for this or that idea or cause. Each of them is impressed by the other's knowledge, rational approach to matters, idealism, and individualism. In effect each admires in the other the qualities each prizes in himself or herself. They have been dating now for several months, and both are pleased with their relationship; they have discovered that they share many ideas, attitudes, and areas of concern. They always have a lot to talk about, they have the same social and political concerns, and they are active in working in local political campaigns, the American Civil Liberties Union, and community projects. Obviously their supplementary relationship is a cohesive one; their similar styles add to each other in a way that enhances their relationship.

Suppose, however, that their supplementarity is divisive rather than cohesive, which might occur, for example, if Kurt's social and political beliefs are different from Nina's. Suppose Kurt is a political conservative: he is passionately opposed to most welfare plans, to a highly centralized government, and to government interference in the free enterprise system. Nina, on the other hand, is a strong liberal: she believes the government should do more, not less, to support and run massive public aid programs; she believes also that the power of the federal government, especially the Congress and the courts, should be used to ensure individual rights. Since both Nina and Kurt are so strongly committed to clashing political (and social) views, the supplementary nature of their styles tends to make their ideological differences more abrasive. In other words, if one (or both) of them was a less ardently committed person, they probably would have a chance of getting along better. In this case, supplementarity works against attraction, since their similar styles put Kurt and Nina in direct confrontation and serve to underscore (and to heighten) their differences of belief. If they agreed, they would agree closely; but they disagree, and because of their styles, they disagree intensely. Thus their supplementarity is divisive.

If Kurt and Nina establish and maintain a relationship in spite of this divisiveness, it will more than likely be marked by a good deal of arguing and disagreement. If each simply wants a good intellectual sparring partner, then the relationship could be a functional one. However, if one (or both) wants a meeting of minds, a closeness built on mutual views and beliefs, the relationship is likely to be dysfunctional; at least one of them is paying some kind of emotional price to stay in the relationship in spite of the clash in views and beliefs.

Mixed. We have discussed the three main types of dynamic equilibrium in relationships—complementary, alternating, and supplementary. In the interest of clarity, we have ignored the innumerable variations possible in these types. However, one basic variation is too important to be totally ignored: the mixed type. The **mixed** type consists of a combination of complementarity and supplementarity; that is, each person's style has some aspects that complement and some that supplement aspects of the other person's style. Using the previous example of Kurt and Nina, who had supplementary independent-intellectual styles, suppose Nina comes from a family that stressed the importance of a woman's being warm and communicative about feelings. Kurt, on the other hand, comes from a family that taught that being a man means being somewhat reserved and not talking about one's feelings. This is an example of a complementary pair of traits in the midst of a basically supplementary relationship. Another example of a complementary pair is if both are articulate, but Kurt is at home expressing his views and rarely holds back, whereas Nina is shy at times and has to struggle with herself to speak before large groups, especially groups of strangers.

In actuality the mixed complementary-supplementary relationship, whatever the particular balance in a given relationship, is a fairly common one.

One other possibility should be mentioned here. There are many people whose personalities and styles are neither complementary nor supplementary but are clashing. If there is no or minimal complementarity or supplementarity and a good deal of conflict, then people are not too likely to establish a relationship. If they do, however, then their relationship is likely to be extremely abrasive (whether overtly or covertly or both) and extremely dysfunctional.

While reading this section on the dynamics of relationships, you may have been struck by the large number of negative examples. One reason for using more negative than positive ones is that negative examples are often clearer because they are sharper and more extreme. Another reason is that you can learn a great deal about relationships by understanding what can go wrong and why. If you do not know what can go wrong, you are not in a good position to fix it.

EVALUATING RELATIONSHIPS

By now it should be obvious that the primary reasons for trouble in a relationship are too much reliance on outsides, too little communication about insides, too little sharing of insides, and a lack of expertise in evaluating relationships. Since many relationships are based primarily on outsides and not much communication about insides, it is important to know how to recognize and identify life-styles.

Identifying life-styles

Since one of the two vehicles that a person has for conveying information about self and for acting on his "selfness" is life-style, the greater your expertise in "reading" life-styles (your own and others') the better your chances of establishing and maintaining more qualitative relationships. Understand, however, that we are not urging you to wander around, subjecting everyone to your penetrating, analytical gaze; rather we are encouraging you to experience life, yourself, and others with sensitivity, alertness, and awareness. All of us must respond to life-styles; we cannot *not* respond. Thus it is important to train yourself to be constructively aware so that you understand and appreciate *what* you are responding to. In addition, by being more aware, you are better equipped to assess the validity of your perceptions of another's life-style. Besides, people watching (and pattern watching) is fun.

Every person has two basic ways of conveying his life-style: communication and action. Every person has two basic means of identifying a life-style: listening and observing. What should you listen and look for? And what should you do with what you hear and see? In optimum terms, you should listen to and observe everything a person says and does; in more human terms, you should take what you notice and try to sort it into categories. Essentially you utilize the **inductive method**—you take those pieces of information and details that you acquire, categorize them, and eventually draw certain general conclusions about them.

The basic way to carry out the inductive method to identify life-style is to watch, listen for, and become aware of those aspects of a person's functioning that are consistent and persistent. For example, if time and time again you hear a person say to himself, "That was stupid of me!" when he makes a mistake, you should listen and be alert for other possible self-depreciating remarks, signals, and actions. If you notice that this same person frequently brushes aside or ignores compliments, you may be looking at a category or pattern of his functioning. When you give a name to a pattern, you are in effect saying that he seems to have a specific personality trait. **Personality traits** are terms describing in a general sense the basic, consistent, identifiable aspects that are characteristic of a person's observable (or inferable) ways of functioning. In other words, personality traits are static descriptions of a person's interpersonal patterns. If you can identify even a few of these traits, you will probably have a fair notion of his life-style. If you look back at the descriptive lists preceding the explanations of each kind of dynamic equilibrium (e.g., complementary), you can see that they are lists of personality traits.

Evaluating the whole person

As most of the examples in this chapter show, the disadvantages inherent in relating primarily on a life-style level can be severe and far reaching. To have a more qualitative and more open relationship, it is necessary to go beyond life-style and to gain some estimate of the self-system, which directs the style. This means evaluating the whole person. The most effective way for each person in a relationship to evaluate the other is for them to communicate and interact openly, but frequently, people's communicational and interactional skills are not highly developed. Therefore it becomes necessary to rely to a degree on factors other than open, conscious communication. This is not an impossible task, since we send and receive many clues about ourselves, and we do tend to indirectly communicate much about ourselves as we interact with one another.

Although it is not feasible to try to cover all the possible ways of evaluating the whole person, it is possible to provide you with a checklist and some sample questions, which will help you to carry out a fairly thorough examination. However, let us point out that nothing—no checklist and no brilliant detective work with clues—can come close to matching good, clear, direct, honest communication as *the* way of evaluating oneself, another person, and a relationship. If this kind of communication is not possible or feasible, then work with what you can get.[16]

We have found that one of the most useful ways to evaluate another person and your relationship with him is to focus on some of the **major components of human interaction**—motivation for growth, expectations, roles, patterns of communication, patterns of interaction, and decision-making processes.

MOTIVATION FOR GROWTH

How does the person react if you try to discuss your relationship or if you say, "Let's talk about our relationship"? Does he put you off? Does he seem angry? Hurt? Bored? Anxious? Annoyed? Interested? What does he *say* about the relationship? Is he content with things just as they are? Is he smug? Is he fearful of change? Is he eager to try new things? Does he act as though he cares what happens to the relationship?

EXPECTATIONS

Is the person loaded with expectations about almost everything? Does he demean whatever does not live up to his expectations? Is he a "the world owes me a living" type? Or does he seem to expect to be hurt or rebuffed by others? That is, does he consistently act hesitant, doubtful, and fearful around others? Does he rarely, if ever, assert himself? Does he seem to expect to be in the wrong?

How does he seem to expect others to treat him? How does he seem to expect to treat others? For example, does he seem hurt and withdraws if you express your anger to him but acts surprised if you seem hurt when he gets angry? Does he say one thing and do another? In other words, does he apply a "double standard" to his expectations?

ROLES

Does the person almost always conform to traditional role ascriptions? Is he a male chauvinist? Is she a believer in "biology is woman's destiny"? Does he act ultramasculine? That is, does he play to the hilt the roles of authoritarian, superior being, ultimate protector of women, and super jock? Or can he take roles with a great grain of salt? That is, he follows some of the broader outlines of a role but feels free to act on his individuality. For example, if he feels like crying, he does so without worrying about the value judgment that "real men don't cry." Does she act ultrafeminine? That is, does she play to the hilt the roles of poor little old helpless me, the passive dependent, and the damsel in distress? Or the coquette, the vamp, and the sex goddess? Or can she take roles with a great grain of salt? Can she follow the broader outline of a role without sacrificing her individuality? For example, can she be assertive when it is appropriate and feel comfortable doing so?

Does the person take an antirole stance, refusing to recognize or abide by any role ascriptions? Does the person criticize others if they do not measure up to the expectations of a particular role? Does he have set notions about men's, women's, husbands', wives', fathers', mothers', and children's roles?

PATTERNS OF COMMUNICATION

Do the person's signals match his verbal messages? For example, does he look angry but act in a friendly way? Does he crack jokes when he looks and acts otherwise depressed or unhappy? What tones of voice does he habitually use? What facial expressions are particular to and consistent with him? Does he usually frown or smile or sneer or pout? Or does he have a wide range of tones and looks? In effect, are his verbal and his metamessages conflictual or congruent?

How does he function on the verbal level? Does he talk mostly about ideas, things, and events? Or mostly about feelings? Or is there a balanced mixture of intellect and emotion? Does he not like to talk much at all but rather to act and do? Is he willing to share his insides? Or does he say such matters are foolishness? Or does he seem frightened by the thought of sharing inside feelings? If he has never done much communicating, is he willing to give it a try?

When he talks, is his tone sarcastic, impatient, peremptory, gentle, ingratiating, warm, distant, whiny, cold, hostile, friendly, emotionless, or flat? Does he consistently put others down? Does he constantly say he is sorry? Is he vague, confused, logical, superrational, suspicious, humorous, superficial, ponderous, talkative, quiet, hesitant, angry, self-depreciating, witty, or compassionate? Is he forever apologizing for his repeated actions and reactions? Is he all talk and no listen? Is he all listen and no talk? Does he listen well? Does he really *hear* others and care about what they say? Does he respond appropriately?

PATTERNS OF INTERACTION

How does he respond to and treat others? Does he treat some people with contempt and others with fawning admiration? Does he act like he does not care if he is always late? Does he do what *he* wants no matter what? Does he try to order others around? Does he demand his own way? Or does he usually say, "You decide, I really don't care"? Is he always trying to be a people-pleaser? Does he let others push him around? Does he agree when agreement is obviously against his best interests? Or is he deceitful? Is he a schemer? A charmer? Does he act indifferent to what others think and say? Or does he usually seek people out, act friendly, ask questions, and listen? Does he act concerned about what others feel? Is he basically considerate?

DECISION-MAKING PROCESSES

How does he reach decisions? Abruptly? Aggressively? Impulsively? Carefully? Thoughtfully? Feelingly? Hesitantly? Is he a power-player? A compromiser? A negotiator?

DRAWING CONCLUSIONS

Suppose, measured by the standards just described, the person you are dating appears to be as follows. He resists talking about your relationship, and if you try to push the issue, he gets anxious and annoyed and tries to change the subject. He seems to expect others, you in particular, to do favors for him, to be patient when he is late (which is often), and to like what he likes. He is a male chauvinist, with conventional ideas about male and female roles. He does not say much and tends to leave the burden of carrying the conversation to you (or anyone else who will take it). When he does talk, he tends to talk mostly about ideas and objects and little about people or feelings. If you try to talk about feelings with him, he tends to clam up or else he makes jokes. He tends to assume that the two of you will do what he wants to do, and if things do not go his way, he tends to become quietly sour about it. He also tends to manipulate others to get them to do things his way. He makes decisions by subtle power playing. For example, he may claim that your choice of activity is not good because of some kind of difficulty. Then he will suggest another activity and urge it on you.

If you draw conclusions from all this, you may decide that you are in a relationship with a person who seems to be basically self-centered, fairly rigid, and closed. Unless you have other indications that he is trying to change or work with himself, you can be fairly certain that he will stay much the way he is now.

Suppose you meet another person and start dating him also. Measured by the same standards, he appears to be as follows. He is willing, sometimes eager, to talk about relationships in general and your relationship in particular. He seems to expect others to treat him with the same respect with which he treats them. He acts as though he expects most people to be basically good-hearted. He also seems to expect that life will usually be an exciting experience; he always seems to be eagerly anticipating whatever will happen next. He tends to follow the broad cultural outlines of the masculine role, but he acts on his feelings even if they do not fit the *machismo* image. In addition, he seems able and happy to accept others for their individuality and does not insist that they fit prescribed roles. He is willing and able to share his insides, and he listens attentively and caringly to you and others. He is basically considerate, but he does not knuckle under or get overpowered by someone who comes on strong. He tends to seek people out, to act friendly, to ask questions, and to listen. But he also will share himself with others. Finally, he makes most decisions by negotiation.

The basic conclusion you may draw from this evaluation is that you should stop dating the first person and concentrate on this one. The second person is warm, vital, caring, honest, and open, and a relationship with him will likely be exciting and growth producing for both of you.

Both of the persons just described represent extremes, but they serve to illustrate the need and the method for evaluating the whole person. Implicit in this discussion is the notion that you will be evaluating yourself as a whole person also. ►IE-2, p. 218.

DEVELOPING MORE OPEN RELATIONSHIPS

Much of this chapter has focused on the ways relationships form and the reasons that so many of them tend to be dysfunctional and that a large number fail. Now it is time to consider the means and methods for developing more functional, more open, and therefore more durable relationships. A set of guidelines follows that will aid you in achieving this end.

Guidelines

The following guidelines will no doubt sound familiar. They should, since they represent a distillation of the ideas and methods presented both in this chapter and in earlier parts of the book. For the sake of clarity, they are divided into three categories.

UNDERLYING PRINCIPLES

1. The less communication there is between two people the more they have to rely on outsides.
2. The more closed a person is the less in touch he is with his insides; thus the more he tends to function in terms of outsides.
3. The more closed a person is the more likely he is to perceive, evaluate, and respond to another's outsides in distorted ways.
4. Outsides alone are usually either poor and unreliable or else incomplete indices of what a person is really like. It is therefore a risky matter to build a relationship primarily or almost totally on outsides.
5. Any time a person experiences, in a flash, a strong feeling of attraction or dislike for another person when there has not been sufficient time for the other person to have earned that response as a result of his actions and reactions, then the attraction or dislike is not realistically based. Technically this phenomenon of the quick, strong, feeling response to another person is known as **transference**[17]—taking one's feelings about an already familiar person or one's feelings based on fantasies or dreams or idealizations and transferring these feelings to a new and unfamiliar person. The reason for this transference of feeling is that the new person seems familiar because he bears some resemblance (no matter how slight) to the already familiar person or to the fantasy. Obviously transference can lead to problems; if a person becomes infatuated with another very early in the relationship (or if there is "love at first sight"), the relationship is based primarily on outsides or on insides that are colored by the transference.
6. To ensure that he will be able to profit most from his dating experiences and be in a position to choose a long-term partner well and wisely, a person should try to get as wide a variety of interactions as possible. If possible, he should have many experiences with many different *kinds* of dating—casual, double, group dating, and going steady. He should have some dating relationships that last for a relatively long period of *time* so that he can experience the weight of repetition of intrapersonal and interpersonal patterns in a relationship. His dating should expose him to a wide *range* of interactions—meeting his dates' friends and family; doing common, everyday things (like studying or shopping or doing the laundry together); and spending nonpassionate as well as passionate time together.
7. Above all, dating should provide practice in communicating effectively and interacting openly. Thus dating should serve as a means for learning and practicing how to share and handle inside material. If a person's dating relationships are based primarily on outsides, then his long-term relationships are likely to be similarly based, and they will tend to be at least somewhat dysfunctional. If, however, a person's dating relationships are based on a sharing of insides and outsides, then these and later relationships will tend to be functional, or he will gradually learn to develop more functional, open relationships.

THE INTRAPERSONAL REALM

A major way of ensuring that your relationships will be based on a healthy balance between insides and outsides is to look within.

1. Get in touch with your own insides. Get to know yourself as well as you possibly can. The way to do this is to use the intrapersonal communication process (Chapter 6).
2. Apply the inductive method (pp. 211

to 214) to yourself to evaluate how you may come across to others. Also drawing on your knowledge of signals, messages, and metamessages, try to determine what you may unwittingly communicate to others. (See Chapters 7 and 8.)

3. Using the process of intrapersonal communication, check out your moment-to-moment thoughts and feelings as you interact with another person. Specifically check out your inside perceptions, interpretations, evaluations, and responses to the other person's outsides (and insides when possible).

THE INTERPERSONAL REALM

As you engage in the interpersonal interaction of a relationship, try to do the following.

1. If you are turned off by your first impressions of another person, try to stick with him anyway. Check out as thoroughly as you can what exactly turns you off. At the least, you will learn more about yourself, and you may come to like the other person.

2. If you are turned on by your first impressions of another person, try to slow yourself down some while you check out as thoroughly as possible what it is that turns you on. As is also true of step 1, you are likely to discover that you are acting on your own feelings of transference. If so, you will need to do a good deal of close checking out to determine whether or not the other person really is the way you first thought and felt he was.

3. Use the process of interpersonal communication. Share your insides with the other person, and try to get him to share his with you. Give and get feedback, and check things out with each other. Try not to function on the basis of assumptions.

4. Check out with the other person the ways you interpret his outsides and insides and the ways he interprets your outsides and insides.

5. Use the inductive method to evaluate your partner. Try *not* to let the relationship develop haphazardly. (Although this may lessen some of the romance, it will also considerably lessen the risks.)

6. If necessary, teach the other person how to communicate and interact more openly.

7. Learn with and from one another. Each of you can teach the other what each of you is like.

8. *Practice!* And—have fun.

Example of an ideal relationship

Since so many of the earlier examples in this chapter have been drawn from the dysfunctional realm, it is fitting to end this chapter with a brief description of an ideal relationship. Although negative examples are helpful in gaining an understanding of how and why relationships can be dysfunctional, it is also helpful to have at least a general idea of what a functional (healthy, more qualitative, more open) relationship is like. Although the following example is one of an ideal relationship, certainly a high degree of its quality and functioning can be achieved.

Diane and Doug have an "ideal" relationship. What does this mean? First, it means that each of them is a reasonably healthy, open individual. For example, Diane (as does Doug) has a pretty good self-concept: she cares about herself and feels generally secure about who she is. She tends to be flexible, relatively free, and freedom granting. Basically she is an autonomous individual. She is skilled at using the intrapersonal communication process and is therefore in reasonably good touch with her insides most of the time. She is aware of her thoughts and feelings on a moment-to-moment basis. Because she has worked carefully and caringly with herself, she is aware of both her strengths and weaknesses, and she works with her insides and outsides on an ongoing basis—implementing what she learns and keeping, modifying, altering, and changing her insides and outsides as she goes through life.

Her perceptions and interpretations of

others are based on a relatively undistorted self-system, but she has the awareness and the expertise to check out whatever distorting she may do from time to time. Since she knows herself well, she is sensitive to her own potential for misperceiving, misinterpreting, or both. She is able to work with her insides and outsides in a constructive way; she knows, understands, and knows how to use The System to change and grow. The same characteristics are true of Doug.

Because they are reasonably healthy and open individuals and because they are willing to work with themselves and with their relationship, Diane and Doug have a reasonably healthy, open, and qualitative relationship. Essentially this means that each of them applies his or her expertise in intrapersonal and interpersonal communication and in the use of The System to their relationship. Their relationship is therefore alive and exciting; they do not take themselves or the relationship for granted but share and work with their thoughts, feelings, and action on a moment-to-moment basis.

They are continually using the intrapersonal communication process with themselves, and they continually use the interpersonal communication process with one another. They tend not to rely on assumptions but check out and give and receive feedback on an ongoing basis. Thus they are usually engaged in sharing information, feelings, and insights. When it is relevant or desirable, they negotiate, develop alternatives, make decisions, and implement their decisions in an open, honest way. Over a period of time, each has built in much of the other person and the relationship; thus they have a reservoir of knowledge and an awareness of one another and feelings for one another so that they do not have to check out everything and can be reasonably certain of one another's basic responses.

Each continually teaches the other by sharing her or his skills and insides and by living The System. In addition, they teach others how to be more open by example.

Although this ideal relationship may seem like an impossible dream, it is not. Granted, no human being is perfect—free from flaws and able to be completely open. However, it is possible to work at and to achieve a relationship that is based on awareness, honesty, trust, caring, sensitivity, and openness. Such relationships do not happen by accident, nor do they fall out of the sky onto the shoulders of a fortunate, chosen few. They are the result of much psychological work and much practice. They are the outcome and the ongoing embodiment of change and growth.

Dating in all its variety is one of the best places for learning how to communicate effectively and interact openly and for gaining practice in the art of relationships.

This chapter has been devoted to providing you with the basics necessary for developing more open relationships. Because it draws on and puts together all that has been discussed before and applies it to relationships, this chapter serves as preparation for the following chapters, in which we look at the dynamics of marriage and the family and see how the principles that underpin relationships and the methods that work in relationships apply specifically to marriage and the family.

Interaction experiences follow.

Interaction experiences

1. Sharing insides with another person (p. 197)

Sharing insides (feelings and perceptions) is important in establishing and maintaining a meaningful relationship. This experience is designed to help you get some practice in sharing insides with your partner.

Complete in writing the following statements with a few words or a sentence and have your partner (your friend, classmate, lover, spouse) do the same.

The thing I like most about myself is ________________________________.

The thing I like most about you is ________________________________.

The thing I like least about myself is ________________________________.

The thing I like least about you is ________________________________.

The thing about myself I would most like to change is ________________________________.

The thing about you I would most like to change is ________________________________.

Now share your answers with each other. Discuss and share your feelings about what your answers mean to each of you and your relationship.

EVALUATION: Can you see any trend in your answers? For example, do you want the other person to be more or less like you? What (if any) disparities did you discover between your perceptions of one another? Do you feel that the differences between you could be reconciled or worked out?

FOLLOW-UP: After a month (or at the end of the course), try this experience again to see if there are any differences in your thoughts, feelings, and relationship.

2. Evaluating a relationship (p. 214)

Using the information and techniques presented in this chapter, evaluate in writing a relationship you have with another person (e.g., friend, date, lover, spouse, parent). Use the specific categories listed on pp. 212 to 214 to make your evaluation (expectations, roles, patterns of communication, patterns of interaction, decision-making processes).

EVALUATION: How do you see your relationship—as open or closed? Constructive or destructive? Is the dynamic equilibrium based on game playing? On open communication? What style does the relationship have? As you were becoming aware of the strengths and weaknesses in your relationship, what feelings did you have about yourself, your partner, and the relationship? Can you see how using The System might help you make your relationship more qualitative? More open?

FOLLOW-UP: Share your evaluation of the relationship with the other person. What does he feel about your evaluation? Does he agree or disagree on specific areas? Ask your partner to do his own evaluation and share it with you. Ask someone who knows both of you to evaluate your relationship. What are the similarities and differences in perceptions among the three evaluations? Can you determine why there may be different perceptions? Do you and your partner have a clear idea of the nature and quality of your relationship? Discuss these questions, and try to use The System to maximize the strengths and minimize the weaknesses in the relationship.

REFERENCES

1. Lambert, B. Geraldine, Rothschild, Barbara, Altland, Richard, and Green, Laurence B.: Adolescence: transition from childhood to maturity, Monterey, Calif., 1972, Brooks/Cole Publishing Co., pp. 79-88.
2. McGinnis, Tom: A girls guide to dating and going steady, Garden City, N.Y., 1968, Doubleday & Co., Inc., pp. 1-4.
3. Howells, John G., editor: Theory and practice of family psychiatry, New York, 1971, Brunner/Mazel, Inc., pp. 30-31.
4. Erikson, Erik H.: Identity: youth and crisis, New York, 1968, W. W. Norton & Co., Inc., p. 73.
5. Jersild, Arthur T.: In search of self, New York, 1965, Teachers College Press, pp. 19-20.
6. Satir, Virginia: Conjoint family therapy, Palo Alto, Calif., 1964, Science & Behavior Books, Inc., p. 13.
7. Ibid., p. 13.
8. Ibid., p. 12.
9. MacKlin, Eleanor D.: Going very steady, Psychology Today **8**:53-59, Nov., 1974.
10. Lewin, Kurt K.: Nonverbal clues and transference, Archives of General Psychiatry, **12**:391, 1965.
11. Lambert and others, op. cit., pp. 77-78.
12. Levy, Ronald: Self-revelation through relationships, Englewood Cliffs, N.J., 1972, Prentice-Hall, Inc.
13. Bach, George R., and Wyden, Peter: The intimate enemy: how to fight fair in love and marriage, New York, 1968, Avon Books, pp. 194-210.
14. Ackerman, Nathan W.: The psychodynamics of family life, New York, 1958, Basic Books, Inc., Publishers, p. 86.
15. Ibid., pp. 62-63.
16. Wolberg, Lewis R.: The technique of psychotherapy, vol. 2, ed. 2, New York, 1972, Grune & Stratton, Inc., pp. 482-492.
17. Ibid., p. 176.

chapter 13

THE DYNAMICS OF MARITAL INTERACTION

This chapter will analyze the **dynamics of marital interaction.** Such an analysis means examining the ways marital partners think, feel, and act in relation to external influences, to each other, to themselves, and to others outside the marriage. A full understanding of the dynamics of marital interaction therefore results from learning about the following: (1) what the essential components of a marital relationship are, (2) how a marital system and marital style develop and how they function, and (3) what the outcomes of marital interaction can be and why they are what they are.

MARITAL RELATIONSHIP: ESSENTIAL COMPONENTS

Marital dynamic equilibrium

Like members of every other human relationship, marital partners always seek to become comfortable with one another in their relationship. They seek to achieve and maintain **marital dynamic equilibrium**—the interpersonal balance that marital partners establish between them, which is based on how each one's self-system and life-style fit with the other's.[1] The way each partner achieves this balance is by adjusting his self-system and life-style in some fashion to the other person's and by making accommodations for the other person's self-system and life-style. These adjustments are made both consciously and unconsciously, and they are based on both verbal and nonverbal agreements that the partners make or that simply occur between them.

The kind of marital dynamic equilibrium (complementary, alternating, supplementary, or mixed) and its quality (functional, dysfunctional; cohesive, divisive) will depend on the specific qualities of each partner's self-system and life-style and on the match-up between them.

The whole marriage

Every couple's **whole marriage** is comprised of two interlocking, mutually influencing parts: its *insides* and *outsides.*

MARITAL INSIDES

Marital insides are the inner thoughts and feelings each partner has about himself, the other partner, and the marital relationship. In addition, insides include each partner's *intrapersonal patterns* (the ways he treats himself). Marital insides are private unless a partner chooses to reveal them by means of communication.[2]

MARITAL OUTSIDES

Marital outsides are each marital partner's conscious and unconscious external expressions and manifestations of his insides. Marital outsides are each partner's *interpersonal patterns* of thinking, feeling, and acting and the interlock between them; they can be observed, sensed, interpreted, experienced, and/or understood by the other partner (and by other people too).[3]

Marital system

Marital system denotes each partner's marital insides plus the interlock between their marital insides (whether it is clashing or harmonious). In effect, marital system refers to the internal functioning of each partner plus the ways each one's insides affect the other's and the marriage's internal functioning. What follows now are definitions and explanations of the various components that make up a marital system.[4,5]

MARITAL PFLs

Marital PFLs are those PFLs (internalized expectations, rules, values) about marriage that each partner brings with him. These PFLs have to do with such matters as marital relationships, marital roles, core characteristics (e.g., intellectual balance), and issues. These PFLs may be societal PFLs about marriage, personal PFLs, or a combination thereof. They are tempered by the specifics of the core characteristics and by the unique background, self-system, and life-style of each partner. Gradually a marital couple usually work out some accommodation among their PFLs if they clash, or they may hold essentially the same PFLs and operate on this merged set of PFLs. These marital PFLs direct and "teach" a person *who* he should be; *what* he should be like; *what* he should think about, feel, and do; and *how* he should think, feel, act, and react *in his marriage*.[6] ►IE-1, p. 235.

MARITAL INTRAPERSONAL PATTERNS

Marital intrapersonal patterns are a person's consistent, private, inner ways that he thinks, feels, and acts within the marriage. They are his consistent ways of treating himself. They become known to the other partner only if the person shares them through communication, although over a long period of time because of repetition a partner may be able to identify the other's intrapersonal patterns.[7]

MARITAL CONCEPT

Marital concept consists of the way each partner sees (perceives) and feels about the marital relationship. Marital concept is naturally based on each partner's self-concept and on the way he perceives and interprets the other's thoughts, feelings, and actions.

MARITAL CHILD/PARENT/ADULT BALANCE

Marital Child/Parent/Adult Balance is the balance created by the interlock between the two partners' individual Child/Parent/Adult balances. For example, if one partner has a Child/Parent/Adult balance that has a large, fearful Child (and small Parent and Adult parts) and the other has a strong, protective, nuturing Parent, the marital Child/Parent/Adult balance is basically a complementary one between the one partner's large Child and the other's large Parent.

IMPORTANCE OF THE MARITAL SYSTEM

The marital system is crucially important to the dynamics of marital interaction, since it is the marital system that underpins all behavior in the marriage. As such it underpins the marital style.

Marital style

Each person brings to the marital relationship his individual life-style (the observable network of consistent interpersonal patterns that determine how he functions—thinks, feels, and acts—in the interpersonal sphere). **Marital style** refers to the interlock between the partners' life-styles; this interlock forms a larger observable network of interpersonal patterns that determine how each partner will function in regard to the other and to their relationship. In other words, marital style is the marital dynamic equilibrium established by the meshing of the partners' life-styles.[8]

Relationships between marital system and marital style

Taken together, marital system and marital style constitute the whole marriage. If the marital partners have little awareness of who they are and what they are like both as individuals and as a marital couple and have little awareness of how they or the marriage functions, then the marital system and style operates in a largely unconscious, automatic, and repetitious fashion. The whole marriage tends to be based on a good deal of misperceiving, misinterpretation, and distortion. The marital system is likely to feed and reinforce the often inappropriate workings of the marital style and vice versa. This kind of marriage naturally tends to be rigid, relatively unchanging, and self-perpetuating. It both encourages and is encouraged by its closed, dysfunctional nature.

If, however, marital partners are fairly mature and relatively aware of who they are and what they are like both as individuals and as a marital couple and if they are relatively aware of how they and the marriage function, then the operations of the marital system and style tend to be fairly flexible, functional, and open; the partners are both in touch with their own and the marriage's insides and can work constructively to make their own styles and the marital style accurately and appropriately reflect those insides.[9,10]

Marital identity

Ultimately just how functional or dysfunctional a marital relationship is can be measured by how aware the partners are of their marital identity and how skilled they are in applying The System to their knowledge of the marital relationship. **Marital identity** can be defined by the answers to the following questions:

Present: Who are we (as a marital couple) and what is our marital relationship like *now?*

Past: How did our relationship get to be the way it is now?

Future: What might our relationship become?

This definition is deceptively brief and simple, but it encompasses an enormous number of complex, interlocking, and mutually influencing factors.[11,12] Breaking the question down into specific components makes the range and scope of these factors evident.

Who are we and what is our relationship like now? These questions involve such matters as the style of the relationship, its degree of openness or closedness, the marital concept, the Child/Parent/Adult balance, the current patterns of communication and interaction, the roles, all the marital PFLs (expectations, rules, values) that apply to the relationship and to each partner's life-style and self-system.

How did our relationship get to be the way it is now? This question involves all the factors just listed as they have contributed to and been a part of the development of the relationship. In addition, it includes an assessment of how the issues in a marriage have affected the partners' ways of interacting and the goals they have set, rejected, and fulfilled.

What might our relationship become? This question involves the answers to the two prior questions as well as such factors as current and future goals, the importance to each partner of the marital investments they have made, the strength or weakness of each partner's commitment to a continuing relationship, what kind of motivation for personal and marital growth each partner has, and the degree of openness or closedness already present in the marital relationship.

THE PROCESS OF DEVELOPING A MARITAL SYSTEM AND STYLE

Being able to determine marital identity means acquiring a good deal of awareness and knowledge. Essentially it means gaining an understanding of what factors influence the interaction in an ongoing marital relationship and how they do so, the ways a marital relationship develops a marital system and style, and what outcomes of marital interaction are possible and how they can be controlled.

Factors influencing ongoing marital interaction

Depending on the interplay among various influencing factors, such as the spouses' self-systems, life-styles, marital core characteristics, and marital issues, each partner may see and respond to the other in terms of one or more roles. The wife may perceive and respond to her husband primarily as an individual and vice versa. Each spouse may see and react to the other primarily as a marital partner. The husband may perceive and respond to his wife as both an individual and a wife, depending on circumstances, and vice versa. Or one partner may see the other as an individual, whereas the other views the first strictly in terms of the marital role.

Whatever the particular role combination in a particular marital relationship, however, five facts are important.

1. If marital partners demand that one another fit or play only one role, then divisiveness may occur unless each agrees to that demand. For example, if Jed demands that Elaine be a wife and submerge her identity in that role, divisiveness will probably occur if she values her identity as an individual and feels that it is being swamped by the role requirements of wifehood. Or if Elaine is not willing to see Jed as anything but a husband, he may object strongly by refusing to go along with many of the role characteristics and by acting more individualistic than he ordinarily might.

2. The more rigid, traditional, and stereotyped the role ascriptions are the more limiting the expectations about that role are and the more closed the relationship is. For example, if Ken can relate to Maureen only as his wife and if "wife" means expectations like "a woman's place is in the home" and "a wife's role is to care for her husband and children," he is not leaving much allowance for Maureen as an individual. What if she does not want children? What if she wants to have a career? What if running a home and staying at home bore her? If Ken's expectations are that she will ignore her own desires as an individual, then there is trouble somewhere ahead for him or her or both of them.

3. If a couple enters a marriage without having thought or verbalized much about roles and expectations, then unless they communicate well about these matters *after* they marry, problems are likely to arise. For example, Beatrice expects Ben to always act like a husband—which to her means that he should support her and the children, spend most of his free time with her and the family, see his bachelor friends only occasionally, and make her and the children the center of his attentions. But suppose Ben brings with him expectations about "husbandhood" that are different from Beatrice's. Ben's expectations of what it means to be a husband are that he should support the wife and children and should pay a certain amount of attention to them. However, he also expects that as a husband his wishes and needs will take precedence (since he is the breadwinner); thus he may feel that he has every right to spend several nights a week at the local tavern with his bachelor buddies and that when he is at home he can spend his time glued to the television, watching sports programs. The conflict between expectations is obvious; how Beatrice and Ben handle both the conflicts and the expectations will have a great impact on the course of their relationship.

4. The role a person is taking tends to "filter" or determine the acceptability of facets of life-style and self-system. For example, Jack may feel that Dinah's patterns of being outgoing, warm, and charming to men are delightful—when he views her as an individual. However, when she is his wife, these same patterns exhibited in the same way and to the same degree may strike him as being outrageously seductive, disgusting, or both. Dinah may feel that Jack's patterns of being cool, reserved, and sometimes withdrawn are signs of strength and fascinating mystery—when she views him as an individual. But when he is her husband and she wants more intimate emo-

tional contact with him in their everyday life, she may be deeply disappointed with and frustrated by these same patterns. In her husband, these patterns may come across as obtuse, difficult, and isolating. Therein lie some of the seeds of divisiveness.

5. The healthiest state of affairs in a marriage occurs when each partner feels and is free to take that role—individual or marital or a mixture of both—which is appropriate to the particular circumstances of the moment. Thus if Scott wants time during the weekend to go off by himself and work on something that interests him, he is free to do so. However, he also feels free to express his concern as a husband about the ways the budget is set up. If Rita, as a wife, feels that she should have more to say about the kind of car they are going to buy, she has the freedom to express her opinions. But she is also free to act as an individual; for example, she may get involved in local politics and use her maiden name so that she will be considered as an individual. This state of affairs is one that exists in an open marriage, a relationship that tends to be cohesive yet freedom granting.

Note two other important concepts. First, although the processes of developing an individual self-system and life-style and marital (and family) systems and styles are somewhat similar, there is a significant difference too. That difference is that the development of an individual self-system and life-style occurs in the child, who starts out with an unformed personality structure. As the child grows toward maturity, he gradually forms his self-system and life-style in response to significant others, events, the environment, and his experiences. The development of a marital system and style, however, begins differently with not one but two already formed personalities. The interaction between these two personalities creates a third entity, which consists of more than the sum of these two parts.[13] This third entity is the marital relationship, and it is comprised of the marital system and style.

Second, of necessity we occasionally use the term "marital style" to designate both the style of the relationship and its dynamic underpinnings—the marital system.

The developing marital relationship: its system and style

MOMENT-TO-MOMENT MARITAL INTERACTION

Marital interaction includes all of each partner's thoughts, feelings, and actions that are occurring from moment to moment. As each partner sends and receives signals and messages and as each responds to the other and to whatever the subject matter is, each begins to get some feel for whatever continuity and consistency exist in each other's ways of communicating and interacting.[14] Over a period of time through what is essentially a long-term process of trial and error (and of question and answer if there is effective communication), each partner begins to learn (consciously or unconsciously or both) which thinking, feeling, and acting responses are acceptable and which are not acceptable to the other partner. Each learns which responses generate approval or disapproval and which responses fit the expectations and values of the other partner. In effect each partner is learning how (and sometimes how not) to match up moment-to-moment thoughts, feelings, and actions with the needs, feelings, desires, ideas, requests, demands, actions, and reactions of the other partner.

By repetitious testing-out of responses, the partners establish and develop their particular ways of relating to one another (and to others). They are effecting some kind of match-up to achieve and maintain dynamic equilibrium in their marriage. Of course, if communication is ineffective, there is little checking out, and the match-up is based mainly on assumptions (accurate or otherwise) about one another's outsides. In this case, the dynamic equilibrium is on shaky ground. If communication is effective, then the match-up and consequent dynamic equilibrium rest on relatively solid ground.

A brief example of how this moment-to-moment interactional process works follows: Emily is not a "morning person." She is grouchy, grumpy, and touchy early in the morning. James is a morning person. When he hops out of bed, he is wide awake, cheerful, and ready to go. He sings loudly in the shower, hums while he is shaving, and plans his day while he is dressing. In the meantime, Emily has groped her way into the kitchen and is numbly waiting for the coffee to finish perking. Early in the marriage, James was likely to bounce into the kitchen and begin a cheerful conversation with Emily. After about the umpteenth time of a pained look and a grumbled greeting from Emily, James decided to withhold his cheer for a while and see what happened. He knows now that if he waits until Emily has had a cup of coffee, he will at least get a civil greeting from her.

By the same token, Emily has learned not to overwhelm James at the end of the day by greeting him at the front door with all the events and disasters of the day. She has learned—by means of the repeated testing-out process—that if she says "Hi," kisses him, hands him the newspaper, and leaves him alone for a half hour, he will usually be in a much better mood for the rest of the evening.

These two examples are simple, but they serve to give some idea of how the process works. Everything is grist for the process' mill: issues, problems, relationships, feelings, attitudes, events, and situations—whatever happens to affect the marital partners in any way has some bearing on their moment-to-moment interaction.

In discussing the process of moment-to-moment marital interaction, we have presented essentially an overview. It is time to examine in more detail the two specific forms of this moment-to-moment marital interaction process: patterns of communication and patterns of interaction.* These represent respectively the moment-to-moment efforts of marital partners to satisfactorily mesh their patterns of communication and interaction.

MARITAL PATTERNS OF COMMUNICATION

As the couple repeatedly interact in terms of their thoughts, feelings, and actions about all kinds of matters, they are communicating with each other. Since each partner brings already formed patterns of communication to the relationship each must do a certain amount of testing out (whether consciously or unconsciously) to determine which communication patterns will be accepted, tolerated, or rejected by the other partner and which of his partner's patterns of communication he will accept, tolerate, or reject. Whether knowingly or not, the couple is learning by trial and error how to mesh their individual patterns of communication so that they can achieve some form of joint communication, which will help them to establish a state of dynamic equilibrium. As they discover which patterns of communication interlock and which ones clash, they are discovering those patterns which help to establish and promote dynamic equilibrium and those which do not; probably they will repeat those that work and drop those that do not. In this way, a couple develop consistent marital patterns of communication, which help them maintain balance in their relationship whether they are communicating privately with each other or publicly with each other and with other people.[15,16]

The following example illustrates the process of achieving a communicational dynamic equilibrium. It is Janice and Harry Johnson's first wedding anniversary, and Harry did not remember.

Janice (Agitated, upset): I don't know *how* you could have forgotten. After all, we've only been married one year, and already you've forgotten we're married! (Her voice rises and takes on an hysterical edge. She is near tears.) You don't really love me. If you did, you would have remembered.

---

*The term "patterns" used throughout the following discussion is intended to refer to all interpersonal marital patterns, whether private (between partners) or public (between partners and others outside the marriage). Breaking patterns into those of communication and interaction is meant simply to highlight these two important facets of interpersonal dynamics.

Harry (Cold, logical, controlled. Speaks through his teeth, which are clenched): That's not true! How many times do I have to tell you—I thought of our anniversary this morning. But then I had two emergency meetings with field salesmen. And the next thing after that, B. S. (Harry's boss) demanded a report on those meetings before I left. There are logical reasons that I forgot. It has nothing to do with not loving you! Can't you understand that?

Janice (Not the least bit impressed or convinced. Her voice gets even sharper and nastier): Oh, you and your reasons. I understand all right—your work means more to you than our marriage. It wouldn't have taken you more than a few minutes to at least get a card and . . .

Harry (His voice rising, interrupting her): But I told you—I forgot. Be reasonable, will you? How could I get a card if I *forgot?* Can't you understand simple facts when . . .

Janice (Sarcastically interrupting): Oh, I understand. Yes, indeed—I understand perfectly. You just . . .

Harry (He is livid. He interrupts in a rage): For God's sake, woman—shut up and leave me in peace! Don't push me any further. If you don't shut up, I'll . . . I'll . . .

Janice (Bursts into tears and runs into the bedroom).

Harry (Yanks open the front door, stomps out, and slams the door behind him).

After this kind of incident occurs a number of times over a period of time, Janice learns that to challenge or criticize Harry directly invariably elicits rage from him. Because Janice is insecure, Harry's rage is too threatening and too overwhelming. It is simply not worth it to communicate with him in this way. So gradually Janice learns not to communicate her criticisms so directly; instead she snipes at Harry, veiling her criticisms under the guise of sympathy for how demanding his job is. With this approach, Harry cannot find the clearly defined "enemy" at which to direct his rage. Instead he becomes and remains irritated and generally irritable. Then Janice gets him by "innocently" asking him if he has had a hard day! Harry then lashes out about someone at work and gets rid of his irritation that way. Thus a kind of balance is established, but it is a dysfunctional kind of balance because it is based on communication that does not deal with the real issues but with distorted substitutes. Nevertheless, it is a balance, one that is worked out in response to the friction from two people's original patterns of communication. As a part of the ongoing interaction in their relationship, Janice and Harry have developed new ways of communicating with each other; they have developed *marital* patterns of communication. (Both can and probably will retain their individual patterns of communication and may continue to use them in other relationships—but not in the marital relationship because they tend to disturb or destroy the dynamic equilibrium of the marital relationship.)

Janice and Harry also develop public marital patterns of communication on the basis of their ongoing marital interaction. They may, for example, have a number of arguments after parties because when Janice is entertaining people with her storytelling abilities, Harry tends to interrupt her to set the facts straight. Finally, if they have enough arguments in which Janice points out how pompous and irrelevant Harry's factual additions are, they may agree on a public communication ground rule: it is okay for either of them to interrupt to set the facts straight when they are alone, but this is not "allowed" in front of others.

Thus through repeated moment-to-moment interactions, couples learn to mesh their individual communication patterns so that they establish some kind of balance. (If they cannot do this with any significant success, the marriage is likely to become divisive.)

MARITAL PATTERNS OF INTERACTION

The same process of establishing dynamic equilibrium operates in regard to patterns of interaction. Each partner brings to the relationship already formed patterns of interaction; therefore each must do a great deal of testing out (consciously and unconsciously) to determine which interactional patterns the other partner will accept, tolerate, or reject and which of the partner's interactional patterns he will accept, tolerate, or reject. As the couple repeatedly interact with one another over a period of time, they are learning by moment-to-moment trial and error how to mesh their patterns of interaction in such a way that they can achieve dynamic equilibrium in their relationship and thereby "get comfortable." They are learning which of their patterns interlock and which ones clash, and they are making adjustments in response to what they are learning. They are likely to keep those combinations of patterns which serve to help establish and maintain dynamic equilibrium and they will probably drop or ignore those which do not. In these ways, they are developing consistent marital patterns of interaction, both private and public.

An example of the process of developing a private marital pattern of interaction follows. When someone gets upset or angry, Della's pattern is to feel that somehow she is at fault and that she should try to be helpful by asking what is wrong and offering to help or fix whatever is wrong. She marries Buddy whose pattern for dealing with things that upset or anger him is to ignore them for as long as possible (meanwhile becoming more and more irritable). Then he blows his stack at some little thing, lets off steam, and feels better. In the beginning of their relationship, when Della noticed that Buddy was irritable, she would assume it was her fault and would immediately ask (and keep asking) him what was wrong. This irritated Buddy even more (because he could not ignore his feelings). If Della kept after him, which she did because his increasing irritation meant to her that she had offended him even more, Buddy's irritation level would rise rapidly and often he would end up getting angry and yelling at her.

At least four alternatives exist at this point.

1. Della and Buddy can continue letting their patterns interlock in this way, but this means war and hurt feelings every time.

2. If Buddy feels annoyed because Della's concern gets in the way of his old pattern or if he feels guilty about taking his anger out on her, he may try to change the interlock to strike a more comfortable balance. Maybe he asks Della just to leave him alone and not say anything when she notices his irritability building up. Or maybe he sees to it that he is not around her when he is ready to blow up (if he is able to foretell that occurrence).

3. Della may try to break into her own pattern by *not* asking Buddy what is wrong or offering to help. Thus she backs off from the situation and lets Buddy run through his pattern unimpeded. That probably would bring about a somewhat more comfortable balance also.

4. The preceding three alternatives leave something to be desired. The fourth is more constructive: suppose Della and Buddy can communicate fairly well and they do so about the clash between their patterns. If they work together and help each other, they can probably help Della interrupt and modify her pattern of overconcern and help Buddy interrupt and modify his pattern of ignoring his anger until he blows up.

Whatever particular choices Della and Buddy make, however, one outcome is certain: they will mesh their patterns in some way and thereby form a private marital pattern of interaction.

An example of a public marital pattern of interaction is as follows: Buddy is an openly affectionate person, and he shows his affection by hugging, patting, pinching, and touching. One of his favorite affection patterns is to pat and pinch Della's rear. Della, however, comes from an uptight family, and at first Buddys' action embarrassed her. Her worst moment came, however, when they were at a party and Buddy patted and pinched her rear as he was walking past her to the kitchen. Della was talking to two old friends at the time; when Buddy did this, she became terribly embarrassed and so flustered she could hardly go on talking.

When they got home after the party, Della exploded, a rare action for her. When the smoke of battle finally cleared, Della and Buddy had reached an agreement and formulated a new marital PFL. Patting and pinching are acceptable (even enjoyable) at home when they are alone. But they are too embarrassing in public, and Della does not want Buddy to do this to her again when they are not in the privacy of their own home. Impressed by Della's anger and argument, Buddy has agreed to limit his pattern in this way. Thus in this case they have established a dynamic equilibrium relating to both private and public marital interaction.[17]

Of necessity we have just "dropped in" on certain moments and decisions in various couples' relationships. This technique tends to freeze those moments and decisions in time, thereby sometimes giving the impression that what is being described is static. Such is not the case. The interactions, the attempts to mesh patterns, the striving for balance, and the decisions—all of these are part of an ongoing process. The process of adjusting to one another in a relationship is one that goes on constantly and is never really finished until such time as the relationship no longer exists.

MARITAL CONCEPT

As a couple communicate and interact from moment to moment over a period of time and form their marital patterns of communication and interaction, they gradually develop a marital concept, which consists of what each partner *thinks* and *feels* about the marital relationship. As each develops his concept, the marital concept in turn influences how each behaves in the marriage.

For example, over a period of time, Carolyn and Lloyd have settled into a dynamic equilibrium that is based on communication patterns of rarely, if ever, discussing or expressing negative thoughts or feelings and on interaction patterns of rarely doing anything negative. In effect they deny or ignore the negative and accentuate the positive as much as possible. In this case both Carolyn and Lloyd have essentially the same marital concept: each *thinks* of the marriage as being pleasant, friendly, and smooth sailing. Each *feels* that the marriage is a secure one, although at times somewhat dull, but essentially it feels comfortable.

As each develops his or her marital concept, the concept exerts an influence on each one's behavior. Since the concept is a pleasing one, both Carolyn and Lloyd are likely to tailor their behavior to fit the concept and to maintain it. In this case therefore both tend to back away from raising negative issues and from acting negatively. In effect, each of them tries never to rock the boat. Thus a circular, self-feeding process occurs.

It is possible for each partner to have somewhat different marital concepts. For example, suppose Carolyn thinks and feels that theirs is a pleasant marriage, secure and comfortable, and she is content with that. Lloyd thinks it is pleasant enough but feels that it is incredibly dull, dull to the point of being stifling. He may then be fair game for an exciting, explosive extramarital affair.

It is probable that the greater the disparity between each partner's concept of the marriage the greater the likelihood of some problem in the future. Of course, if the partners have good communication with each other and are aware of their own and the other's views and feelings, they may be able and content to maintain a satisfactory relationship. However, if each partner thinks and feels differently about the relationship but assumes that they both hold the same concept, then the potential for divisiveness is there.

MARITAL CHILD/PARENT/ADULT BALANCE

The efforts of a marital couple to establish a marital dynamic equilibrium in the course of their moment-to-moment interaction extend to their attempts to achieve a marital Child/Parent/Adult balance. That is, each partner brings to the marriage his own individual Child/Parent/Adult balance; each partner then consciously and/or unconsciously teaches and learns from the other how to mesh their individual balances to create a new marital Child/Parent/Adult balance.

For example, Jack has patterns of being cautious, hesitant, and of planning ahead; these are the outgrowth of a large and harsh *Parent*, which constantly "lectures" him that if he is not careful and does not plan ahead he will be sorry.

Dinah perceives Jack's patterns in a positive light: his caution and his tendency to plan ahead impress her as being mature and intelligent. She is impressed because her large *Child* often gets her into trouble because she acts first on impulse and only later does she look to see what has happened or what she got herself into.

Dinah has patterns of being impulsive, fun loving, playful, and spontaneous; these are the result of her large *Child*, which is constantly urging her to be wild and free, daring her to kick up her heels and make the world her playground.

Jack responds to Dinah's patterns with amused tolerance and affection. At times, her spontaneity and her impulsive fun-loving nature absolutely delight him. His responses are based on two parts: his stern *Parent* and his blighted *Child*. His Parent wants to temper Dinah's impulsivity and protect her from whatever troubles she gets into because of it. His blighted Child is enchanted by the chance to have some fun, by the implicit invitation to come out into the world and play, and by the freedom and vitality of her spontaneity.

Their marital Child/Parent/Adult balance is complementary in two ways: Dinah's wild Child/Jack's stern Parent and Dinah's fun-loving and free Child/Jack's blighted Child. Things will probably be fine as long as they can maintain this particular balance. However, suppose Dinah is a little more boisterous, talkative, and impulsive than usual (perhaps as a result of a couple of drinks). If she acts this way at a backyard barbecue, that may be fine, and Jack's Child may encourage him to be wild with her. But suppose she acts this way at a cocktail party given by Jack's boss at the company. Then Jack's Parent part may prompt him to become angry and punitive toward Dinah, and he may act coldly to her after the party and tell her to grow up and act her age. (It is also possible that Dinah may simply act like her usual self in both situations but that Jack will perceive her differently and react differently.) In either case, however, the effects tend to be divisive.

Suppose Jack and Dinah go to the boss's party, where she allows his caution and reserve to set the tone of her actions: she is more restrained and not boisterous but is quietly pleasant and outgoing. Her Child is responding to his parental tempering. But suppose Jack acts like the heavy Parent whenever Dinah starts being the least bit impulsive. He has to plan everything to the last detail, and he is consistently disapproving and condescending. If he acts this way at their backyard barbecue where they are with old friends who are having fun, Dinah's Child may begin to feel restricted and extremely irritated by Jack's heavy Parent. She may begin to perceive Jack as dull and plodding—a wet blanket. Unless each of them deals constructively with these negative feelings, the results will be a marital Child/Parent/Adult balance that is divisive rather than cohesive.

OUTCOMES OF MARITAL INTERACTION

As a result of marital partners' moment-to-moment interaction over a period of time, they gradually develop certain overall outcomes: a specific marital system and style, which have a particular quality, that of being open or closed.

Marital system and style

As a couple develop their marital relationship, the relationship itself takes on a style of its own, which is the result of a merger between the partners' individual life-styles. Since to establish and maintain a relationship the partners must mesh their own styles in some way, the marital style of the resulting relationship usually reflects the combination of the strongest, most dominant elements of each partner's life-style (and self-system).

The specific name given to marital style identifies the dominant element of each partner's life-style that puts his stamp on the marital dynamic equilibrium. For example, if one partner's style is predominantly sadistic and the other's is predominantly masochistic, more than likely their marital style is a sadomasochistic one. If both partners are essentially independent and individualistic, their marital style is independent/individualistic. But if the main thrust of one's style is independence and the other's is dependence, then obviously the marital style is independent/dependent. Harry and Janice Johnson's style would technically be termed as obsessive-compulsive/hysteric style. However, in more down-to-earth terms, it could accurately be called a thinker/feeler style or an overly rational/overly emotional style.

Open or closed style

Not only does the couple's moment-to-moment interaction shape the system and style of the marriage, but it also determines the *quality* of the style. In other words, the ways that the couple interact are governed by the degree of openness or closedness present in their individual life-styles and self-systems, and the ways they interact determine the degree of openness or closedness of the marital style and system that they are developing.

In an **open marital relationship,** ideally each partner has the freedom to be who he is; he does not have to make himself over to meet the expectations of the other partner. Each partner is able to get in touch with his thoughts and feelings (his insides) and can and does share them with the other partner. Each can and does communicate effectively. Each is aware of his own patterns (his style), he knows how they work, and his patterns are not automatic and repetitious; rather they operate appropriately. Thus the open relationship is freedom granting, allows for and encourages sharing of inside material, and functions on the basis of accurate information, insight, and appropriate responses. For these reasons, the particular style of the relationship (e.g., extrovert/introvert) reflects a constructive blending of each partner's uniqueness, self-system, and life-style.[18] The **open marital style** represents an essentially harmonious meshing of personal styles, which results in a healthy and functional dynamic equilibrium.

In a **closed marital relationship,** each partner has little freedom to be himself; instead he suits his personality to the expectations of the other partner or rebels against those expectations. Neither partner is much in touch with his insides. Neither partner communicates effectively. Neither partner is very aware of his own patterns (his style). Neither knows much about how his patterns function—they operate in an automatic and repetitious and therefore inappropriate manner. The patterns rather than the person tend to run his life. Thus the **closed marital style** allows little freedom, does not promote the sharing of inside material, and functions on the basis of minimal or distorted information and insight and frequently inappropriate responses. Thus the particular style of the relationship is either the outcome of a disharmonious jamming together of two styles that conflict (e.g., aggressive/aggressive) or of a harmonious but nonconstructive blend of neurotic styles (e.g., obsessive-compulsive/hysterical), which results in an unhealthy or dysfunctional dynamic equilibrium.

Marital identity is the outcome of the developmental process. It consists of a detailed perspective on that process and on the functioning of the components of that process. Those marital partners who have a good grasp of their marital identity are those who have a fairly high degree of self-awareness and marital awareness and therefore usually have relatively open, functional marital systems and styles. Conversely, those partners who have little or no conception of their marital identity generally have rather closed, dysfunctional marriages.

Games couples play

Married couples who have little or no conception of their marital identity tend to communicate and interact in a rather limited fashion. One primary way is to play games. As you will remember, **games** are a person's specific but distorted application of intrapersonal and/or interpersonal patterns of communication and interaction, which set up a series of preprogrammed (automatic, repetitious) reactions and interactions to achieve certain psychological ends—basically the establishment and maintenance of intrapersonal and interpersonal dynamic equilibrium no matter how dysfunctional these may be.[19]

Marital games arise out of the harmonious and/or disharmonious interlock between the partners' self-systems and lifestyles. The outer form or flavor of the game reflects the marital style, but the psychological ends of the game are determined by each partner's self-system and the marital system. That is, each partner plays a particular game to satisfy his own inner thoughts and feelings in relation to the other partner and to the marriage.[20]

For example, Jack's and Dinah's marital style is passive (Jack)/aggressive (Dinah). Thus the games that Jack initiates have a passive quality, whereas the games Dinah initiates have an aggressive quality. The psychological ends of Jack's games are to protect him against intimacy and others' depending on him, whereas the ends of Dinah's games are to seek greater intimacy, to protect herself against loneliness, and to establish and maintain emotional dependency.

Following are some of Jack's games: "Anything you say, dear"; "Of course I love you, but do I always have to say it?"; "We'll talk about it later"; "Nothing bothers me"; and the "Silent Treatment." Some of Dinah's games include "You never listen to me"; "There you go. You're cold and unfeeling—just like your father!"; "Look, I do the best I can. Heaven knows, I do the best I can to please you"; and "Max (her best friend's husband) at least acts like he *knows* Dorothy when they're out together!"; and a mind-blowing, "nonstop stream of talk."

Games are always based on a certain amount of truth or fact (that is, a person plays a specific game because something in the reality situation touches him off). Nevertheless, although somewhat reality based, games are dysfunctional in nature. Like rigid patterns, they are repetitious, automatic, and ordinarily inappropriate and are largely controlled by unconscious forces. In addition, games are attempts to manipulate self, others, reality, or all of these. However, although they are dysfunctional, games can be either cohesive or divisive.

In a marriage, through moment-to-moment interactions over a period of time each partner learns how to match up his thoughts, feelings, and actions with his partner's desires, expectations, demands, needs, fears, and responses. In effect, partners learn (both consciously and unconsciously) enough about one another to know or to sense or both, for example, what turns the other on, what angers the other, what interests the other, what upsets the other, and what bugs the other. For example, a wife may come to know that all she has to do to send her husband up in angry smoke is to say, "You never remember my birthday or our anniversary." Or a husband may come to know that the fastest way to put his wife down is for him to ask, "Can't you ever be on time?" Each learns little tricks like playing dumb or withdrawing or whistling softly while the other is talking. Games are a kind of verbal and nonverbal interactional shorthand—one signal, one phrase, one look, one move, or one sentence is often so loaded with assumptions or implications or accusations that it will set off a torrent of reactions and will involve the other person plus the game initiator in an automatic, repetitious, and usually inappropriate series of preprogrammed interactions.[21,22]

If the games' match-up serves the particular "needs" or desires of each partner's self-system (no matter how distorted those needs or desires may be), then the games will be cohesive. If, however, the games' match-up serves one partner better than the other, the one who is less well served may pull back, pull out, yield, or fight; divisiveness will probably result. If one partner changes and grows but the other continues playing the same old games, then divisiveness will probably occur. For example, consider Garrett, a punitive, hostile alcoholic, and Cleo, his long-suffering, masochistic wife. If Garrett joins Alcoholics Anonymous, stops drinking, and becomes less hostile and more responsible, Cleo's "Look how badly you treat me—feel guilty" game may lose its power. Or if Cleo joins Alanon (a group designed to help relatives and friends of alcoholics) and learns to detach herself from Garrett and his drinking, then his game of "Punish but forgive me" may lose its force.

In effect the cohesiveness or divisiveness of games depend on two interlocking factors.

1. An interpersonal game requires at least two players who are willing to play the game. If one will not play, the game collapses at least on the interpersonal level.

2. Games exist because they are psychologically purposeful; they enable people to achieve certain psychological ends. For example, games can protect people from learning bitter truths, from getting in touch with anxiety-producing emotions, or from getting to know one another. They can serve as a means of controlling or dominating or as a means of yielding or knuckling under. They can be used to prove superiority or inferiority, to get something from the other person, or to get the other person to think or feel or do something. If one partner will not play or if the game stops achieving its psychological ends or if the price of playing the game becomes too high for one or both partners, the game may collapse or become extremely divisive. ►IE-2, p. 236.

Marital identity crises

Many couples may go through their whole married life playing games and having little or no awareness of their marital identity. Usually, if this is the case, it is possible because the marriage is not subjected to a major stress or change that exercises enough impact to jolt the couple out of their automatic and repetitious ways. If, however, something does happen that really challenges or shakes up the couple's usual ways of maintaining their dysfunctional dynamic equilibrium, then one or both of them is likely to experience a **marital identity crisis.**[23]

Many different occurrences can precipitate such a crisis:

1. The breadwinner may lose his job, and the couple have to change their accustomed style of living.
2. One (or both) of the partners may have a personal identity crisis that moves him to evaluate not only himself but also the marriage.
3. When the children leave home, the

couple may suddenly have a lot of unfilled time and may begin to assess their marital identity.

4. The "marital menopause" may jolt them into appraising their relationship.
5. One (or both) of the partners may have an extramarital affair, which may cause him to take a long, hard look at the marital relationship.
6. The discovery of the other partner's infidelity may jolt both the discoverer and the discovered into a reassessment.

Other crisis-precipitating factors may consist of physical problems, psychological problems, or both besetting one (or both) of the partners. For example, one partner becomes excessively dependent on the other. One (or both) of the partners sloshes across the line between heavy social drinking and alcoholism or becomes addicted to drugs. One (or both) partner's alcoholism or drug addiction becomes evident as it affects the marriage. The wife is (or becomes) truly "frigid" and cannot or will not have sexual relations. The husband is (or becomes) impotent. One (or both) of the partners becomes physically disabled, or a serious physical disease or condition occurs (e.g., cancer, heart attack, senility). One (or both) of the partners suffers a psychological breakdown (e.g., severe depression, psychosis, frank paranoid behavior, attempted suicide). One (or both) engages in criminal behavior (e.g., embezzlement, armed robbery, homicide—attempted or accomplished).

Obviously any of these events or problems would be adequate occasion for an evaluation of marital identity. Of course, one of the surest ways to set the assessment process in motion is for one partner to announce to the other that he or she wants a separation or divorce. Whatever the precipitating factors may be, however, evaluating the marriage may reveal shocking disparities in the partner's perceptions of one another and in the partners' perception of the marriage.

DISPARITIES IN PARTNERS' SELF/OTHER PERCEPTIONS

One particular aspect of partner perception is especially vulnerable to the shock of recognition. This aspect involves how each partner perceives the other and how each partner *thinks* the other perceives him. If there is a disparity between their perceptions, there is distortion. Such distortion is not only divisive per se but can be especially divisive when it suddenly becomes evident—often through direct confrontation and revelation.

For example, Jack's self-concept is that he thinks of himself as intelligent, thoughtful, responsible, reserved, and pleasant but not too exciting. He feels that he is uptight, insecure, too passive, dull, shy, cold, and aloof. He believes that these are essentially the ways that Dinah perceives him too. Thus he may feel puzzled about why she would want to marry someone like him, he may feel flattered, or he may feel somewhat disdainful of her for marrying him when she should know better.

But suppose Dinah really perceives Jack in another way. She perceives him as strong, mysterious, "deep," shy but not dull, independent, and self-sufficient. However, if he acts on his self-concept and on the way he *believes* she perceives him, Jack may send off many distorted signals and messages. For example, if he assumes Dinah sees him (as *he* sees himself) as insecure, too passive, and dull, he may start acting overly aggressive to counteract what he *thinks* is her low opinion of him. His move to overaggressiveness may confuse, disappoint, and upset her, and she may react with her own aggressive style. The result is likely to be a tangle of distortions, crossed signals and messages, ruffled feathers, hurt feelings, and faulty assumptions. If enough disparity exists between how Jack believes Dinah perceives him and how she actually does perceive him and if that disparity lasts for a long time, their relationship may be in for serious trouble.

For example, Dinah may one day get tired of the whole business and tell Jack off.

She may accuse him of being a phony, she may demand to know why he is being so aggressive, or she may ask why he acts as though he thinks she does not respect him. Or Jack may get angry at Dinah and accuse her of not caring about him because even though she *knows* he is insecure, she acts like he is the Rock of Gilbraltar. She probably will be startled by Jack's outburst and feel that somehow he has changed from the pleasant, independent, strong person she married.

DISPARITIES IN MARITAL CONCEPT

Another potential source of shock and trouble will exist if the partners have differing perceptions of the relationship (marital concept). If an event or problem prompts an assessment that reveals a disparity between the partners' marital concepts, then trouble may ensue. (If a marked disparity does exist, trouble has been there all along but underneath the surface.)

Suppose, for example, Janice and Harry Johnson share essentially the same concept of their marital relationship: each thinks of it as being fairly pleasant, solid, durable, although a bit dull and disappointing. Each feels vaguely dissatisfied—as though surely there is more to marriage than this, but what is it? Each feels a certain amount of anxiety about the relationship—that in some mysterious way they are always on the edge of some unknown trouble. Suppose Harry goes through a seven-month period of great problems and troubles at work, and during that time he withdraws into himself, becomes irritable, and treats Janice rather badly (is sarcastic to her, aloof, cold, distant, generally hostile).

After about six months of Harry's rough treatment, Janice feels beaten down, hurt, and terribly lonely. Distraught and miserable, she tells her troubles to their mutual friend, Alex (one of Harry's business associates), and he responds with concern and caring. Gradually they become more intimate, and, finally, they have an affair. In the course of their relationship, Alex treats Janice with gentleness, teaches her something about communicating, and is warm and loving to her.

As a result of this experience, Janice's concept of her marital relationship changes. When she checks out what she thinks and feels about the relationship, she decides that she really does not like the off-hand, hostile, cold way Harry treats her. Perhaps she realizes that she has never liked Harry's refusal to deal with anything emotional. Although she may not ask for a separation or divorce, Janice will probably react in new and different ways—so Harry, who has been acting on his same old patterns (only more so), is in for a shock.

Another way that shock can occur is if one (or both) of the partners assumes that both he and the other partner have essentially the same concept of their relationship when this is not the case. For example, Dinah's marital concept is that Jack's and her realtionship is satisfying, fun, warm, affectionate, and secure. However, Jack thinks and feels that the marriage is okay, fun at times, but mostly it is a drag because Dinah wants too much togetherness, affection, and attention. Furthermore, he feels that the relationship is a trap (because Dinah is dependent on him and their relationship). Should Jack decide he wants out because he cannot stand feeling trapped and because he considers the marriage a disaster, when he announces his desires and feelings to Dinah, she will be shocked because she has been unaware of Jack's position and of the disparity between their marital concepts.

Obviously the potentials for trouble arising from faulty perceptions are great, and those troubles can be divisive. Such divisiveness can come as a shock to one or both partners when the disparity suddenly comes to light. Even if the revelation of a disparity does not accompany or lead to a request for separation or divorce, such a revelation in itself can be both an indication of long-term trouble in the relationship and a terrific jolt to the current relationship.

By now it is obvious that the more aware a couple are of their marital identity, that is, the better their understanding of and feel for it is, the better their chances are for developing, maintaining, and enjoying a healthy, functional marital relationship. Conversely, the less aware a couple are of their marital identity the greater the chances that they will develop, maintain, and be dissatisfied with or break up an unhealthy, dysfunctional, and frequently divisive marital relationship.

CONCLUSION

This chapter has focused on many different aspects of marriage: the essential components of the marital relationship, the process of developing a marital system and style, the outcomes of marital interaction, and effects of those outcomes. In essence, this chapter has examined the basic dynamics of the marital relationship—the components of the relationship and how those components work.

This examination naturally leads to a final step—a consideration of the connections between the dynamics of marital interaction and closed and open marriage. However, instead of treating the subject here, we have chosen to wait and discuss it at the same time that we discuss closed and open family (Chapter 14).

Our principal reasons for doing so are as follows:

1. Since the marital relationship is the essential building block and key determinant of the family relationship, any discussion of the ultimate outcomes of their dynamics should include both of them.
2. Since the qualities of closedness and openness remain the same whether applied to marriage or the family, to discuss them separately would be repetitious.
3. To treat the closedness or openness of one of these relationships without reference to the other is to present only a partial picture. You cannot get an overall understanding of marriage without some grasp of the family's influence on it; similarly, you cannot fully comprehend the family relationship without understanding the influences that marriage exerts on it.

For these reasons, we will discuss closed and open marriage and family life in Chapter 14 so that you can gain an overall perspective on these two crucial relationships.

Interaction experiences

1. Working with marital PFLs (p. 221)

Select a partner. Each of you write down and then discuss five marital PFLs that you feel influence your parents' marriages. What are the effects of these PFLs on the marital relationship? In what ways do they influence the marital partners' thoughts, feelings, and actions:

With your partner, role play a pair of interlocking PFLs about a specific question relating to an issue (e.g., money). Try to get in touch with how these PFLs prescribe, define, and direct the ways you think, feel, and act during the interaction.

EVALUATION: What happens if the PFLs are in conflict? Did you get into a power play? Did one of you give in or compromise? Was it possible to negotiate and come to a respectful settlement? Could you feel the power of these PFLs? Did acting on them lead to a gap between your insides and your outsides? What effects might these PFLs have on your parents' marriage?

FOLLOW-UP: Would you say that your parents' PFLs tend to be closed or open? Try to rewrite the list to make the PFLs more open. For example, if you father has a marital PFL that says, "A wife should put her husband's interests first," then a more open version might be "it's good if a wife takes her husband's interests into consideration and tries to help him out when possible." Do this for all the PFLs on the list, and then role play one of them in relation to a particular issue (perhaps the same one that you did before).

Try this same experience with your own PFLs about relationships or marriage (if you are married).

2. Getting the feeling of a marital game (p. 232)

This interaction experience is designed to help you get in touch with what a marital game "feels" like. Select a partner, and together role play Jack and Dinah, with their passive/aggressive marital style, handling a particular aspect of an issue. For example, Dinah wants Jack to take her to a movie tonight, but Jack is tired and wants to stay home and watch television. (See p. 231 for some indications of the types of games they play.) Try to experience what it feels like to be Jack or Dinah as he or she slips into the defensive marital game. Who wins? Who gives in? What happens later on? Then discuss the experience with your partner.

EVALUATION: What did the particular style (passive or aggressive) feel like to you? Could you identify any anger, fear, guilt, etc., as you played the game? Could you feel the power of the game? Could you feel its automatic quality? Try to imagine other games Jack and Dinah might play. How might they handle other problems, situations, and issues?

FOLLOW-UP: Switch with your partner and play the other role. Could you feel the difference? Were there any similarities in your feeling response to each role? Could you empathize with one role more than the other?

REFERENCES

1. Ackerman, Nathan W.: The psychodynamics of family life, New York, 1958, Basic Books, Inc., Publishers, p. 152.
2. Ruesch, Jurgen, and Bateson Gregory: Communication: the social matrix of psychiatry, New York, 1951, W. W. Norton & Co., Inc., pp. 278-279.
3. Ibid., pp. 279-280.
4. Ackerman, op. cit., p. 155.
5. Ruesch and Bateson, op. cit., pp. 280-281.
6. Montague, Ashley: The humanization of man: our changing conception of human nature, New York, 1962, Grove Press, Inc., p. 173.
7. Bell, Robert R.: Marriage and family interaction, Homewood, Ill., 1967, Dorsey Press, pp. 288-290.
8. Howells, John G.: Theory and practice of family psychiatry, New York, 1971, Bunner/Mazel, Inc., p. 32.
9. Gillies, Jerry: My needs, your needs, our needs, Garden City, N.Y., 1974, Doubleday & Co., Inc., pp. 1-15.
10. Smith, Gerald Walker, with Phillips, Alice I.: Me and you and us, New York, 1971, Peter H. Wyden/Publisher.
11. Ackerman, op. cit., pp. 22 and 83.
12. O'Neill, Nena, and O'Neill, George: Open marriage: a new life style for couples, New York, 1972, M. Evans & Co., Inc., pp. 205-223.
13. Ackerman, op. cit., p. 150.
14. Larsen, C. E.: Interaction patterns and communication effectiveness in the marital context, Journal of Communication **17**:342-353, 1967.
15. Clinebell, Charlotte H., and Clinebell, Howard J.: The intimate marriage, New York, 1970, Harper & Row, Publishers.
16. McGinnis, Thomas C.: Joint interview counseling and psychotherapy with married couples, unpublished doctoral dissertation, New York, 1962, pp. 101-106.
17. Bach, George R., and Wyden, Peter: The intimate enemy, New York, 1968, Avon Books, pp. 17-34.
18. McGinnis, Thomas C., and Ayres, John U.: Open family living: a new approach for enriching your life together, Garden City, N.Y., 1976, Doubleday & Co., Inc., Chapter 4.
19. Berne, Eric: Games people play: the psychology of human relationships, New York, 1964, Grove Press, Inc., p. 48.
20. Ibid., pp. 92-109.
21. Drakeford, John W.: Games husbands and wives play, Nashville, Tenn., 1970, Broadman Press.
22. Mazdzierz, Gerald J., and Lottman, Thomas J.: Games married couples play: Adlerian view, Journal of Individual Psychology **29**: 182-194, Nov., 1973.
23. Peterson, James A.: Married love in the middle years, New York, 1968, Association Press, pp. 60-80.

chapter 14

THE DYNAMICS OF FAMILY INTERACTION

The move from a closed to a more open society has encouraged people to seek answers to the following questions: What contributes to and helps determine the quality of family relationships? Why are the relationships in so many families dysfunctional rather than functional? Why are so many families bedeviled by divisiveness? Why is a given family a battleground or a hostile camp or an indifferent shell? Why do many families that seem placid or happy or loving nevertheless have members who are unhappy or emotionally troubled? Why is a given family happy and productive, and how does that come about?

The answers to these and other similar questions are to be found in an understanding of the **dynamics of family interaction.** What determines the specific nature of any given family and its life is the way its members interact within the structure of the family. Just why a given family interacts as it does depends on its kind of dynamic equilibrium, its members' relationships, its system and style, its identity, the degree of its openness or closedness, and its members' communicational and interactional abilities.

An understanding of the dynamics of family interaction results from analyzing and learning about the following: (1) what the essential components of a family relationship are, (2) how a family system and family style develop and how they function, and (3) what the outcomes of family interaction can be and why these outcomes are what they are.

The definitions that follow will be familiar to you, since they are logical extensions of the definitions of the same components in the individual and marital realm. Since they are extensions, it would be misleading to try to make these family definitions different or different sounding from the individual and marital ones. Furthermore, the repetition will help you build in all of these definitions.

PARENTAL RELATIONSHIP: KEY TO THE FAMILY RELATIONSHIP

The dynamics of family interaction is a complex form of interaction because of the larger number of people involved, because of the greater number of possible roles and relationships, and because of the interplay among individual, marital, parental, and family systems and styles.[1] The marital-parental systems and styles are the primary determiners of family system and style; therefore an understanding of the dynamics of family interaction requires some knowledge of the influences exerted by the marital-parental relationship on the how and the why of family functioning. Thus it is imperative that you have a basic grasp of the parental relationship, its components, and its functioning. The following discussion is not extensive or detailed, however, because the parental relationship is built off the marital relationship, which has been closely examined in Chapter 13. The couple tends to work out their parental relationship along lines and in a manner similar to those of their marital relationship.

Because we wish to focus primarily on the dynamics of the interaction of the family as a unit, after briefly examining the parental relationship, we will (wherever possible) assume the parental relationship as a given, as already established and functioning.

Parental dynamic equilibrium

Every marital partner probably brings to the marriage some thoughts and feelings about being a parent. As soon as a child becomes a likelihood, certainly when pregnancy and then birth occur, marital partners seek to get comfortable with one another in their new parental relationship. That is, they seek to establish and maintain **parental dynamic equilibrium**—the interpersonal balance between them. Parental dynamic equilibrium is more complex than the marital balance, since it is based not only on the match up between the marital partners' individual self-systems and life-styles but also on their marital system and style. In addition, the parental balance may *seem* to be more fluid than other kinds of dynamic equilibrium because it is often subjected to more obvious, more clearly observable influences that demand readjustments.[2,3] For example, the birth of a second child, a child's illness, and even just a child's presence are not influences that can be ignored but that force the issue of adjustment. This kind of "pressure" is far more obvious and overt than, for example, the passing of the second year of marriage.

The whole parental relationship

The **whole parental relationship** is comprised of **parental insides** (each parent's private, inner thoughts and feelings about self, the other parent, and the parental relationship and his intrapersonal patterns) and **parental outsides** (each parent's interpersonal patterns of thinking, feeling, and acting in regard to the parental relationship).

Parental system

Parental system is comprised of each person's parental insides plus the interlock between those insides. In essence, parental system refers to the internal functioning of each parent plus the ways each one's insides affect the other's and the parental relationship's functioning. The components of the parental system are parental PFLs (PFLs about parenthood), parental intrapersonal patterns, parental concept, and parental Child/Parent/Adult balance.[4]

Parental style

Parental style (which is underpinned by the parental system) is the observable network of consistent interpersonal patterns that determine how each parent will function in regard to the other, to their relationship, and to the children. In other words, parental style is the parental dynamic equilibrium established by the meshing of the parents' individual life-styles and by the contributions of the marital dynamic equilibrium to the parental relationship.[5]

Parental identity

Parental identity consists of the answers to the following questions:

Present: Who are we (as parents) *now?* What is our parental relationship like *now?*

Past: How did our relationship get to be the way it is now?

Future: What might our relationship become?

If people lack awareness of their parental identity, their parental relationship is likely to be somewhat dysfunctional and closed. But if they are aware of their parental identity and are able to utilize that awareness, their relationship is likely to be basically functional and at least moderately open.

Because parental identity sets the tone for and helps determine the content, quality, and nature of family identity, if the parental identity tends to be dysfunctional and closed, so will the family's identity. Contrarily, if the parental identity tends to be functional and open, so will the family's identity.

Development of parental system and style

Parental system and style are pivotal entities that begin to develop prior to but continue to develop along with the family system and style. Thus parental system and style are distinct entities that coexist with, form a part of, and act as a primary determinant of family system and style.

The process of developing a parental system and style is the same as that for any other kind of system and style (e.g., individual, marital). This process consists of the onging, moment-to-moment interaction between the two parents in which they deal with themselves, each other, and the influences on them, such as core characteristics and issues. For various reasons, this process is considerably more complex than the development of marital system and style.[6] First, now the couple must handle not two but three roles: individual, marital, and parental. Second, they must deal with a complex interplay among marital, parental, and family situations and influences. Third, they must work out their parental relationship and its system and style. Finally, they must continue to adjust their developing parental system and style to the shifts and changes that the family life cycle* and circumstances subject their parental relationship to. In effect the couple must work out a complex balance among individual, marital, parental, and family factors and circumstances.

*Every family follows a **family life cycle**: infancy (when the children are infants), youth (when the children are young until puberty), adolescence (when the children reach and go through their teenage years), young adulthood (when the children leave the home to get a job, enter the armed services, go to college, get married), maturity (when the children are independent of the family of origin and/or become parents themselves), and old age (when the children's own families are well into *their* life cycles).

EXAMPLES OF PARENTAL INTERACTION

Two examples will provide some notion of the complexities of developing a parental system and style. Suppose both a husband and wife have marital PFLs that weekends are for sleeping late, then waking up about the same time and making love. When they become parents, the husband holds to these same PFLs, but the wife's PFLs dictate that both parents should get up and be with the children. The conflict depends on various factors. The husband may continue to hold to the original PFLs and try to ignore the children, to sleep late, and then to make love. Or he may keep the sleeping late PFL for himself and grudgingly or willingly allow his wife to get up early according to PFLs that say that husbands (and fathers) have the right to sleep late on weekends but *mothers* should tend to the children.

If the partners communicate effectively and are fairly open with one another, they probably will be able to work out a functional and cohesive arrangement. For example, they may agree that they can appropriately share or divide the parental role: one weekend he may get up early and let her sleep late; the next weekend she may get up early. Or the husband may sleep late but watch the children while the wife catches a nap later in the day.

Whether a couple develops a dysfunctional and cohesive or divisive or a functional and cohesive parental relationship, certain outcomes are inescapable. Parental and marital relationships are interlocking and mutually influencing. Thus ordinarily if the marital relationship is dysfunctional, the parental relationship is also likely to be dysfunctional. However, one relationship may be more dysfunctional than the other.

The following example illustrates the process of developing and meshing parental communication and interaction patterns to achieve dynamic equilibrium. When Sophia and Andrew were first married, they had some rough times because they operated on numerous PFLs that led them to make faulty assumptions about one another. They have been able to get along all right in their marriage, but now they are parents, and they must work out their communication and interaction as parents. By this time, Sophia knows that Andrew feels she makes a big to-do over little problems and that he is at least partially correct. She also recognizes that he backs off and withdraws. In turn, Andrew knows (perhaps through the experience of several big crises) that he tends to play down almost everything that Sophia gets upset about. He has also learned that although she sometimes exaggerates, she has also been right on occasion about the seriousness of some matters.

Their child David starts running a slight temperature, acts cranky, and cries a lot. Sophia becomes upset and wants to call a doctor. But it is a weekend. Andrew keeps telling her that it is nothing, that it will go away, and that she is making a mountain out of a molehill. Then late Sunday night David's temperature shoots way up, and they have to rush him to the hospital, where the doctor determines that David has a strep infection.

Shocked by this frightening experience, Sophia and Andrew decide—after some angry words—that they need to do something about the ways they communicate and interact as parents. So they sit down and talk about what has happened. They agree that each will hear the other out fully and will listen as carefully and as sensitively as possible. Sophia identifies her feelings: she gets frightened when matters seem to be going wrong, and as she tries to evaluate the situation realistically, her fears and her sense of being alone in the midst of a crisis get in the way of clear evaluation. In addition, she says that when Andrew ignores her fears or makes light of them, she feels terribly alone and helpless, and then she panics and loses her sense of proportion. She also identifies some of her PFLs such as "always think the worst; then you'll be prepared for any emergency."

Andrew identifies his feelings: when matters seem to be going wrong, he tends to ignore them and hope they will go away. The more panic he feels the more he backs off to lessen his anxiety. Thus when Sophia gets more and more upset, Andrew's usual move is to not listen or to tell her she is exaggerating. He also identifies some of his PFL's such as "mothers always exaggerate" and "if you don't get swept up by emotion, you can deal better with whatever happens."

As they reveal and work with their feelings and PFLs, Sophia and Andrew begin to understand how each one's patterns of communication and interaction tend to clash with and intensify the other's patterns: her panicky exaggerations evoke annoyance and withdrawal from him; his annoyance and withdrawal evokes exaggeration and panic from her. By using intrapersonal and interpersonal communication techniques, Andrew and Sophia have acquired an important set of insights, and just acquiring insights helps them achieve a certain new dynamic balance.

By using other communication techniques, Sophia and Andrew can discover viable alternatives to their previous ways of communicating and interacting and work on implementing the alternatives. One possible alternative might be for either or both of them to identify the exaggeration or panic or withdrawal when these become evident and then to openly talk about and evaluate the feelings and circumstances that are occurring. A further step in this alternative might be for Andrew to consciously try not to withdraw, to try to stick with it, to try to feel Sophia's position and help her clarify it, and to offer some support when she feels panicky. Sophia might try to slow down and evaluate, try not to exaggerate so much, try to feel Andrew's position and help him modify his withdrawal, and try to see that his withdrawal is not necessarily a rejection of her as a person.

Although their original marital patterns of panic and withdrawal meshed and thereby created a dynamic equilibrium of sorts, it was a dysfunctional (and potentially divisive) one. Now, however, as they work to alter their old patterns of communication and interaction, Sophia and Andrew are establishing a new and more functional parental and marital dynamic equilibrium.

The establishment and maintenance of parental dynamic equilibrium (whether functional or dysfunctional) depends then on the partners' moment-to-moment interaction —how they react to it, how they communicate about it, how they allow their patterns to mesh, and how they work with and deal with their communication and interaction. Seeking and achieving parental dynamic equilibrium is therefore not a static but an ongoing process. It depends on what is going on inside of each partner, what is going on between them and between them (or one of them) and others (e.g., the children), what is going on in their other relationships (e.g., in their marriage), and what is going on around them (MIFs) from moment to moment. This process of establishing and maintaining parental dynamic equilibrium by means of moment-to-moment interaction lies at the heart of developing a parental relationship, its system, and its style.

FAMILY RELATIONSHIP: ESSENTIAL COMPONENTS

As soon as one child is born and an actual family unit exists, the process of developing the family relationship begins. This process includes the development of family dynamic equilibrium, family system and style, and family identity. The definitions of these components follow.

Family dynamic equilibrium

Like members of every other human relationship, family members seek always to get comfortable with one another in their relationship. They seek to achieve and maintain **family dynamic equilibrium**—the interpersonal balance that family members establish between them, which is based on how each one's self-system and life-style fit with those of the others. The way each member achieves this balance is by adjusting his self-system and life-style to those of the other members and by making accommodations for the other members' self-systems and life-styles. These adjustments are made both consciously and unconsciously, and they are based on verbal and nonverbal agreements that family members make or that simply occur between or among them.[7]

The kind of family dynamic equilibrium (complementary, alternating, supplementary, or mixed) and its quality (functional, dysfunctional; cohesive, divisive) will depend on the specific qualities of each member's self-system and life-style and on the match-up between or among them.

Specifically, the kind of dynamic equilibrium a family has is basically determined by the kind of dynamic equilibrium established by the parents primarily in their marital relationship and secondarily in their parental relationship. This does not mean, however, that the kind and intensity of the original marital-parental balance will remain exactly the same for the family. Although it seems highly unlikely that the basic kind of balance would change radically with the advent of children (e.g., from a passive/aggressive balance to an obsessive-compulsive/hysterical balance), the presence of one or more children will inevitably affect the balance in some way.

For example, suppose a couple has a passive/aggressive marital relationship. However, the woman who is passive as an individual and wife may become more aggressive when she has a child and experiences new feelings of protectiveness. The man who is aggressive as an individual and husband may be gentled by his new experiences with a helpless infant and become less aggressive. It is also possible that a passive woman may be frightened by her new maternal role and become even more passive and dependent, or an aggressive man may become jealous of his wife's attention to the child and become even more aggressive.

When a child arrives on the scene, he does not choose a partner as did his parents; perforce he must make-do with the parents he finds himself with. In some way or another, he must accommodate himself to a preexisting relationship. Thus he is not likely to develop a style that is radically different from that of at least one of the parents. Essentially three different outcomes are possible. The child may develop a style that is primarily the style of one parent (e.g., the child of a passive/aggressive couple might develop either a predominantly passive or a predominantly aggressive style). He may develop a style that represents a mixture of the parent's styles. Or using one or both of their styles as a base, he may develop a somewhat different style as the result of a strong outside influence. For example, he might be shy and retiring like his passive mother but warm and friendly like his grandfather on his father's side. Whatever route the child follows, however, one result is certain—his presence will affect the original balance between his parents and the developing family balance. His presence may strengthen the existing balance, it may tip the balance in favor of one style, or it may alter the balance by introducing outside influences or by challenging the existing styles.

We have been focusing on the effect of one child. What happens if a second child arrives on the scene? A third? A fourth? Matters become more complex, and the original balance may change a number of times. Suppose, for example, the passive/aggressive couple has four girls. The father travels a great deal, and the major responsibility for rearing the children falls to the passive mother. Under these circumstances, it is conceivable that the family's basic dynamic equilibrium will become markedly passive in nature.

All kinds of variations are possible. Thus to understand the kind of family style and equilibrium that exists, it is necessary to look closely at the alignments between or among family members. One must pay close attention to the dyadic, triadic, sometimes quadradic, or more subrelationships* to determine what goes into the makeup of the overall dynamic equilibrium. It is also important to realize that by definition and nature, dynamic equilibrium is not a static, once-and-for-all matter. Many different factors can affect the dynamic equilibrium and can create a need for renegotiating the balance or for finding a new one. If a new member is born or adopted, if a present member temporarily or permanently leaves (e.g., because of going away to school, hospitalization, job requirement, service in the armed forces, separation, divorce, death), if a grandparent or other relative comes to live with the family—any one of these engenders the need for a new balance. Other agents also can create the need for new balances. For example, if a member becomes emotionally ill, if a member becomes addicted, if a member changes jobs, or if a member wants more privacy or freedom, then new balances must be worked out. Other influences can result from the natural life cycle of a family. For example, at certain ages a child is often closer to the same-sex parent; at other ages the child is often closer to the other-sex parent. As parents get older and gain more life experience, many become more relaxed about parenting. Those factors affecting the dyads or triads or whole family relationships of necessity generate shifts in the dynamic equilibrium.

*These are useful, shorthand terms for designating the number of people engaging in a given relationship or interaction: e.g., dyadic means two people, triadic means three people, and so forth.

The whole family

Every **whole family** is comprised of two interlocking, mutually influencing parts: its insides and outsides.

FAMILY INSIDES

Family insides are the inner thoughts and feelings each member has about himself, the other members, and the family relationship. In addition, insides include each person's intrapersonal patterns (the ways he treats himself). Family insides are private unless a person chooses to reveal them by communication.

FAMILY OUTSIDES

Family outsides are each member's conscious and unconscious external expressions and manifestations of his insides. Family outsides are then each member's interpersonal patterns of thinking, feeling, and acting and the interlock between them. They can be observed, sensed, interpreted, experienced, and/or understood by the other members (and by nonmembers too).

Family system

Family system denotes each family member's insides *plus* the interlock between or among those insides (whether it is clashing or harmonious). In effect, family system refers to the internal functioning of each member plus the ways each one's insides affect each other member's and the whole family's internal functioning.[8,9] Definitions and explanations of the various components that make up a family system follow.

FAMILY PFLs

Family PFLs are those PFLs (internalized expectations, rules, values) that each member has about the family. These PFLs have to do with such matters as the family relationship, family roles, core characteristics (e.g., intellectual balance), and issues. These PFLs may be societal PFLs about family, personal PFLs, or a combination thereof. They are tempered by the specifics of the core characteristics and by the unique background, self-system, and life-style of each member. Gradually family members usually work out some accommodation (whether functional or dysfunctional) among their PFLs if they clash, or they may hold essentially the same PFLs and operate on this merged set of PFLs. These family PFLs direct and teach a person *who* he should be; *what* he should be like; *what* he should think, feel, and do; and *how* he should think, feel, act, and react *in relation to his family*.[10,11]

FAMILY INTRAPERSONAL PATTERNS

Family intrapersonal patterns are a person's consistent, private, inner ways he thinks, feels, and acts within the family. They are his consistent ways of treating himself. They become known to the other members only if the person shares them by means of communication, although over a long period of time because of repetition, other members may be able to identify some of a person's intrapersonal patterns.[12]

FAMILY CONCEPT

Family concept consists of the way each person sees (perceives) and feels about the family relationship. Family concept is naturally based on each member's self-concept and on the way he perceives and interprets the other members' thoughts, feelings, and actions.[13]

FAMILY CHILD/PARENT/ADULT BALANCE

Family Child/Parent/Adult Balance is the overall balance created by the interlock among the members' individual Child/Parent/Adult balances. For example, if one parent and two children have large, fearful Child parts (and small Parent and Adult parts) and the other parent has a strong, protective, nurturing Parent part, the family Child/Parent/Adult balance will be basically a complementary one between the three members' large Child and the one parent's large Parent.

IMPORTANCE OF THE FAMILY SYSTEM

The family system is crucially important to the dynamics of family interaction, since it is this system that underpins all behavior in the family. As such it underpins the family style.

Family style

Each parent brings to the family relationship his individual life-style—the observable network of consistent interpersonal patterns that determine how he functions (thinks, feels, acts) in the interpersonal sphere. Each child develops his individual life-style within the family environment. **Family style** refers to the basic interlock among members' life-styles; this interlock forms a larger observable network of interpersonal patterns, which determine how each member functions in regard to the others and to their relationship. In other words, family style is the family dynamic equilibrium established by the meshing of members' life-styles.

Family identity

Ultimately just how functional or dysfunctional a family relationship is can be measured by how aware the members are of their family identity and how skilled they are in applying The System to their knowledge of the family relationship. **Family identity** can be defined by the answers to the following questions:

Present: Who are we (as a family) now? What is our family relationship like now?

Past: How did our relationship get to be the way it is now?

Future: What might our relationship become?

This definition is deceptively brief and simple because it encompasses an enormous number of complex, interlocking, and mutually influencing factors.[14] Breaking the questions down into specific components makes the range and scope of these factors evident.

Who are we and what is our relationship now? These questions involve such matters as the style of the relationship, its degree of openness or closedness, the family concept, the current patterns of communication and interaction, the roles, all the family PFLs (expectations, rules, values) that apply to the relationship, and each person's life-style and self-system.

How did our relationship get to be the way it is now? This question involves all the factors just listed as they have contributed to and been a part of the development of the relationship. In addition, it includes an assessment of how the issues in the family have affected the members' ways of interacting and the goals they have set, rejected, and fulfilled.

What might our relationship become? This question involves the answers to the two prior sets of questions plus such matters as current and future goals, the importance to each person of the family investments they have made, the strength or weakness of each person's commitment to a continuing relationship, the kind of motivation for personal and family growth each person has, and the degree of openness or closedness already present in the family relationship.

ONGOING FAMILY INTERACTION: THE DEVELOPING RELATIONSHIP

One step in determining family identity involves perceiving and understanding the dynamic equilibrium of the developing family relationship. This dynamic equilibrium is established and maintained or reestablished in the course of the ongoing interaction between or among family members. This section therefore focuses on (1) the contributing components of ongoing family interactions, (2) the possible ways family members can interact with one another and how these ways of interacting affect the dynamic equilibrium of the developing family relationship, and (3) how particular kinds of dynamic equilibrium are established according to the patterns of communication and interaction that develop between or among family members.

Contributing components of ongoing family interaction

Both family core characteristics and issues are constantly contributing to family interaction: the core characteristics provide and give shape to the specific circumstances with which family members must deal; the issues provide the specific content of their interaction. Furthermore, there are the family members themselves, each of whom must relate to each other member. To these relationships, each person contributes the complexities of his individual self-system and life-style. In addition, the parents bring to the family interaction their already established marital system and style and their developing parental system and style.

Complexities of ongoing family interaction

IMPORTANCE OF ROLES

Essentially the role that each family member assumes at any given moment and member's interactions with one another in terms of particular roles help to determine the kind, nature, and quality of the family dynamic equilibrium, of the whole family relationship, and of the subrelationships within it. Because roles can be so important, it is necessary here to comment on them.

Different roles and role interlocks have different significances within their particular context. Husband-wife, parent-parent, and sibling-sibling role interlocks are basically peer relationships, whereas the parent-child role is essentially an unequal one, ascribing responsibility, nurturance, and giving to the parent role and ascribing need, dependence, and taking to the child role. The individual role is the least classifiable one but certainly connotes freedom, flexibility, uniqueness, and probably openness.

IMPLICATIONS OF ROLES AND THEIR INTERLOCKS

It is instructive to examine the roles and role interlocks in family interaction because an understanding of them can help establish guidelines for assessing family dynamic equilibrium and interaction.

Family roles. The roles most basic to the family relationship and interaction are the **family roles:** parent (mother, father) and child (daughter, son). It is a virtual necessity for the health and welfare of young children that these roles be the predominant ones. The young child is totally dependent on others for his very existence; just to live, and hopefully to flourish, he must be **parented:** cared for, protected, socialized, and given physical and emotional nurturance.

If one (or both) of the parents will not or cannot assume the parent role, then at best there will be difficulties ahead; more likely, problems will ensue. Suppose a couple who have been married about two years have a child whose conception was the result of a slipup. Neither the wife nor the husband really wants or is ready for the child; neither wishes to be a parent. Although each may fulfill the minimal requirements of parenthood, primarily they are enamored of each other and tend to give most of their energies to their marital roles and interaction. Needless to say, the child's position is not an enviable one, and the family relationship is a dysfunctional one.

If, on the other hand, the family goes to an extreme and holds its members to family roles almost to the exclusion of other roles, then the family tends to be fairly closed—rigid, not flexible, limiting, restrictive, and probably authoritarian. This family's demands that members stick strictly to family roles allow little freedom to sibling-sibling, wife-husband, or individual role assumption.

Peer level roles. The wife-husband and sibling-sibling role interlocks, although they are not as fundamental in some ways as family role interlocks, are nevertheless vitally important to the health of the family. One reason is that these roles and interlocks acknowledge and encourage each generation's need for experience and interaction with peers. Another is that these roles and interlocks allow and provide for the differences in age; interests; intellectual, emotional, social, and physical abilities; tastes; life experience; and maturity.

If, as often happens, the wife pours most of her time and energies into being a good mother, values this role above others, or retreats into this role, the effects on the marital relationship may be divisive. Without the balancing and tempering effect of the marital peer relationship, she may become almost childish, or she may "overmother" the children.

Contrarily, if family members overemphasize these peer role interlocks to the neglect of family roles, the result is likely to be an overly permissive, often fragmented, and directionless family. For various reasons, the husband and wife are likely to do little parenting. They may be so intent on their marital relationship that they are detached from or indifferent to what their children do. They may back off from asserting parental authority as a form of rebellion against their stricter upbringing, or they may have been persuaded by current cries from the young (and some parents) for noninterference in their children's business. Or they may try to be their children's "buddies" rather than authority figures. Whatever the reasons for this kind of neglect of family roles, the results tend to be dysfunctional and divisive; separating off almost exclusively into peer level roles creates a generation gap with a vengeance. There is likely to be minimal communication and interaction between the marital-parental and sibling dyads.

Individual roles. The need for and value of individual roles are great indeed. Without the freedom or opportunity to step into these roles when appropriate, family members tend to be stifled by the demands of other-oriented roles. The freedom to fill one's role as an individual is basic to personal and interpersonal growth. The allowance for and encouragement of individual roles assure family members of respect for their individual differences, that is, for their uniqueness. Essentially these are the marks of the basically open family.

If family members do not give or receive respect for one another's individuality, then they tend to lock themselves into more group-oriented and more masklike roles. Frequently, failure to respect individuality becomes a major sore point between adolescents and parents. If the young person has been boxed into family and peer roles and not granted much individual freedom or recognition, he may at the time of an adolescent identity crisis rebel and demand that his parents stop treating him like a child and regard him as an individual. Many younger children also experience anger and frustration because their parents cannot seem to step out of the parent role and treat them like individuals—because the parents do not act much like individuals either. Conversely, many parents feel frustrated and angry when they feel that their children stereotype them and treat them as fuddy-duddies or "horns of plenty" or hopeless idiots.

As is true of the other roles, if individuality is taken to an extreme, trouble will probably ensue. Since each person would tend to go his own way and "do his own thing," the result would likely be a fragmented, disunified, divisive, and dysfunctional family relationship. In effect, family members would be denying their actual and emotional kinship.

• • •

This discussion has examined both the negative and positive sides of each set of roles and the whole question of balance among the sets. As is true of most matters having to do with the dynamics of human interactions, the basic tenet of the Interactional Therapeutic System of the balanced blend applies to roles also. It is not sufficient to operate from one role only or even from two. All three are important if the family and its members are to be healthy, open, and growth producing. Without the freedom and flexibility to move from one role to another (or to have a mixture) when appropriate, family members are limited and restricted by rigid and stereotyping role ascriptions.

Family dynamic equilibrium: some typical variations

The intent in the following discussion is not to give a detailed discussion or explanation of family dynamic equilibrium, but rather to provide some typical variations. The perspective used for evaluating the dynamic equilibrium is that of the consistency and quality of the communication and interaction between or among family members.*

*We use a four-person nuclear family for our examples for the sake of simplicity and therefore greater clarity; a larger unit would unnecessarily increase the complexity of the discussion.

When there is consistent and meaningful communication and interaction between or among all family members, the dynamic equilibrium is likely to be healthy, well balanced, and functional. This is the **ideal family type dynamic equilibrium.**

Conversely, the **precarious family type dynamic equilibrium** is unhealthy, dysfunctional, and, if not divisive, then certainly negative. Family members communicate and interact in only the sketchiest manner. The dynamic equilibrium is therefore extremely precarious; a serious problem or crisis tends to result in the family coming unglued.

If each (or both) of the parents has (or attempts to have) a powerful, often controlling influence on each child, this is one form of **authoritarian family type dynamic equilibrium.** For example, the parent (or parents) gives many orders to each child, conveys numerous rather strict PFLs, and expects obedience. Each child has little to say about these parental influences and is obedient (willingly or not). On the sibling level, not much sharing goes on, perhaps because each child must look to his own interests with the parents.

Another kind of authoritarian family type dynamic equilibrium is the "united parental front." In this type, the parents have agreed never to disagree about their treatment of the children at least not in front of them. In this kind of equilibrium, the parents tend to come across as a monolithic entity; they have yielded up their parental individuality. This means that the children cannot even hope to get one parent to intercede with the other. Nor do they fight back against the parents. The children have little impact on the united parental front. There is no alliance between the siblings.

When the two parents are wrapped up in their own marital relationship and tend to ignore or barely tolerate and relate to the children, this is known as the **tight marital bond type dynamic equilibrium.** Thus whereas the parents have each other, the children exist in a kind of limbo.

In the **generation gap family type dynamic equilibrium,** the children have banded together, whether in scorn or rebellion or fear or loneliness. Perhaps a better term for this situation is a "generational communication and interaction gap."

In the **parent-child alliance family type dynamic equilibrium,** each parent is allied with one child, an alliance based perhaps on identification between the parent and the child or on male/female role divisions. The indication is also that the marital relationship is dysfunctional and perhaps divisive.

Then there are the powerful but lonely (and loneliness-producing) matriarchy and patriarchy. In the **matriarchal family type balance,** the mother influences everyone else, but no one influences or "makes a difference with" her. She holds the power, calls the shots, and runs the whole show.

In the **patriarchal family type balance,** which is supported by the mother, the father calls the shots but may share the decision-making powers with the mother. He and she exert reciprocal influences, but if the mother wants to get through to the children or order them around or exert some influence on them, she has to work through the father because he is the only one who communicates and interacts with them in a strong or significant way.

Perhaps one of the saddest family balances of all is the **left-out member family type balance.** One member is not included in the family's significant communication and interaction. The left-out member could be any member. The exclusion may result from factors such as the person is rebellious, mean, and nasty; introverted; much smarter or stupider than the other members; or sickly when the others are strong and athletic. ►IE-1, p. 264.

THE PROCESS OF DEVELOPING A FAMILY SYSTEM AND STYLE

To determine and appreciate family identity, it is necessary to be able not only to evaluate what the present family relationship is like now but also to understand how it got to be that way. Thus we will examine how a family relationship develops a system and a style. Keep in mind our earlier statement that, whenever appropriate, we will start with the parental relationship as an established entity.

The developing family relationship: its system and style

MOMENT-TO-MOMENT FAMILY INTERACTION

Family interaction includes all of each member's thoughts, feelings, and actions, which are occurring from moment to moment. Over a long period of time and as a result of innumerable moments of experience with one another, family members begin to get some feel for the continuity and consistency that exists in their ways of communicating and interacting. At the same time, by means of a long-term, testing-out procedure, each member begins to learn (whether consciously or unconsciously or both) which of his ways of responding are acceptable and which are not acceptable to other members. Each person therefore learns which responses generate approval or disapproval and which responses fit the expectations and values of the other members. In effect each person is learning how (and sometimes how not) to match up his moment-to-moment thoughts, feelings, and actions with the needs, feelings, desires, ideas, requests, demands, actions, and reactions of the other members.

As a result of much repetitious testing out of responses, members establish and develop their particular ways of relating to one another (and to others). They are effecting some kind of match-up to achieve and maintain family dynamic equilibrium. Of course, if communication is ineffective, there is little checking out, and the match-up is based mainly on assumptions (accurate or otherwise) about one another's insides and outsides. In this case, the dynamic equilibrium is on shaky ground. If communication is effective, then the match-up and consequent dynamic equilibrium rest on relatively solid ground.

A brief example of how this moment-to-moment interactional process operates is as follows. In their marital relationship, Janice and Harry Johnson established a balance in which Janice let Harry give the orders, but she usually got what she wanted from him by acting weak and helpless. This arrangement carried over into their parental relationship and worked fairly well for them.

Harry became the patriarch of the family, Janice supported him, and she wielded most of her power over the children through Harry's authoritarian rule. That is, she complained to him if they stepped out of line, and he ordinarily issued the orders and disciplined them. As Mike and Sally were growing up, they soon learned that if they wanted something from Harry or if they wanted to avert his wrath, Janice was the person to see and Harry was the person to avoid. Mike and Sally learned to cultivate their influence on Janice so that she would help them out. However, Janice had relatively little impact (in terms of direct authority or control) on either Mike or Sally just as they had little impact on their father.

Even now, Mike has little significant communication and interaction with his father. Mike may rage at his father, but he cannot change him or get around him. So Mike still relies on (and manipulates) Janice. Sally, however, because of what she has learned from Janice and Harry *plus* the Thompsons, the parents of Sally's best friend (see Appendix A), has established a good, working relationship with Harry and therefore has little need for Janice to intervene with Harry. If Sally wants something from Harry or if she wants simply to talk to him, she deals directly with him. Thus a family establishes its dynamic equilibrium by means of its moment-to-moment ongoing interaction.

This discussion of the process of moment-to-moment family interaction is essentially an overview. We will examine in more detail the two specific forms of the moment-to-moment family interaction process: patterns of communication and patterns of interaction.* These represent respectively the moment-to-moment efforts of family members to satisfactorily mesh their patterns of communication and interaction.

FAMILY PATTERNS OF COMMUNICATION

As family members repeatedly interact in terms of their thoughts, feelings, and actions about all kinds of matters, they are communicating with each other. Since the parents bring with them their already formed marital patterns of communication, they must do a certain amount of testing out (whether consciously or unconsciously) to determine which of their individual communication patterns and which marital communication patterns will work in the parental and family relationship. That is, which patterns will the other partner accept, tolerate, or reject and which of his partner's patterns of communication will he accept, tolerate, or reject? Knowingly or not, the parents are learning by trial and error how to mesh their individual and marital patterns of communication so that they can achieve some form of parental and family communication, which will help them to establish a state of dynamic equilibrium. In addition, as each child joins the family, he starts developing his individual patterns of communication by copying one or both parents and then testing out his ways of communicating to determine (consciously, unconsciously, or both) which ones are acceptable and which are not and which ones help him to get comfortable with himself and other family members and which ones do not. In effect he is trying to achieve personal and family dynamic equilibrium.[15]

An example of how family members develop family patterns of communication follows. Janice and Harry bring their already developed marital patterns of communication to their parental-family relationship. In the course of their marital interaction, Janice has learned not to criticize (and in fact not to approach) Harry directly when she wants him to change. She has discovered (probably unconsciously) that veiled sniping or lavish, idolizing praise (depending on the circumstances) get results with Harry. In the family relationship, she feels justified in manipulating Harry in certain matters because she is doing it for "the good of the family" or the children. Because Harry has been taught to feel guilty if he gets irritated, he tends not to yell at Janice when she snipes at him, but he often replies with sharp sarcasm. If Janice flatters him, Harry tends to become warmer and more cooperative. He may even listen carefully for a while, and he tells her what she wants to know or usually says what she wants him to say or does what she wants him to do.

Because he is the first born and a male, Mike has received an overabundance of attention from Harry. In turn, when he was young, Mike worshipped Harry, and after that he identified closely with Harry. Thus it was only natural for Mike to copy Harry. One of Harry's communication patterns attracted Mike because it seemed to be masculine and adult—this is Harry's tendency when frustrated or angry to lash out at others, yell a lot (sometimes bellow), and make direct and pointed comments about what displeases him. Early in the game Mike used this same approach when he got angry at Harry, Janice, or Sally. But he soon learned (the hard way) that this pattern of communicating was the sole prerogative of Harry the authoritarian. After

*The term "patterns" used throughout this discussion refers to all interpersonal family patterns, whether private (between or among members) or public (between or among members and others outside the family). Dividing patterns into those of communication and interaction is meant simply to highlight these two important facets of interpersonal dynamics.

Harry blasted him often enough with comments like "don't you ever talk to me that way again!" Mike just stopped using this pattern. To replace it, he uses sarcasm veiled by innocence (copied from Janice). By and large, Mike and Harry do not do much direct communicating. If Mike wants to get something from Harry, he asks Janice to intercede for him. Mike uses another of Harry's ways with her: he compliments her; she melts and agrees to help, whereupon she manipulates Harry into helping Mike or allowing him to do something.

Originally Sally copied Janice's pattern of pleasant manipulation; when she wanted something from a family member (especially Harry), she would smile artlessly when asking or pout or cry if thwarted. Usually she got her way—both with Harry *and* Janice. However, as Sally has come to know the Thompsons and has witnessed a good deal of honest, open, respectful communication, she has dropped the manipulative pattern because she began feeling so uncomfortable when she used it. She now tends to copy Mrs. Thompson's style when communicating with Janice: she is gentle, firm, and as open as she feels Janice can stand. If Janice tries to manipulate Harry for Sally, Sally firmly blocks her mother from doing so. With Harry, Sally uses Mr. Thompson's direct, honest, bantering, logical pattern. (She also learned to be logical by copying Harry and knows he responds best to and feels least threatened by a logical approach.)

In these ways, the family establishes its dynamic equilibrium. Originally it was one of Janice and the children manipulating Harry the ogre. Now Janice and Mike (through Janice) still manipulate Harry, but Sally plays it straight. Therefore when the chips are down in a tight situation or crisis, the others look to her as chief mediator and the voice of reason.

Thus through repeated moment-to-moment interactions, family members learn to mesh their communication patterns so that they establish some kind of balance. If they cannot do this with any significant success, the family relationship is likely to be or become divisive.

FAMILY PATTERNS OF INTERACTION

The same process of establishing dynamic equilibrium operates in regard to patterns of interaction. Each parent brings with him to the relationship his already formed individual and marital patterns of interaction. As the couple repeatedly interact with one another over a period of time, they are learning by moment-to-moment trial and error how to mesh their patterns of interaction in such a way that they can achieve dynamic equilibrium in their parent-family relationship and thereby get comfortable. They are learning which of their patterns interlock and which ones clash, and they are making adjustments in response to what they are learning.

As each child joins the family, he begins developing his own patterns of interaction by copying one or more Significant Persons' patterns or combinations of those patterns. By means of the family's ongoing interaction, he tests out the acceptability and practicality of these patterns and keeps those which are useful to him. He is learning in effect to bring about a comfort-producing interlock of his patterns with his parents' patterns and any other siblings' patterns and is thereby achieving dynamic equilibrium.[16]

An example of how family patterns of interaction develop follows. Originally in their early marital years Harry and Janice had some troubles when trying to mesh some of their patterns. Harry the perfectionist used to give Janice a hard time whenever she made a mistake. He would criticize her for being disorganized and illogical (which she is), and he would impatiently show her how to "do it right." But this created such a ruckus between them (Janice would cry, sulk, and/or criticize sharply and at length) that Harry finally gave up trying to change Janice (except in emergencies). Harry now treats Janice's disorganization with bemused, mild contempt. She puts up with this because Harry's logic and organization help her keep her chaotic emotions at arm's length.

When Mike was born, Harry turned his perfectionistic patterns on Mike and has taught him to be a driving perfectionist also. Harry has always tended to pick at and criticize Mike when he failed (which is also Harry's way of treating himself). Now Mike treats himself that way too. During the time he was growing up, Mike tried to please Harry by performing well and thereby tried to get Harry's approval. However, that was not easy to get, and when he could not bear the feeling that Harry was disappointed in him, Mike would turn to Janice for comfort. Although Mike's responses to Janice are tinged slightly with contempt, by and large he likes her and needs her reassurance (which she readily gives him, since she idolizes him). Mike and Janice are not extremely close, but there is some comfort in their dyadic relationship.

When Harry becomes too perfectionistic and too demanding, Mike becomes extremely angry and blows his stack at him. Ever since the age of 15, Mike has argued vigorously with Harry, and presently Mike is overtly rebelling against Harry.

Sally's interactions with Harry tend to be much less stressful. One reason is that Harry has never demanded as much perfection from her as he did from Mike because of her sex. Yet Harry has always been proud of her accomplishments, perhaps because he felt he did not have to feel so responsible for her achieving. So Sally has developed patterns that are more relaxed about driving herself and getting ahead. Because Sally is fairly accepting of herself (as were both Harry and Janice), she can go her own autonomous way, yet at the same time she can interact with each family member in a meaningful way. Her basic patterns are those of caring, being accepting, and respecting others' individuality. Thus when Janice gets panicky and disorganized, Sally's help and presence are soothing to Janice. With Harry, Sally tends to be logical, but she is not a perfectionist and accepts herself as she is. She has learned to tease Harry the way Janice does to get him in a good mood, and she enjoys entertaining him. Sally performs much the same function for Mike.

All in all, Sally tends to be the balance wheel in the family relationship. Her patterns are those of the appropriate middle ground (except when she gets really angry and lets her hot temper run wild). By and large she acts as the person who tempers the more extreme patterns of the others.

FAMILY CONCEPT

As family members communicate and interact from moment to moment over a period of time and form their family patterns of communication and interaction, they gradually develop a family concept, which consists of what each member thinks and feels about the family relationship. As each develops his concept, the family concept in turn influences how each behaves in the family relationship.

For example, Harry sees his family as being good, right, and essentially moral, and he thinks they are a credit (mostly) to the American way of life. He feels that his family is pleasant, a little dull, but at the same time too demanding of his time, emotions, and energies. Janice sees the family as being tightly knit, loyal, and almost clannish. She feels it is a wonderful family—secure and emotionally close. Mike sees it as too clannish, too demanding of perfection, and too nosy. He feels that it is a family of good but dull people, and he feels frustrated when he is around them. In a way, he feels like an outsider. Sally sees the family and its ways as disunified, limiting, and limited. But she feels a certain fondness for its comfortable familiarity and for the foibles and strengths of the other members.

As each member develops his family concept, the concept exerts an influence on each one's behavior. Harry tends at times to back off and seek time away from the family. Janice tends to press for togetherness. Mike wants out; he wants his freedom and his own life. Sally works to lessen the disunified and limiting quality of the family, and she tends to enjoy its comfortable familiarity and to work hard at maintaining this comfortable state. She also attempts to inject some fun and humor into the family atmosphere.

FAMILY CHILD/PARENT/ADULT BALANCE

The efforts of family members to establish a family dynamic equilibrium in the course of their moment-to-moment interaction extends to their attempts to achieve a family Child/Parent/Adult balance. That is, each person brings to the family relationship his own individual Child/Parent/Adult balance; each person then consciously, unconsciously, or both teaches and learns from each other person how to mesh their individual balances to create a new family Child/Parent/Adult balance.

The Child/Parent/Adult balance of the Johnson family is built on the following parts. Harry's balance consists of a very large Parent (perfectionistic, moralistic, overly intellectual), a minuscule Child, and a small Adult. Janice's balance is composed of a large Child (fearful, overly emotional, romanticizing, fun loving), a fairly large Parent (critical, moralistic), and a small Adult. Harry's and Janice's marital (and then parental) Child/Parent/Adult balance is comprised of a large, basically fearful Child, a somewhat larger, strong and harsh Parent, and a small Adult. Mike does not really change this basic balance, since he develops a strong, harsh Parent like Harry's (and somewhat like Janice's), which overbalances his small Child and Adult. Sally, however, does alter the balance somewhat; she brings to it a good-sized fun-loving Child and a fairly large Adult. Since her communication and interaction within the family is fairly good, she is able to have a significant influence on the family balance. The basic outcome for the Johnsons then is a large Child (that is about one-third fearful Child, two-thirds fun-loving Child), a somewhat larger harsh Parent, and a fairly small but still influential Adult part.

OUTCOMES OF FAMILY INTERACTION

As a result of family members' moment-to-moment, ongoing interaction over a period of time, they gradually develop certain overall outcomes: a specific family system and style, which have a particular quality of being open or closed.

Family system and style

As family members develop their family relationship over a period of time, the relationship itself takes on a style of its own, which is the result of a merger among the members' individual life-styles. Since to establish and maintain a relationship the members must mesh their own styles in some way, the family style of the resulting relationship usually reflects the combination or synthesis of the strongest, most dominant elements of each members' life-style (and self-system).

The specific name given to family style identifies the dominant elements in the family dynamic equilibrium. For example, if one member's passive style dominates the family dynamic equilibrium, the family style is termed "passive." If, however, more than one element predominates, then the name of the family style reflects this combination or synthesis. For example, the Johnson's family style is characterized as obsessive-compulsive/hysterical.

Open or closed style

Not only does the family's moment-to-moment interaction shape the system and style of the family, but it also determines the *quality* of the style. In other words, the ways that the family members interact are governed by the degree of openness or closedness present in their individual life-styles and self-systems and the combinations thereof. Conversely, the ways they interact determine the degree of openness or closedness of the family style and system that they are developing.

The **open family style** represents an essentially harmonious meshing of personal styles, which results in a healthy and functional dynamic equilibrium.[17] In contrast, the **closed family style** is the outcome of a disharmonious jamming together of styles that conflict (e.g., aggressive/aggressive) or of a harmonious but nonconstructive blend of neurotic styles (e.g., obsessive-compulsive/hysterical), which results in an unhealthy or dysfunctional dynamic equilibrium.

Family identity is the outcome of the developmental process. It results from a detailed perspective on that process and on the functioning of the components of that process. Those family members who have a good grasp of their family identity are those who have a fairly high degree of self-awareness and family awareness and therefore usually have relatively open, functional family systems and styles. Conversely, those family members who have little or no conception of their family identity usually have rather closed, dysfunctional family relationships.

Games families play

Family members who have little or no conception of their family identity tend to communicate and interact in a rather limited fashion. A primary way is to play games.[18]

The number and variety of games families can play are enormous because there are at least three players, because there are more kinds of relationships in a family group, and because there are simply more interactions going on. The particular kinds of games a family will play depend, on the particular life-styles of the members and the overall family style. For example, if the overall family style is hostile/aggressive but one member is rather passive, the specific games he will play are likely to be subtly hostile, delivered as covert attacks.

Family games*—preprogrammed sets of signals, messages, and/or responses between or among family members, which evoke preprogrammed responses—can be divided into six categories: games parents play with one another, games parents play with the children, games children play with the parents, games children play with one another, games any member can play, and games the whole family plays as a unit.[19]

PARENT-PARENT GAMES

In games parents play with one another, the husband and wife shift out of their marital roles and relate to one another in their parental roles. What often occurs is that one spouse plays "Stern Parent" to the other's "Bad Child," or one spouse as "Good Parent" berates the other as "Bad Parent."

The "Stern Parent-Bad Child" category includes such games as the following: "There you go—spoiling him (her)—just like your mother spoiled you"; "She (he) is just like you—stubborn and lazy"; and "Why do you always have to act more like a child than your children do? When are you ever going to grow up?" In the "Good Parent-Bad Parent" category are the following games: "Why do you always give in to the children?"; "How come you're never around when they have to be disciplined?"; "It's just too bad they get on your nerves. Who was it wanted to have children in the first place?"; "*Your* child just wrote his name in crayon on the living room wall!"; and "It's a pity they didn't take after my side of the family."

PARENT-CHILD GAMES

These games may be played by one parent alone or by both parents. These include such games as "I (we) don't know why

*Not surprisingly, many family games consist essentially of "PFLs in action." PFLs are the ultimate basis of all games, but they are usually more evident in family games because the family is the chief originator and teacher of PFLs.

you act that way. We never did such things when we were children"; "You're older than your sister (brother), so you should know better"; "Children should be seen but not heard, so stop interrupting"; "If you can't speak civilly to me (us), then don't say anything at all"; "If you don't do your chores, you can't watch TV"; "Denial" ("I never said you could do any such thing; whatever gave you that idea?"); and "Hostile Power" (the parent picks or nags at or harrasses a child until the child gets angry and fights back; then the parent pounces on the child for being rude or disrespectful).

Other parent-child games are "United Front" ("Your mother (father) and I agree—there's no use arguing about it"); "Because we're you're parents—that's why"; "How can you say (do) that (or feel that way) after all we've done for you"; and "We're only doing this for your own good."

In "Dumping," one parent "dumps on" the other parent by way of the children: "Your father (mother) wouldn't like that"; "Just wait till your mother (father) hears about this"; "Go ask your father (mother); if he (she) says it's okay, then it's okay with me"; "Stop complaining; you sound just like your mother (father)"; "Don't tell your father (mother) I said so—but go ahead and do ________"; and "Well, I don't approve, but I suppose your mother (father) will overrule me."

CHILD-PARENT GAMES

Often the games a child plays with his parent(s) serve as a covert means of getting back at the parent(s), as a means of expressing disapproval, as a means of asserting independence, or as a means of getting something from the parent(s). These games can take the following forms: "You don't love me—if you did, you'd let me ________"; "Well, I didn't *ask* to be born into this family"; "Interrupt the Adults"; "Temper Tantrum" (holding the breath, screaming, making animal noises); "Sullen Silence"; "Foot-dragging"; "Play Mama Against Papa"; "________'s parents don't make him do that"; and "You never let me do anything."

SIBLING-SIBLING GAMES

Siblings play games not only with their parents but also with each other. These include such games as "I never could stay up that late when I was your age. It's not fair"; "How come Dad (Mom) always favors you? That's why you're such a pain"; "Get lost!"; "No, you can't play with me"; "Why don't you grow up? (You're such a baby!)"; "Mother! ________ hit me!"; "Wish I was a boy—you have all the fun"; "Dad always lets you off the hook 'cause you're a girl"; "Blackmail" (If you don't give me ________ or do ________, I'll tell Mom (Dad) about the time you did ________); and "Secrets."

GAMES ANY MEMBER CAN PLAY

So far we have described games that are played by family members when they are in specific roles. However, there are other games that do not depend so much on role or position; these are the games that any family member can play at any time it suits his purposes, and he can play it with any other member of the family. These include such games as "Fake-out" ("While you're up, please get me ________"); "Criticism" (criticize someone and when he gets upset, act surprised at his irritation or hurt and ask, "What's the matter with you?"); "Challenge" (challenge or attack all the other members and get the whole family in an uproar); "Pass the Word" (complain to one member about something another member has done, thus ensuring that the word will get passed along to the offender); "Outraged Innocence" (claiming not to know something after having acted on ignorance: "How was I supposed to know you were saving ________ for later on?"); "No Bones about It" (revealing personal secrets about another member to someone outside the family); "Dawdling" (dragging the feet when asked to do something); "How Come?" ("How come I'm always the last to know? How come nobody understands me? How come no one ever listens to me?"); and "Negation" ("You wouldn't understand; you're just a—child, parent, adult, woman, man").

FAMILY GROUP GAMES

Whereas games any member can play are instigated by one person, family games are instigated by all (or many) members and pit the "group" against the individual. These consist of such games as "Stereotype" in which the whole family stereotypes a member and then acts toward him on the basis of that stereotype. For example, families may develop stereotypes like "The Bungler," "The Monster," "Sulky Face," "The Roarer," "The Whiner," "The Martyr," "The Giggler," "The Dumb One," "The Awkward One," "The Dull One," "The Tactless One," "The Brain," and "The Weeper." Other games include "Gang Up" (everyone gets angry at one member and gangs up on him, or everyone tries to persuade a member that he should or should not do something); "Ostracize" (members punish one of the group for not conforming); and "Invisible" (family members act as if a particular member is the same as everyone else even though the member is *not* the same; for example, he may be deaf, retarded, crippled, antisocial, hostile, or seriously disturbed).

Games and family dynamic equilibrium

The kinds of games the members of a particular family play strongly depend on the dominant, overall style of the family plus the specific styles of the individual members. The purpose of these games is to establish and/or maintain personal and interpersonal dynamic equilibrium. The reasons therefore that a person plays a game are generated and dictated by his thoughts and feelings—his self-system. In short, the chosen game will receive its "shape" and expression from the player's life-style and from the style of the "group" to which he belongs, but it will receive its impetus, its meaning and significance, and its reason for being from the player's self-system. Thus although we have been discussing the dynamic equilibrium sought by three or more people, it is important to remember that the key to all games, all interactions, and all relationships is the individual—his life-style and his self-system. In viewing family interaction, it is equally important to remember, however, that the determining factor in the creation and continuation of family system and style is the marital-parental system and style.

Family identity crises

Many families may go through their whole life playing games and having little or no awareness of their family identity. Generally, this is possible only because the family is not subjected to a major stress or change that exercises enough impact to jolt the members out of their automatic and repetitious ways. If, however, something does happen that really challenges or shakes up the family's usual ways of maintaining their dysfunctional dynamic equilibrium, then one or more of the members are likely to experience a **family identity crisis.**[20]

Many different occurrences can precipitate such a crisis.

1. The breadwinner may lose his or her job, and the family has to change their accustomed style of living.
2. One (or more) of the members may have a personal identity crisis that moves him to evaluate not only himself but also the family.
3. When one or more of the children leave home, the parents may suddenly have a lot of unfilled time and may begin to assess their family identity.
4. The "marital menopause" may jolt the parents into appraising their family relationship.
5. One (or more) of the children may establish a close relationship with another family, which causes him to take a long, hard look at his family relationship.
6. The discovery of another member's major flaws (e.g., lying, cheating) may jolt both the discoverer and the discovered into a reassessment.

Other crisis-precipitating factors may consist of physical problems, psychological problems, or both besetting one (or more) of the members. For example, one member becomes excessively dependent on the other. One (or more) of the members crosses the line between heavy social drinking and alcoholism or becomes addicted to drugs. One (or both) parent's alcoholism or drug addiction becomes evident as it affects the family. One (or more) of the member's sexual behavior affects the family relationship (e.g., one of the parents has an extramarital affair; one of the children impregnates or is impregnated; one of the members contracts venereal disease; one of the members announces or reveals his homosexuality). One (or more) of the members becomes physically disabled, or a serious physical disease or condition occurs (e.g., cancer, heart attack, senility). One (or more) of the members suffers psychological breakdown (e.g., severe depression, psychosis, frank paranoid behavior, attempted suicide). One (or more) engages in criminal behavior (e.g., embezzlement, armed robbery, homicide—attempted or accomplished).

Obviously any of these events or problems would be adequate occasion for an evaluation of family identity. Another sure way to set the assessment process in motion is for one member to announce to the others that he rejects one or more of them or the whole family relationship. (For example, a teenager rebels and renounces—at least temporarily—his family ties; a mother leaves in order to fulfill her nonbiological destiny). Whatever the precipitating factors may be, however, evaluating the family may reveal shocking disparities in the members' perceptions of one another and in the members' perception of the family.

DISPARITIES IN MEMBERS' SELF/OTHER PERCEPTIONS

One particular aspect of family member perception is especially vulnerable to the shock of recognition. This aspect involves how each member perceives the others and how each member *thinks* the others perceive him. If there is a disparity between their perceptions, there is distortion. Such distortion is not only divisive per se but can be especially divisive when it suddenly becomes evident—often through direct confrontation and revelation.

For example, Josh's parents have always been (at least in Josh's eyes) law-abiding, God-fearing, morally upright people (as have his two much older sisters). Josh perceives them as never doing much wrong and never making moral mistakes. In his view, they are surely incapable of lying, cheating, and stealing, and he is basically correct. But his perception of them goes beyond this: he thinks they are all morally perfect. Surely none of them ever does or wants to do anything "bad," none of them thinks mean or petty thoughts, and none of them ever feels lustful or angry or jealous. Surely none of them is ever curious about sex.

The problem for Josh is that he has had *all* these thoughts and feelings at one time time or another. He feels angry at his parents and sisters frequently; sometimes he fantasizes taking petty revenge on one or more of them. When he was 7 or 8 years old, Josh stole two dollars from his father's savings jug, and he stole other small amounts at other times until he was 10 years old, when he father caught him at it and punished him. In addition, Josh cannot remember *not* being curious about sex: playing doctor was his favorite game when he was younger. His wet dreams have always bothered him but at the same time intrigued him. From time to time, whenever he can get past his guilt feelings, he masturbates.

Partly as a result of the vast disparity between the way he perceives the other family members and the way he knows himself to be, Josh has developed a rather negative self-concept. He sees himself as a bad person, perhaps immoral. He feels unworthy of belonging to this good family, since he feels that he is dishonest, sinfully fascinated by sex, and morally weak and corrupt. Josh is convinced that this is really the way his parents and sisters perceive him, since that is the way he is, isn't he?

His behavioral response to his self-concept has long been one of overcompensation. He tries never to show anger, to be helpful to his parents, and to do well in school. He is polite, quiet, pleasant, hard working, responsible, and trustworthy (now that he is past his "stealing years"). He goes to church every Sunday, sometimes twice.

It is primarily on this behavior that his family bases their perceptions of him. They see him as a "good" boy—indeed as being morally superior by far to most of his peers. They have come to expect this kind of behavior from him, and they are always amazed if he says something negative about himself.

Suppose Josh meets a girl he really likes and starts spending a great deal of time with her. She was originally attracted to him by the challenge he presented. She wanted to see if his goody-goody behavior was for real, and she wanted to see if behind his moral exterior there lurked a red-blooded American male. She introduced him to marijuana and got him to drink and smoke with her; finally, in response to a lot of seductive teasing, they began sleeping together.

The stage now is fully set for a personal and family identity crisis. Perhaps the girl gets pregnant. Or maybe his mother finds a condom in the pocket of Josh's jeans. Perhaps after drinking and smoking, Josh racks up the family car. Maybe he, his girlfriend, and several others get busted for a pot party, and his parents are called to post bail for their son.

Whatever the particular precipitating event, the family confrontation with the realities of Josh's identity and behavior may be devastating. Josh when questioned may fling at them that they are hypocritical; that he is just doing openly what they have always known about him. His feeling and accusation may be, "You've always known what I'm really like; why do you act so surprised now?" The other family members, of course, are indeed shocked, since "this isn't the boy we've always known!" They may be wondering at the sudden "appearance" of this stranger in their midst. Josh's parents especially may be asking themselves the heart-wrenching question: "Where did we go wrong? Why did this happen?" Needless to say, Josh's troubles have severely shaken the family's dynamic equilibrium and have provoked a family identity crisis.

DISPARITIES IN FAMILY CONCEPT

Another potential source of shock and trouble will exist if the members have or develop differing perceptions of the family relationship (family concept). If an event or problem prompts an assessment that reveals a disparity between or among members' family concepts, then trouble may ensue. (If a marked disparity does exist, trouble has, of course, been there all along but underneath the surface.)

For example, one kind of disparity and shake-up may occur if all the members do hold essentially the same family concept, but then one person's perceptions change. Suppose Felicia, like other members of her family, sees the family as tolerant, liberal, and dedicated to humane principles. She feels proud to be a member of such a group. When she goes to the state university and is exposed to others' views, feelings, and experiences, she realizes with a jolt that her family *talk* tolerance and liberal ideas but do not practice what they preach. Her realization has come about through encounters with her roommate Jill and Jill's family. Jill's family believe in equality and civil liberties, and they act on their beliefs. Jill and her parents took part in many civil rights protests and demonstrations and were once jailed for their activity. All the family members have friends from all kinds of different ethnic, religious, and racial backgrounds.

When Felicia goes home over Christmas vacation, she sees that although her parents and two brothers deplore the terrible conditions in their city's ghettos, none of them has ever tried to *do* anything about those conditions. Felicia also notices that when she talks about her friend Stanley—who is black—her parents get nervous and tend to ask a lot more questions than they ordinarily would.

When Felicia realizes the disparity between the rest of the family's concept and her concept of the family, she gets angry and accuses them of being two-faced or of being pseudoliberals. She may refuse to discuss social issues with them, and she may see to it that she does not spend much time at home. The rest of the family may be shocked by Felicia's reactions and feel angry toward her. They may accuse her of becoming a fanatic. Whatever the eventual outcomes of this may be, Felicia's experiences have jolted her into a family identity crisis. The whole family may also be so jolted. Whether the effects of this crisis are divisive depends on how the family members deal with the crisis and with one another.

Another way that a crisis can occur is if one (or more) of the family members assumes that all the members have basically the same concept of the family but then discovers that such is not the case. For example, suppose the father and children perceive their family life as being happy, secure, individually rewarding, and generally pleasant and comfortable. They assume that Eve, the wife and mother, feels the same way. However, in fact, she has had her consciousness raised and now has a different concept of their family life. She regards it as a trap; she feels that she does an inordinate amount of household "junk work." Eve feels that the happy, secure, pleasant comfort that the rest of the family experiences is due largely to the fact that she has provided good "hotel service." The children do not help much with the chores and getting them to do even the barest minimum is more of a hassle than it is worth. For her husband to wash or dry one dish or to help with any of the "woman's work" is apparently inconceivable to him.

One sunny day in suburbia, something snaps for Eve: she has had it. She wants time for herself; she wants to go back to school and have some creative life of her own. At dinner she quietly announces that she is going to start taking courses at the community college in the next term and that she is no longer going to make the others' beds or do their laundry. In fact, she is going to stop doing many chores that the others are capable of doing for themselves. She announces that from now on there is going to be a fairer division of labor, and in response to the family's loud and vehement protests, she blasts them as being lazy parasites and says they can either start cooperating or she is leaving. Obviously this shocking announcement will bring on some kind of family identity crisis and some kind of reassessment of the family's identity. Whether Eve's new attitudes and plans will be divisive or cohesive depends on how the family responds to and deals with this newly revealed disparity in family concepts. If the family does not make a large effort to understand Eve's feelings and does not cooperate in working out a viable and agreeable course of action, Eve may detach herself and go her own emotional way. Or she may go off and get a job to finance her plans. If, however, the other family members and Eve work with the disparity in their perceptions, then the evaluation of the family's identity may have a constructive outcome for the whole family. But whatever the outcomes, the revelation of this disparity is an indication of long-term dissatisfaction and provides a terrific jolt to the current family relationship.

By now it is obvious that the more aware family members are of their family identity, that is, the better their understanding of and feel for it is, the better their chances are for developing, maintaining, and enjoying a healthy, functional family relationship. Conversely, the less aware the members are of their family identity the more likely they are to develop and then become dissatisfied with or break up an unhealthy, dysfunctional, and frequently divisive family relationship.

CLOSED AND OPEN MARRIAGE AND FAMILY: AN OVERVIEW

This chapter and the one preceding it have focused on many different aspects of marriage and family life: the essential components of the marital and family relationships; the process of developing a marital, parental, and family system and style; the outcomes of marital, parental, and family interaction; and the effects of those outcomes. In essence, these two chapters have examined the basic dynamics of the marital and family relationships—the components of the relationships and how those components work.

The last section of this chapter provides an analytical overview of how these dynamics relate to closed and open marriage and family living. This overview includes a comparison of closed and open marriage and family, which draws on all that has been discussed; a detailing of the essential attributes of openness; and a presentation of guidelines for working constructively toward openness.

Comparison of closed and open marriage and family

Most certainly, the topics of open marriage and the modern open family are relevant ones. People discuss these ideas on radio and television talk shows; innumerable magazine articles talk about them; and the book *Open Marriage*[21] has become a best-seller. However, it is one matter to talk and read about open marriage and family and openness in general; it is another to determine *how* to be a more open person and *how* to develop and maintain open relationships. Some people try to achieve these things and are successful; others try and are disappointed by or become anxious about the results. Some would like to try but are fearful of the risks; others would like to try but do not know how to go about it. To say the least, the subjects of openness and of open marriage and family in particular are not terribly clear. Therefore the following comparison of closed and open marriage and family is an attempt to clarify this somewhat vague and confused subject.

A list of what we consider the most important characteristics of closed and open marriage and family follows on pp. 260 to 262. To make the two kinds of marriage and family and the differences between them clear, we have presented the extremes of each kind. The list is organized so that both sides follow a particular matching order: (1) the individuals (their self-systems), (2) motivation for growth, (3) roles, (4) communication, (5) patterns of interaction (behavior), (6) intellectual climate, (7) emotional atmosphere, (8) relationship to the "outside world," and (9) marital and family system.

Essential attributes of openness

When you read this comparative list, you may respond with horror and awe at how incredibly crippling and distorting extreme closedness can be. Openness may appear to be an unbelievably idealized state, one that is impossible to attain. However, let us remind you that we presented extreme forms of openness and closedness.

Even if we make these states more credible by looking at their less extreme forms, a relationship between or among two or more fairly closed or semiclosed people is a combination of fragmented people struggling and scrambling to make one Humpty-Dumpty–like whole. The relationship between or among two or more fairly open or semiopen people is different. It is a union between or among whole people who retain their individual identity but at the same time join together to create a relationship that is greater than the sum of its partners or members.

The sad truth is, however, that closedness is familiar to almost all of us—it has been a part of our cultural heritage (as discussed in Chapter 1) and, for many of us,

Comparison of closed and open marriage and family

CLOSED MARRIAGE AND FAMILY	OPEN MARRIAGE AND FAMILY
1. Individuals (self-systems)	**1. Individuals (self-systems)**
Condition Unhealthy; not in touch with insides; live in future and/or past; operate on basis of hang-ups from past	*Condition* Healthy; in touch with insides; live in the present but with an appreciation of the past and an eye on the future; operate on basis of realistic appraisals of past, present, and future
PFLs *Expectations* Unrealistic (too high or too low)	*PFLs* *Expectations* Realistic; appropriate to abilities, feelings, situations, and circumstances
Rules Limiting; inflexible and often harsh or absent or not meaningful; rule breaking elicits punishment and rejection by self and others and feelings of guilt	*Rules* Flexible, relevant, and appropriate; serve as guidelines, not flat injunctions; can be questioned and changed if changing them is appropriate (if rule breaking does occur, each person attempts to understand and communicate about the matter and does not reject or try to produce guilt)
Self-concept Poor, undermining, low ego strength, and conflictual or inappropriately inflated self-concept	*Self-concept* Good ego strength; acceptance of self based on realistic assessment of weaknesses and strengths; caring, nurturing, and loving attitude toward self (which is the opposite of selfishness or self-centeredness); a celebration of self
Child/Parent/Adult Child or Parent (or both) rigid; Child or Parent inappropriately large (imbalanced); conflict between Child and Parent; impotent, weak, ineffectual, underdeveloped Adult	*Child/Parent/Adult* Child, Parent, and Adult flexible and maintain a healthy balance; Adult effectively mediates between demands of Child and Parent
2. Motivation for growth Limited; discouragement of experimentation; resistance to change	**2. Motivation for growth** Strong, steady, and unlimited; encouragement of experimentation; deep and abiding interest in change and growth
3. Roles Rigid role prescriptions (each has specific roles and must play them); role behavior stereotyped, restricted, and limiting; role requirements usually assumed, i.e., "unwritten"; deception and game playing based on roles; unequal status (top dog and bottom dog) with top dog running the show	**3. Roles** Flexible role prescriptions (each is free to cross role lines, to step out of usual roles, and to reject traditional stereotyped role ascriptions; each is free to act as individual, as husband/wife, as parent, as child, as sibling, or as a mixture in keeping with his or her feelings and appraisal of the situation); role attributes not stereotyped, not predetermined, and not assumed—members discuss and negotiate their own role ascriptions; no deceptions or game playing; members have status appropriate to the realities of the situation and run the show together through process of negotiation

CLOSED MARRIAGE AND FAMILY—cont'd	OPEN MARRIAGE AND FAMILY—cont'd
4. Communication Little if any intrapersonal in-touchedness; poor listeners; little or no checking out of assumptions; poor and inadequate feedback; distorted signals and messages sent and received; little if any negotiation; decision-making—either by compromise or power play	**4. Communication** Excellent intrapersonal in-touchedness; alert and caring listeners (each really hears what the other communicates); thorough checking out of assumptions and feelings; full and thorough feedback; clear signals and messages sent and received; much negotiation; decision-making—no power playing, minimal compromising, and maximum negotiating
5. Patterns of interaction (behavior) Automatic, repetitious, unconstructive, directed at maintaining status quo, and antichange (a person who goes against established marital or family patterns, is considered as having problems or being a troublemaker); productive of state of bondage—insistent on tight togetherness, possessive, locked together, caught in the couples or family game, and intolerant and fearful of autonomy	**5. Patterns of interaction (behavior)** Under each person's conscious control; neither automatic nor repetitious; constructive—directed at maximizing individual, marital, and family growth by means of constructive, appropriately shared change; members dedicated to helping one another realize individual potential; freedom granting—able to enjoy coupleness or familyness without being bound by it; interdependent but not caught in couples or family game; tolerant, respectful, appreciative of autonomy but at same time open to one another and welcoming of intimacy
6. Intellectual climate Rigid, narrow ways of thinking; emphasis on thoughts over feelings; use of reason as a weapon; intellectual arrogance or anti-intellectualism	**6. Intellectual climate** Free, wide-ranging ways of thinking; emphasis on balance between thoughts and feelings; use of reason as instrument for making realistic evaluations; commitment to intellectual curiosity, freedom, and integrity
7. Emotional atmosphere Marked by extremes—authoritarian, tight, controlled or impulsive, irresponsive, or indifferent; basically negative—distrustful, angry, passive, aggressive, fearful, critical, callous, demanding, denying, intolerant, punitive, not very affectionate or loving, and shallow; dull and boring because lacking in spontaneity	**7. Emotional atmosphere** Accepting of emotions as natural to the human condition; open expression of feelings; marked by balance in emotional reactions, i.e., no inappropriate extremes; basically positive—trusting, friendly, caring, accepting, tolerant, reassuring, supportive, affectionate, loving, warm, life-celebrating, gentle, deep, sensitive, understanding, and empathetic but capable of anger, sorrow, reserve, regret, and distrust when appropriate; vital and exciting because spontaneous
8. Relationship to "outside world" Tend to shut out others or to let them in too much of the time; relate to others in terms of coupleness and familyness or marital-family roles	**8. Relationship to "outside world"** Tend to be open to others, i.e., to stimulate and to be stimulated by encounters with world outside the marriage and family; free to let others make a difference; able to make emotional room for others; relate to others in terms of family, marital, and individual roles

Continued.

Comparison of closed and open marriage and family—cont'd

CLOSED MARRIAGE AND FAMILY—cont'd	OPEN MARRIAGE AND FAMILY—cont'd
9. Marital and family system Self-perpetuating rigidity: static, restrictive, and limiting—trust and love conditional on "good behavior" (e.g., absolute fidelity); live not so much in the present as in the past and/or future; subordination of selfhood to couplehood or familyhood with sharp limitations and restrictions on individual potential; discouragement of moves toward or expressions of autonomy; significant disparity between or among members' marital-family concepts; marital-family relationships either cohesive or divisive but always dysfunctional; minimal awareness of marital-family identity	**9. Marital and family system** Expanding and growing; dynamic, vital, permissive (within appropriate, agreed on limits), and democratic—trust and love freely given (not conditional); live primarily in and for the present; balance between selfhood, coupleness, and familyness; no limitations or restrictions on individual potential; encourage moves toward and expressions of autonomy; no significant disparity between or among members' marital-family concepts; marital-family relationships cohesive and functional; strong and clear awareness of marital-family identity

a part of our family heritage as well. The concept and state of openness are new, somewhat confusing, somewhat threatening, often alluring, yet elusive to many of us. One problem has been that openness received much of its original publicity by way of the drug, sexual, and counterculture revolutions and from the attitudes of the so-called permissive society. Thus openness has frequently been viewed as suspect and has been felt as threatening (and dangerous). At the same time, however, openness is alluring because it holds out a promise of more qualitative and meaningful ways of living.

The elusiveness of openness—even as a clear concept, much less as an attainable state—derives partly from not enough clarity about the *what* of openness and greatly from almost no information about the *how* of attaining it. Therefore we will touch briefly on the *what* and then give guidelines relating to the *how*.

What are the central, irreducible attributes of openness? Essentially openness means just that—being open to self, to others, and to life. Thus **openness** means the following:

1. Being willing to try new and different experiences; trying not to "shut up intellectual and emotional shop" when you encounter thoughts, feelings, actions, events, and people that are different from those you are used to; choosing not to close your mind, harden your heart, shut your eyes and ears, stay your hand from, or turn your back on newness and difference
2. Being willing to experiment and to risk and deal with the anxiety inherent in experimenting
3. Being willing to feel, to reveal, and to be honest with yourself and others
4. Being willing to share yourself with yourself and with others
5. Being willing to reach out, to risk intimacy—to see, hear, smell, touch, taste, and feel your own and others' humanness
6. Being willing to accept and respect your own and others' weaknesses and strengths and your own and others' autonomy; being willing to cherish and celebrate your own and others' uniqueness
7. Being willing to be available to and to work at changing and growing; being willing to commit yourself to

change and growth with the recognition that they constitute an ongoing process—the process of a lifetime

8. Being willing to recognize that the process of changing and growing *is* life ►IE-2, p. 265

Guidelines for working constructively toward openness

We recognize that full openness is perhaps an unattainable ideal, a state of perfection—but ideals are not for attaining; they are for striving toward. It is the *process* of striving, of doing, that constitutes life.

The following discussion is a distillation of ideas already presented in this book. These are guidelines to the process of becoming more open: if you follow them out in detail and in terms of their full implications, they will help you travel a long way down the open road.

1. Since individuals are the building blocks of relationships, start with yourself. Apply The System to *you*—which means gathering information (and gaining awareness), acquiring insights, implementing your insights (e.g., breaking into the automatic quality of PFLs and patterns), and building in your competence.

2. Learn about, practice, build in, and *use* the methods of intrapersonal and interpersonal communication; in many ways effective communication is the golden key to opening the doors of self and others.

3. Work on gaining a thorough awareness of your own past and on developing respect, appreciation, and empathy for those (including you) who have played a part in it. This means looking back, remembering, recreating, and being willing to relive not only pleasant but also painful past incidents. It means realizing that those who raised and influenced you probably did the best they could. It means recognizing that any psychological scars you may have from the past were inflicted on you by others because they too have psychological scars. At the same time, it means acknowledging that often these same people have given you not only scars but strengths also.

Dealing constructively with the past means then leaving behind or exorcising the negative aspects of the Parent (whatever was hostile, punitive, disturbed, distorted, domineering, limiting, controlling, critical, or rejecting in your parent models) and keeping and cherishing the positive aspects (loving, caring, encouraging, guiding, teaching, supporting, reassuring, empathizing). Dealing constructively with the past also means leaving behind the negative aspects of the Child (blind rebellion, temper tantrums, mindless impulsivity) and keeping and nurturing the positive aspects (playfulness, creativity, humor, joy, spontaneity). It means learning to accept, to empathize with, to value, and to love the child that you were and the Child that you carry within you to this very day and hour.

4. Awareness of and respect and empathy for the past do not mean, however, inordinately dwelling on or inappropriately living in the past. Becoming more open means concentrating primarily on your own and others' moment-to-moment thoughts, feelings, and actions as they occur. The open life is not yesterday and back *there*, not tomorrow and out *there*—it is today, *now* and *here*. As the Sanskrit proverb states:

> Look to this day,
> For it is life,
> The very life of life.
> . . . .
> For yesterday is but a dream
> And tomorrow is only a vision.
> . . . .
> Look well, therefore, to this day.

Living in the here and now involves a willingness to acknowledge ownership of and to take responsibility for yourself—for your thoughts, feelings, and actions—in the present. In effect this means not blaming others or external circumstances for what is really your responsibility, it means not denying your real feelings, and it means being willing to accept and take responsibility for whatever consequences are built into and result from your actions and choices.

5. Concentrating on the here and now does not mean ignoring the future. Rather it includes recognizing and accepting that what you do in the present (e.g., whether you risk intimacy; whether you work on changing a destructive PFL or merely sit back and let it control you) affects not only the present but the future as well.

6. Although we say to start with yourself, we are not suggesting leaving others out of your moves toward openness. Quite the contrary, people not only need people, but people can be good for people. Apply The System to yourself; teach it to others; practice it with others. If you do, both you and they will benefit.

7. Become as conversant as you can with the dynamics of human interaction—the what, the how, and the why. Apply this knowledge to yourself and to your relationships.

If you implement these guidelines in detail and in terms of their full implications, you will be strengthening your Adult and moving toward greater autonomy. The outcomes of such moves are greater personal and interpersonal competence, greater personal openness, and an increased capacity for establishing and maintaining healthy, functional, open relationships.

The open road is not an easy road to travel; it involves hazards, risks, and hard work. If you work to become more open, you may grow away from some of your partners in some of your relationships (e.g., friendships, marriage, dating). If you use the techniques of becoming more open in your family and marriage, you could grow apart. However, we feel that far greater risks are involved in *not* trying to change, grow, and become more open. One risk is that you might just drift away from your partner(s), or you might split because of misunderstandings resulting from distorted communication. You also risk contracting *rigor mortis in vivo*—living a life and having relationships that are rigid, limited, repetitious, dull, and perhaps quietly desperate.

The open road beckons. Why not follow the guidelines and go?

Interaction experiences

1. Examining the dynamic equilibrium in your family (p. 247)

One way to get a feel for the dynamic equilibrium in your family is to give yourself the following experience. Get together enough mugs or tea cups to match the number of members in your family. Put the mugs on the floor or on a table and name each mug (e.g., Mom, Dad, Tim, Judy). The handle of the mug represents the person's nose. Now arrange the mugs according to the ways family members characteristically relate to one another. For example, if Mom and Dad have a warm and loving relationship, you might put their mugs "nose to nose." If Mom loves Judy, but Judy acts cool and distant toward Mom, you could put Mom's handle pointing toward Judy, but Judy's pointing away from Mom. In addition, you would probably put their mugs far apart. Do this for all family members.

EVALUATION: When you have arranged all the mugs, examine the meanings of their placement. Who is close? Who is distant? Who is hostile? Who is warm and loving? Do any family members seem to be allied with each other? Who communicates with whom? Do any family members seem to be alone, that is, to stand outside the family circle? Is the whole family close? Does the family group consist only of a loose and somewhat alienated confederation? What is your emotional response to your arrangement? Are you sad or happy about it? Are you surprised by your arrangement? What have you learned from this experience?

FOLLOW-UP: After you have examined and evaluated your family relationships as they are now, rearrange the mugs to eliminate all alienated relationships. Try to feel the differences between the two family arrangements. Do you feel it would be possible to bring about such a change? Would you want such a change? Ask other family members to arrange the mugs according to the ways they see the family's dynamic equilibrium and then discuss the experience with them.

2. Evaluating your family in terms of openness and closedness (p. 263)

Using the categories (e.g., roles, emotional atmosphere) on the list comparing closed and open families (see pp. 260 to 262), evaluate in writing how open or closed your family is. Try to draw on all that you have learned to make your evaluation as complete and as accurate as possible.

EVALUATION: Was it difficult for you to make this evaluation? Was it a painful experience? An exciting one? A boring one? An instructive one? What were you thinking and feeling as you did it? Did this experience help you become more aware of your family and its dynamics? Did you become more aware of characteristics you would like to see changed? Were you surprised by any of your observations? Did you discover any strengths or weaknesses you had not realized before? Do you see any ways that you and other family members might work on minimizing the weaknesses and maximizing the strengths?

FOLLOW-UP: You might share your evaluation with one or more family members and see if they perceive the family in the same or different ways.

REFERENCES

1. Howells, John G.: Theory and practice of family psychiatry, New York, 1971, Brunner/Mazel, Inc., pp. 30-31.
2. Ackerman, Nathan W.: The psychodynamics of family life, New York, 1958, Basic Books, Inc., Publishers, pp. 159-161.
3. Foster, R. M.: Parental communication as a determinant of child behavior, American Journal of Psychotherapy **25**:579-590, 1971.
4. Ibid., 162-164.
5. Callahan, Sidney Cornelia: Parenting, Garden City, N.Y., 1973, Doubleday & Co., Inc., pp. 32-63.
6. Mulford, C. L.: Socialization, communication, and role performance, Sociological Quarterly **13**(1):74-80, 1972.
7. Ackerman, op. cit., pp. 23 and 74.
8. Ackerman, op. cit., p. 342.
9. Costello, A. J.: Scientific investigation of relationships and communication within the family, Proceedings of the Royal Society of Medicine **62**:900-901, 1969.
10. Ferreira, Antonio J.: Family myth and homeostasis. In Howells, John G. editor: Theory and practice of family psychiatry, New York, 1971, Brunner/Mazel, Inc., pp. 358-366.
11. Pollay, R. W.: Intrafamily communication and consensus, Journal of Communication **19**(3):181-201, 1969.
12. Odum, L.: A study of family communication patterns and personality integration in children, Child Psychiatry and Human Development **1**(4):275-285, 1971.
13. Murdock, George P.: The universality of the nuclear family. In Bell, N. W., and Vogel, E. F., editors: A modern introduction to the family, Glencoe, Ill., 1960, Free Press, pp. 37-44.
14. Erikson, Erik H.: Identity: youth and crisis, New York, 1968, W. W. Norton & Co., Inc., pp. 47-48.
15. Ruesch, Jurgen, and Bateson, Gregory: Communication: the social matrix of society, New York, 1951, W. W. Norton & Co., Inc. pp. 280-281.
16. Howells op. cit., p. 41.
17. McGinnis, Thomas C., and Ayres, John U.: Open family living: a new approach for enriching your life together, Garden City, N.Y., 1976, Doubleday & Co., Inc., Chapter 1.
18. Berne, Eric: Games people play: the psychology of human relationships, New York, 1964, Grove Press, Inc., p. 48.
19. Ibid., pp. 58-60.
20. Ackerman, op. cit., pp. 117-118.
21. O'Neill, Nena, and O'Neill, George: Open marriage: a new life style for couples, New York, 1972, M. Evans & Co., Inc.

EPILOGUE

Janus, the ancient Roman god with the two faces looking in opposite directions, is a fitting symbol for this book's perspectives on time and human life. To the Romans he was the god particularly concerned with time and destiny; from his vantage point in the present he looks back at what has occurred up to the present moment, and he looks ahead at what is to come. Because the two faces are joined back to back, Janus aptly symbolizes the interconnection between the world of what is already formed and the world of future potentialities.

A key perspective of this book is that the individual is caught in the conflicts between PFLs of an earlier, more closed time and the more open situations and new PFLs of the present. This dilemma is the result of the rapid changes in society and its institutions.

Whether any of us like it or not, the worldwide closed systems (e.g., government, religion) that have held sway from time immemorial are breaking up or are at least undergoing vast shake-ups and changes. Originally, within the framework of these closed systems, the focus was not on openness or attempts to develop it; by and large there were few attempts to challenge or break down or get out of these closed systems. However, as the framework has been shaken or broken into, the stability offered by the restrictions of closed systems has been weakened or eroded or destroyed.

The results of shaking the foundations of a rigid, stable, closed system are lack of direction, confusion, sharp clashes among seemingly innumerable interest groups, struggles among conflicting (and often nebulous) belief systems, conflicts between closed and more open PFLs, and seeming (sometimes actual) chaos. These results tend to elict feelings of ambivalence, uncertainty, confusion, alienation, anxiety, and/or fear in many of those caught up in a world and time they no longer know or understand.

In the midst of this confused and confusing opening up of society stand the individual and his personal institutions of marriage and the family. Stripped of the stabilizing influence of the limitations imposed by a closed society and stripped of the traditional external support systems and frames of reference provided by a closed society, man's existential dilemmas stand out in raw, high relief. The eternal questions demand to be answered: Who am I? Why am I who I am? Where have I come from, where am I now, and where am I going? How do I get there? Who goes with me? Who is he or she? Who are they? Who are we in relation to one another? What do our relationships mean? How and why did they form, what are they like now, and what will become of them and me?

In response to the potential and actual discomfort, anxiety, or pain inherent in the opening up process, many people become defensive; many withdraw; many ignore the changes as best they can and try to call back "the good old days"; many try to get the original rigid system back into balance and operation. Others float in a sea of confusion and uncertainty; lacking fixed stars or familiar landmarks by which to determine their position or course, they drift along, going wherever a new wave takes them. Others, although perhaps anxious or scared, evaluate the conditions and alternatives as best they can, look within for guidance, search for new directions, and set out on the long life's journey into self and new meanings. They turn inward to find the way to the outer limits of their human potential.

In previous times, versions of the journey into self were generally deemed to be the cultured prerogative of the nobility, the rarefied activity of the scholar, the Christian duty of the clergy and thoughtful layman, the God-given glory of the Christian mystic, the satanic carryings-on of the insane, or the mythic function of the folk hero. The common folk ordinarily had neither the affluence nor the time for such matters. Generally, journeys into self (or introspection or concentration on the inner self) were considered an activity that was privileged or selfish or strange or exotic or disturbed. Ever since the time that psychology became a significant influence, however, the journey into self has gradually gained a place (albeit until recently a suspect place) in the lives of the general population. In the second half of this century, awareness of and in-touchedness with one's inner self has finally gained general, although certainly not total, respectability and acceptance.

Along with many others, we believe that the journey into self is *the* way to achieve psychological health; only by being in touch with his insides and being willing and able to work constructively with them can a person effect significant, long-term change and growth in himself. We contend, furthermore, that the most effective way to bring about constructive change and growth in society is for its individual members to first bring it about in themselves. In our view, true change and growth toward openness are determined not from without but from within.

This point of view may help to explain why we have tended only to briefly mention such specific subjects as alternate forms of marriage and family (e.g., homosexual marriage, the unmarried parent, communes, group marriage) or such concepts as Margaret Mead's proposal that couples should qualify for children licenses before they can legally become parents. Ultimately we are interested not so much in how to build better institutions but in how to build better human relationships. If individuals are basically healthy and open, then the particular form of institution they choose to develop is likely to be healthy and open too.

For these reasons, the other major objective of the book has been the specific and detailed examination of an individual's, a marriage's, and a family's past, present, and future—in effect, their identities. The results of this examination form a conceptual and practical framework within which to analyze the dynamics of individual, marital, and family interaction. These analyses make possible the understanding of and feeling for the dynamics of human interaction, which can enable a person to modify, alter, or change the ways he interacts with and relates to himself and others. These changes encourage and potentiate growth toward greater autonomy and openness.

This book presents both the theory and techniques of communicating and interacting in ways that are often different from those specified and required by a closed society. Thus the interactional approach set forth, developed, and explained in this text offers a major alternative to the traditional, limited, restrictive ways of living, which have been fostered and perpetuated by a closed society. This alternative approach is synthesized by the Interactional Therapeutic System.

A primary strength of The System is its flexibility, which results from the incorporation of the best of many different approaches. Its two hallmarks are its insistence on the importance of, the absolute necessity for, being in touch from moment to moment with insides and its emphasis on communication as the golden key to being in touch with self and others, to sharing insides and outsides, and to implementing The System.

The Interactional Therapeutic System is a flexible but systematic approach to developing, establishing, and maintaining healthier, more open individual, marital, and family relationships. Although The System is systematic, it allows for enormous variety of experience, since it is not prescriptive. In addition, it does not dictate outcomes but teaches how to evaluate alternatives, decisions, and outcomes in terms of appropriateness and inappropriateness, health and lack of health, and happiness and unhappiness.

The System is teachable and learnable; it can be built in and made an integral part of the way a person lives. The Interactional Therapeutic System provides the tools for processing human experiences in honest, open, constructive, life-enhancing ways. Once a person begins to make conscious and deliberate use of The System, he has begun the never-ending process of a lifetime—the process of journeying into self and out to others.

If you look at them individually, the concepts and techniques of The System may strike you as extremely simple and familiar. They are. The reason they are so simple and familiar is that these concepts and techniques naturally belong to and are a constant part of all of us. From the moment of birth, we are all naturally involved in the twin processes of communication and interaction.

Since these processes are our natural heritage, you may wonder why most of us have to be taught how to use them effectively. The reason is that unfortunately until recently a closed society has taught and insisted that we learn *not* to be in touch with many of our insides and *not* to be too free and open in communicating and interacting.

The Interactional Therapeutic System is offered as a means of helping you to get in touch with your natural heritage. We would hope that as T. S. Eliot wrote:

> . . . the end of all our exploring
> Will be to arrive where we started
> And know the place for the first time.*

If you have tried to use the material provided in this book constructively (e.g., attempted to become more aware of your identity and to develop the tools and skills set forth in the Interactional Therapeutic System), then we hope that you have become turned on to the possibilities of living a more open life and having more open relationships both with yourself and with others. We trust that you have gained some, if not all, of the following benefits:

1. That your use of The System has helped you replace old characteristics like fuzziness about your feelings and your identity with greater awareness and in-touchedness
2. That you have been able to work through and abandon self-contempt, blame, and punishment
3. That you have developed self-respect and greater feelings of confidence, adequacy, and competence, and that you have established a more positive self-concept
4. That you have moved away from any tendency to hold the outside world responsible for your inside anxiety, hurts, and pain
5. That you have worked well enough with yourself that you can feel the differences between your former fragmentation and your present feelings of greater integration and wholeness and between the former imbalance in your blend of thinking, feeling, and acting and your present, more balanced blend of thinking, feeling, and acting
6. That your Adult part is larger, stronger, and more autonomous and that it now helps you to enjoy the pleasurable and helpful aspects of your Child and Parent

*From Eliot, T. S.: Little Gidding. In The complete poems and plays (1909-1950) of T. S. Eliot, New York, 1952, Harcourt, Brace & Co., p. 145.

7. That you have become aware of many of your PFLs and the part they may play in creating conflicts, confusion, or double binds in your life and that you can use The System to live a fuller, more meaningful life
8. That you realize that being a mature, responsible adult need not mean living a life of complacency, conformity, and boredom but instead can mean growth, excitement, and joy as you fulfill your potential as a human being
9. That you have become more alive to yourself and others and that you now have a sense of outreach, which means that you can and will experiment with the rich and varied experiences that life offers in such sharp and vivid profusion

We hope that we have given you—with The System—some new and helpful tools and guidelines for functioning with greater health, greater openness, and greater aliveness. Above all, we hope that we have been able to help you gain a new interest in yourself and others, a new feeling of commitment to change and growth, and the truly thrilling knowledge not only that you can change and grow but that you can also help in a larger sense to make significant alterations in your society and the world. Although all of us are to one degree or another subject to outside forces that we cannot control, we no longer need to feel so helpless or hopeless in the face of societal pressures and demands. By gaining in-touchedness with and the ability to work constructively with the forces inside us, we can then better manage the forces outside us.

We hope that you are pleased by your involvement in life's most exciting and rewarding experiences—communicating and interacting honestly and openly with yourself and others. Welcome to the celebration of your own and others' uniqueness, to the celebration of your membership in the human family, and to the celebration of life.

appendix A
THE JOHNSON FAMILY

HOW THE COMMUNITY PERCEIVES THE JOHNSONS

The members of the Johnson family are Harry (father), Janice (mother), Mike (son), Sally (daughter), Brandy (dog), and Samantha (cat). On the surface, they are a typical middle-class WASP family. Beneath the surface, the Johnsons are nothing of the kind; they are a collection of unique individuals who are related to each other and who are joined together in a rather uneasy union. The following is a brief description of the community they live in and a description of how people see the Johnsons.

The community in which the Johnsons live is a commuting town, a suburban satellite of a big city to which 85% of the men commute to work. The population (approximately 18,000) is essentially middle class with family income ranging from about $15,000 to $50,000 a year. The racial and religious makeup of the town is 90% white and 10% black and 3% Jewish, 15% Catholic, and 82% Protestant. Most of the women do not work and have some domestic help. About 60% of the adults have attended college, and about three fourths of that group completed four years of college. About 80% of the high school graduates go to college.

The community as a whole perceives the Johnson family as somewhat of a model family: they are law-abiding and constructive citizens, all four members seem to get along peaceably, and the children will grow up to be solid citizens. Close friends of the Johnsons know that they have their troubles. The friction between Mike and his father is evident. Harry and Janice tend to do a fair amount of in-fighting; she nags and picks at Harry, and he either snarls at her or withdraws and does not speak to her for periods of time. Their friends also realize that Harry is demanding of the children—either they measure up to his standards or they get a tongue-lashing, sometimes in front of visitors. Janice comes across as sort of fluttering through life: she is pleasant enough, but she is forever making a crisis out of something. The children strike the Johnson's adult friends as nice and polite but sometimes as a little sullen and withdrawn. However, by and large, most of the adults regard the Johnsons as having a minimum of troubles.

Most people who come into the Johnson's home with any frequency begin to sense (whether unconsciously or consciously) an atmosphere of friendly tension mixed with a kind of indifference. It is as though the family members are constantly on guard and are always on their best behavior (except perhaps Harry who, as king of the roost, is free to have outbursts of temper). Even when Harry lets loose, Janice responds with undercover sniping, and Mike and Sally sullenly and silently move away. The air of indifference in the home springs from the fact that much of the time, family members seem either to not listen to each other or to kind of drift by the other members without making any meaningful contact. They all live together in the same house, but they live in different worlds.

A CLOSER, IN-DEPTH VIEW OF THE JOHNSONS

Although a few people have a fairly clear understanding of what the family is like, no one knows the Johnsons as they really are either as individuals within the family group or as a family. This is because every family and every member in it has an inner life that an outside observer cannot know about unless he is told about it. Thus even though outsiders can see parts of the truth, they are usually not in a position to put all the pieces together to get a coherent, accurate, and full picture of another family's inner life. Ordinarily only family members themselves have sufficient information to be able to know about and understand their family's inner life.

The analysis of the Johnsons presented here and in other parts of the book is intended to help you to gain a fuller understanding of them and thereby to develop some skill in working with family dynamics. Hopefully this experience with the Johnsons will enable you to learn to use the information you acquire about your own family to evaluate and understand the meaning of your family's identity and functioning.

The analysis of the Johnson family is set up as follows. Harry and Janice (the parents) are analyzed in terms of their PFLs and patterns and the outcomes of their interactions based on their PFLs and patterns. The descriptions of Mike and Sally are somewhat less structured because they are still growing and forming their self-systems and life-styles.

The parents

HARRY *Basic life-style:* Obsessive-compulsive
Age: 43 *Occupation:* Chemical engineer
Race: White *Annual salary:* $35,000
Religion: Protestant

A. Pattern and PFLs:

Pattern: Aggressive; sometimes hostile
PFLs: Attack is the best defense; might makes right; never deal from a position of weakness.

Pattern: Perfectionistic
PFLs: Work hard; don't fail; achieve; don't tolerate weakness or failure (in self or others).

Outcomes

People who are passive, dependent, or both and who do not like to make decisions or to lead are drawn to him. He irritates them, but he gives them the leadership, guidance, and strength they need and want. Aggressive, stronger personalities tend to not like working with or under him because the almost inevitable results are personality clashes and conflicts between them. His bosses value him because he gets the job done and does it well. His wife admires and "adores" him for his self-assertiveness and strength. His children resent his demands for perfection and often feel inferior because they cannot live up to them. He pushes them too hard to achieve. His friends admire his drive, but they do not like to work with him on boards or committees because he is hostile and domineering.

B. Pattern and PFLs

Pattern: Conservative; resistant to change
PFLs: The status quo is best; newness, difference, strangeness, and change are dangerous and will probably lead to trouble; deviations from the time-tested ways threaten the stability and order of life; don't rock the boat.

Outcomes

His employees try not to cross him because that means trouble. When someone has to suggest changes to Harry, he does so hesitantly and fearfully. Those above Harry respect his abilities, but his resistance to change makes them wary of promoting him any further or of putting him in a top management position even though he is an ace organizer. His family and friends try not to rock the boat but instead try to minimize changes or new ways. His son has rebelled against

Harry; consequently they are eternally fighting with each other. Harry does not approve of (and vocally expresses his disapproval of) young Mike's friends, some of whom are long-haired and different. Mostly Harry feels uncomfortable and angry when he considers the world around him, especially the young people in it. Mike's and Sally's friends therefore consider him overly conservative and avoid him whenever possible.

C. PATTERN AND PFLs

Pattern: Rigidly authoritarian; moralizing
PFLs: Always do your duty; always be upright, moral, and honest; everything is either right or wrong—there is no gray in-between; respect and obey authority; those who deviate from societal norms and conventions are contemptible.

OUTCOMES

Many people feel uncomfortable around Harry because they know he is critical and intolerant. His friends avoid talking about such subjects as civil rights, politics, religion, the women's liberation movement, young people, or foreign or domestic policy with him because they know he will hold forth at length in his intolerant and moralizing way. His wife Janice tends to be conservative in her actions—she does not drink or smoke to excess and she conforms to his wishes—so that she will not give her husband cause to criticize her. His children cringe when they make mistakes and hope he does not find out because they know he will immediately criticize them and start muttering about the younger generation. Their defense is to try to deceive him or to cover up their mistakes.

D. PATTERN AND PFLs

Pattern: Intellectual; antiemotional
PFLs: Always be logical and rational—that is the only way to deal with the chaos inherent in life; don't trust or fool with emotions—they will get you into trouble because they are chaotic.

OUTCOMES

Few people are eager or willing to tangle with Harry intellectually, since he can beat most people in any kind of intellectual argument. One quality that gives him an edge is that he argues on the basis of cold logic, not emotions. He seems to enjoy winning arguments and tends to act intellectually superior about his ability. This tendency turns a lot of people off. Either they feel inferior and inadequate or they get mad. However, if people want problems solved in a logical way, they often come to him even if they do not like his style.

JANICE — *Basic life-style:* Hysterical
Age: 41 — *Occupation:* Housewife; volunteer worker at local hospital
Race: White
Religion: Protestant

A. PATTERN AND PFLs

Pattern: Great difficulty being close; emotionally shallow
PFLs: If you show people what you really feel, they will hurt you or disapprove of you; don't concentrate on any one feeling for very long because it will overwhelm you.
Pattern: Stereotyping; idealizing but critical
PFLs: If you look too closely at another person, you will be very disappointed; ignore people's flaws and glorify their good points.

OUTCOMES

She leads an extremely limited kind of life. Although she is sociable and friendly with many people, she tends not to have any really close friends. She may think she is close to someone, but she is not able to be. Her stereotypes block her from seeing the other person as a person, and her friends get little notion of what she is really like. Therefore her relationships for the most part are rather shallow. People tend to sense this, and although many people like her, few people look to her for a close, meaningful relationship. She stereotypes her husband as "wonderful" and as her "Prince Charming"; at the same time, she feels much hostility toward him because he treats her with condescension and indifference. He takes her for granted. Since her stereotype prevents her from dealing directly with her hostility, she expresses it covertly by nagging and belittling him in subtle ways. She regards her children as she thinks they ought to be—as paragons of intelligence and virtue and talent. When they fail to live up to her expectations or when they express doubts about their abilities (something they have done less and less often as they began to realize how she feels), she cannot accept this and performs a kind of magic on their problems. She denies their existence, and for her the problems disappear.

Her husband, her children, and her friends do not try to share their deeper emotions with her; they know that her emotional responses will be shallow and superficial. Mike and Sally learned this lesson by the time each of them was about 10 or 12 years old. Sally especially experienced despair when she was younger because when Sally turned to her mother for emotional guidance and comfort, Janice failed her emotionally. Janice's discomfort about deep feelings makes others uncomfortable, so they look and go elsewhere when they want a strong and straight emotional response. Consequently Janice is always on the emotional fringes of life.

B. Pattern and PFLs

Pattern: Overdramatizer; crisis mentality
PFLs: Life is one long series of emergencies; always be prepared for the worst; life is full of trouble and can overwhelm you if you don't watch out.

Outcomes

Because she is a natural entertainer, Janice is often the life of the party, although friends who have known her for years are bored when they hear her tell the same stories over and over. Her tendency to see everything as a crisis makes her appear superficially as an exciting, because excited, person. But people tend to back away from her after a while because they sense a falseness in her crisis mentality. Strangers are frequently put off by her seeming insincerity. Her husband is proud of her socially, although his pride is tinged with condescension. Her children often write her off as a phony because so many things are such a big deal for her.

C. Pattern and PFLs

Pattern: Disorganized, illogical, and scatterbrained
PFLs: Men don't like smart, logical women; intellectual women are masculine; always trust your hunches; it is no fun to think things out ahead of time; life is confusing.

Outcomes

Because she is so disorganized and illogical, Harry considers her his intellectual inferior and does not even try any more to share with her ideas that are important to him. At the same time her scatterbrained quality makes him feel protective toward her. Mike shares his father's contempt for his mother's lack of intellectual sharpness; Sally mostly feels annoyed because she feels her mother perpetuates the stereotype of the stupid female. Her friends and casual acquaintances find her scatterbrained nature rather charming, but because she has so little actual content to give to conversations—mostly she just gives opinions—most people do not take her too seriously and she frequently feels out of touch with situations.

D. Pattern and PFLs

Pattern: Naive; innocent
PFLs: A woman shouldn't be interested in sex; a woman shouldn't know much about sex; most men don't like overly

sophisticated women; innocence equals purity and goodness; sex is dirty and bad.

Outcomes

Her naivete and innocence are two qualities that originally attracted Harry to Janice because he felt masterful, superior, and protective. Although he is still protective of her in social situations and likes the image of innocence that she projects to others (an image that fits well with his strong feelings of right and wrong), Harry is bothered by the results of her naivete and innocence. These two characteristics tend to mask a good deal of prudery and feelings of disgust about sex. In the early years of the marriage, Janice dutifully submitted to Harry's sexual advances (and sometimes in spite of herself enjoyed them), but gradually she withdrew behind a cloud of excuses. Now they rarely have sexual relations, and the act is a rather mechanical one.

In many ways, Mike and Sally have given up on Janice. They long ago learned that she was the last person to ask about sexual matters or about the ways of the world. Janice simply does not (or cannot let herself) know about such matters. Janice's friends are amused by her naivete; although some think it is a pose, by and large they just regard her as being out of touch with both the sexual and emotional facts of life. Since she actually is out of touch, she feels inadequate and falls back on her stereotypes and opinions. She avoids topics she feels naive about and thus limits her range of interests and conversation. If she cannot avoid them, she becomes uncomfortable and conveys that discomfort to others. Since they react by catching some of her discomfort, they tend to avoid these topics too.

The children

MIKE *Occupation:* College student (junior) majoring in political science

Age: 20

Because he was the first child and a male child, Mike received a great deal of attention from his father when he was growing up. Harry spent as much time with Mike as he could: he became an umpire for the Little League when Mike joined, and he became an assistant scout master when Mike went into the Boy Scouts. Because Mike was *his* son, Harry did not encourage others to take any major role in Mike's upbringing; in fact subconsciously Harry was jealous of others who might exert an influence on the boy. Therefore there were not many outside influences on Mike when he was growing up.

Although Janice naturally has an influence on Mike, Harry tended to negate much of her positive influence simply through his own attitudes toward her. Since Mike saw his father treat his mother with only slightly veiled contempt and condescension, Mike gradually learned (unconsciously and partly consciously) to devalue her as someone to listen to or to view with great respect. Thus Harry's style has been the one dominating Mike's life. Inevitably Mike's personality is much like his father's, but because Mike is not Harry and because Janice, Sally, a few peers, and a few teachers have exerted some influence on Mike, he is not as tightly locked into his father's personality style as is his father.

MIKE'S PERSONALITY

Mike has a strong sense of right and wrong, and he finds it difficult to see or allow any gray in between the black and white. Thus he frequently is critical in his judgments of his own and other people's actions. He is, for example, uptight about sexual matters. His PFL is that any girl who sleeps with a guy before she is married to him is bad or loose. Yet his peer culture says this is not necessarily so. Mike swings back and forth between the two sets of values;

occasionally he sleeps with one of the girls he takes out, but this causes him much conflict. He feels guilty, and also he tends to reject the girl and not date her again even if he is attracted to her.

Mike is basically a loner. He is a successful cross-country runner in college track. He has never been interested in team sports. He knows many people on the campus and comes across to them as a nice enough person. However, he has few close friends, and he finds it difficult to talk with them about anything that is emotionally important to them or him. He is vaguely aware that he is missing something in life; sometimes he feels cut off from other people, and he wonders uneasily why this is so. Occasionally he tries to understand how his friends feel, but he usually ends up acting impatient with them because he feels they bring most of their problems on themselves. Also he cannot understand why they cannot simply will themselves to get their work done on time, for example.

He himself is strong-willed and self-controlled. He stopped smoking because he could will it. His "better judgment" (his logical turn of mind) keeps him from taking drugs. He uses alcohol to relax, but he rarely drinks to excess.

Another trait of Mike's is that he is rather rigid and compulsive. He studies too much (and makes excellent grades), and he does not have much fun. It is almost as if he does not know how to have fun. He is extremely neat; his room, car, clothes, and everything he owns are always in order.

He is a perfectionist who is especially demanding of himself. Like his father, he has a tremendous inner drive that forever keeps him on the go. He cannot let himself be passive or inactive. If he rests or sleeps or plays or just takes time off, it is not long before he begins to get anxious, nervous, and restless. The only way he knows to quiet his anxiety is to work as hard as he can or else go out to the track and run a mile or two. (According to his PFLs, this kind of release from tension is acceptable because it fits the category of useful activities.) His perfectionism is the monkey on his back: he fights to get the highest grades; he fights to win every race; and he finds it extremely difficult, almost impossible, to accept a position of second best. If he does fall short, that is a signal to him to work even harder. When he succeeds, however, he has trouble enjoying his success for any length of time or with any kind of deeply rewarding emotional satisfaction. It is as if each success is simply a demand for him to seek and conquer another obstacle.

MIKE'S HERE AND NOW

Mike is glad to be away at college, since now he does not have to hear his father's constant lectures on getting ahead and making something of himself. Mike feels that he has made an almost complete break with his father. Although he writes home faithfully once every 2 weeks, he feels as though he has cut loose from the family and can go his own way.

Mike's rebellion against his father is just about complete. He is now a pacifist, and he despises his father's militaristic stand on United States foreign policy. (Harry thought we should have dropped atomic bombs on North Viet Nam years ago, and he believes the federal government is "soft" on Communists.) After college, Mike would like to work with underprivileged children.

On the surface, Mike and his father seem radically different from each other. Mike rejects Harry's values of being materially successful, making money, and getting ahead. They obviously disagree violently on political matters.

Whenever Harry and Mike are together, they quarrel. Harry is forever referring to Mike's friends as "weirdoes" and Communist-inspired. Mike defends his long-haired, barefooted, bearded friends and tells his father he is intolerant. What Mike cannot admit and what Harry probably would not believe is that Mike has to force himself to be tolerant of the more extreme people he knows because Mike has trouble handling that which is new or different to him.

Although Mike is pleased that he is free

now that he is in college and not around his family often, especially his father, Mike is bothered by a vague and fuzzy feeling that this freedom is not as good as he thought it would be. For example, Mike thought that once his father was off his back, he would not feel so pressured to achieve. However, the pressure is still there, just as real and demanding as it ever was. Although Mike is glad to be out and away from his home environment, he is puzzled at the lack of satisfaction in his newfound freedom.

Why is Mike's freedom not satisfying to him? Because he is not free. Mike is not likely to be free of his family's and especially his father's influence until he realizes that his father (i.e., his father's attitudes toward himself and toward Mike, his father's patterns, and his father's PFLs) is built into him. In essence, Mike carries his father around inside of him. Until Mike becomes conscious of this, he cannot realize how strongly his father influences so much of what Mike thinks, feels, and does.

If someone were to ask Mike if he is like his father, he might answer, "Yes, in some ways, I am." How? Mike might point out that like his father he is independent, hard working, strong-willed, and somewhat perfectionistic. However, he would probably also protest that in matters that really count, he is different from his father. Harry is conservative, militaristic, intolerant, and "square," whereas Mike sees himself as liberal, pacifistic, tolerant, and generally "with it." How different can you be?

Mike is measuring and comparing his father and himself by the surface. However, although their activities, their outlooks, and some of their values and feelings are different, they both have similar life-styles. Mike's life-style may be a little less tight (constricting) than Harry's, but essentially it is the same style.

It is to Mike's credit that he had the guts and the drive to rebel and to challenge his father's positions. But at this point in his life, Mike is nevertheless in many ways merely the flip side of Harry. Harry holds blindly and stubbornly to his conservative political beliefs. Mike has liberal beliefs, but he holds to them just as blindly and stubbornly. Both are committed to their beliefs; both will hold onto those beliefs to the bitter end. Harry has always been goaded by his own inner drive to achieve perfection; he channeled that tremendous drive into his work and became a success in business. Mike has channeled his own inner drive for perfection and achievement into his schoolwork, into his athletic activities, and now into pacifism.

This does not mean that Mike is a mindless robot or a carbon copy of his father. However, Mike is operating in essentially the same way as his father. At this point, Mike's autonomy resides in *what* he applies the style to, not in the *way* he operates. One major problem is that Mike is unaware of the tremendous similarities between his father's and his own styles.

MIKE'S CHILD/PARENT/ADULT BALANCE

In terms of Child/Parent/Adult balance (pp. 99 to 101), Mike's personality is clearly dominated by the Parent (almost all of it from Harry) built into him. The Child in Mike has long since yielded to the dominance and control of the Parent. Mike's Child—his spontaneity, his direct emotional responses, his desire to explore new and strange territories, his desire to be free of restrictions, his urge to mess around in mud puddles (i.e., to be happily disorganized), and his creativity—all these qualities (which belong to everyone's Child) have been and are stifled, cramped, organized, blocked out, or stomped on by Mike's strict, hostile, unyielding, and unforgiving Parent.

Much the same situation has happened to Mike's Adult. The Parent has in effect forbidden his Adult to develop (don't explore; don't question my rules or values; do what I tell you to do; my style of life is best for you). Even in the face of such hostile forces, however, Mike's Child has survived, and he does have an Adult part. His Adult is nurtured fortunately by his own uniqueness: although he is like his father, Mike is *not* his father. Even though he has his father's styles, at least Mike has applied them in some degree to other ways of seeing life. Hopefully, with knowledge, understanding, and know-how, Mike will be able to strengthen and enlarge his Adult to the point where it will be able to promote a healthy balance between his Parent and Child and to the point where the Adult will function with autonomy and freedom.

• • •

SALLY *Occupation:* High school student (junior)

Age: 16

Since Mike's life-style and personality are more rigid than Sally's, they are more clear cut and easier to identify. Therefore we have purposely described and analyzed Mike more fully than we will Sally because he better served our purpose of teaching about the transmission of the Parent part.

A primary reason Sally is not as clear cut as Mike is that her full personality is still forming. Her life-style and her personality are not so tightly locked into the family system either; consequently she is a freer and more flexible person. The next five to ten years will be a crucial period in her life, since it will be a time of transition and new experiences (college among them). How she blends the various life-styles she has seen in her parents and others and how she manages her experiences will have much to do with whether she can fulfill her potential for growth toward emotional maturity.

Her chances for growth and development into a mature, autonomous adult, however, are good. Although she has her difficulties and problems, she has a good self-concept, she has good ego strength, she is mature for her age, and she has both the capacity and the motivation for emotional growth.

Why is Sally—child of the same parents as Mike—so different from Mike? One important reason is her position as the second child in the family. As the first child, Mike bore the brunt of his parents' apprehensions and anxieties about their new and unaccustomed role of parents. By the time Sally arrived on the scene, Harry and Janice had gotten used to being parents and were able to relax and be less anxious or fussy. Thus their attitude toward Sally started out and has continued to be a more casual and relaxed one. Another effect of Sally's second child position is that, coming after Mike who is so strong-willed and at times rebellious, she inherited the freedoms he had to fight for. Thus as a young child, she was able to go to bed later because Mike had fought to gain that privilege for himself. In effect, Mike helped to clear the path for Sally by breaking down some of the restrictions his parents had applied to him.

Another extremely important reason for the difference is that she is a girl. Harry tends to demand a lot from his *son,* but because Sally is a girl, Harry does not expect or demand as much from her. Although Harry puts a high premium on her intellectual achievement, he does not demand the same levels of performance. This is, of course, a male chauvinist attitude, but it has protected Sally from her father's perfectionistic demands and allowed her greater freedom to grow. Also, because Sally is not a male, Harry is able to relax more with her and be softer toward her; he does not perceive her as a potential competitor. Another effect of her being a girl is that she naturally spends more time with her mother who is not a demanding person. Janice's flighty nature and her disorganization can be irritating, but they do not make Sally feel inadequate. One other positive effect of being a girl is that the whole culture allows and tacitly encourages her to have feelings. Although there is a price attached to being a woman in this culture ("she's only a female"), there is also a distinct advantage; women are allowed to feel and to express their emotions with a freedom that is traditionally denied to men.

Another major reason Sally is different from Mike is that she has had the benefit of knowing, spending time with, and being accepted by the Thompsons, the parents of her best friend. Mr. and Mrs. Thompson have a basically solid, warm, and affectionate relationship both with each other and with their children. In this home there is love, companionship, respect, and acceptance of others as unique individuals. Sally has known this open family for eight of her sixteen years; she ordinarily spends at least an afternoon or evening a week at their house (usually more) and has been strongly influenced by her experience with this family. The Thompsons provide other adult models for Sally; thus she has more alternatives from which to draw as she shapes her own personality and life-style. She has access to something Mike does not—a happy family atmosphere.

SALLY'S PERSONALITY

What is Sally like, and how did she get to be this way? Basically she is the steadiest and most well balanced member of the Johnson family. The overall reason for this is that she has been able to take the best that each parent has to give and to avoid the more negative patterns they employ. One strong influence that enabled Sally to do this was the supportive atmosphere she found in the Thompson home. Also Sally's own uniqueness—made up in part of her position as the second child and her role of female—has helped her to adopt the more positive features of her family background and dynamics and to slough off the more negative aspects.

One of Sally's traits is that she does her work and does it well (like her father and Mike), but unlike Harry and Mike she enjoys her work and her achievements. Essentially what she has done is to copy Harry's work patterns (concentration, logic, energy, drive, organization). Although she rejected Janice's disorganization, she did adopt her mother's PFL that work isn't everything. Thus Sally takes a far less serious view of work and feels that people should gain feelings of satisfaction and even fun from doing a job well. Part of this more positive attitude rubbed off on her from the Thompsons. Both Nancy and Paul Thompson approach work with a certain zest and delight. He enjoys his job as an architect; Nancy enjoys running a lively household and working part-time as a high school guidance counselor. Both of them are creative people; frequently, they go antique hunting, and the whole family spends time together refinishing their treasures.

Another of Sally's traits is her ability to feel things deeply but within a rational context. Here again she is a mixture of the best of her parents plus some of the Thompsons. Sally picked up her mother's quick emotional responses to situations, but she learned about sustained and deep emotional responses from Mr. and Mrs. Thompson, who are able to feel deeply about life. Sally gained the rational context from her father (and the Thompsons). Sally is a sensitive, aware, alive person who listens, sees, and feels with a good deal of perception and caring. But she is not all seriousness. She is the fun person in the Johnson family. She has some influence with each person in the family. For example, she tends to tease her father and try to get him to loosen up. She also tends to not take him as seriously as most other people do. As a result, Sally is one of the few people he feels comfortable with. He can even let himself go enough to be a little bit kooky with her.

Another quality characterizing Sally is the way in which she manages her sexual role. When Sally was about 13 years old, she consciously rejected the naivete she perceived in her mother because she felt it was phony and because she already had sensed her father's contempt and condescending protectiveness toward her mother's naivete. Since Sally could not turn to her mother for any direct information about sexual matters and questions, she had to go elsewhere. Fortunately, her junior high and high school provided excellent sex education courses taught by mature and well-trained teachers. In addition, Sally's best friend, Barbara Thompson, has acquired from her parents healthy attitudes toward sex, attitudes that she shares freely with Sally.

Although Sally rejects her mother's naiveté about sexual matters, she has a certain admiration for her mother as a social success. She sees her mother move with pleasure and a good deal of grace in social situations: her mother is able to talk with guests, give smoothly operating parties, and be extremely entertaining. Furthermore, her mother knows how to dress to good advantage, and she is a good-looking woman. Therefore Sally has copied her mother's social and feminine style to some extent, especially because this is one quality about her mother that her father seems to admire. To a fair degree then Sally tends to copy the way her mother dresses, talks, and acts. However, Sally does not have just her own mother as a social and feminine model; she also has Barbara's mother, whom she also admires. To the group of qualities that Sally can copy, Nancy Thompson adds warmth, sincerity, grace, gentleness, dignity, and strength.

At 16 years of age, Sally is still in the process of fully realizing her sexual identity, but she is well on her basically healthy way. She is fairly realistic about her role as a woman: she is a supporter of the women's liberation movement, but she is not a fanatic. She recognizes that women have been put down by this culture in many ways, but she also sees and appreciates the advantages of being a woman—one of them being the freedom to feel and to express emotions. Her relationships with others tend to reflect this same sort of levelheaded and open approach to life: she has many friends, both boys and girls. She dates some but is not at this point going steady with any one boy; if she were to find someone, she would be only too happy to go steady with him. All this is not to say that Sally does not have her doubts and her problems and her worries, but by and large she feels basically adequate and happy as a young woman.

SALLY'S CHILD/PARENT/ADULT BALANCE

Sally's Child is much larger than Mike's because she did not receive the same restrictive attention from her father and because she did not have to live up to the demands of perfection and all the rules and values that go with it. Sally is freer than Mike to express her basic and direct emotions: her Child is more accessible to her and is freer to operate. Her Parent is smaller than Mike's because although she has built in many qualities from her parents and other adult models, these qualities are not as restrictive as those that Mike took. Her Parent is in better balance with her Child; they tend to complement each other rather than exist in a slave/master relationship. Her Adult is fairly strong; she is used to making autonomous choices about what she will copy and what she will reject. Her Adult part will likely continue to grow stronger as she gains more like experiences.

This construction and analysis of the Johnson family is detailed and thorough. However, this kind of thoroughness is necessary to really understand how and why a family functions as it does and how and why the children in a family get to be who they are.

appendix B

WAYS OF WORKING CONSTRUCTIVELY WITH DISTORTED COMMUNICATION AND INTERACTION

Communication and interaction are delicate and complex processes. We have, however, intentionally simplified our examples of these processes; thus there are many more things going on in and influencing the communication than we take into account. We have deliberately chosen to ignore many of these subtleties and intricacies to avoid confusion and to gain clarity. In effect, we present stripped-down examples so that we can highlight particular problems and solutions.

We treat each example of distorted communication and interaction in the following ways:

1. The situation existing between the two people is described.
2. The verbal messages and signals that each person sends are given.
3. A running account of at least one person's inside operations (what he is thinking and feeling but not necessarily reporting) is presented. In a sense, these are metamessages.
4. Analyses and explanations of what is contaminating or blocking clear communication are given.
5. Suggestions are made about how these problems might be more constructively handled.

To avoid breaking the flow of dialogue any more than necessary, we have used parentheses and brackets to designate three specific kinds of occurrences: parentheses enclose descriptions of *signals,* brackets enclose *inside operations*—what a person is thinking and feeling inside, and double parentheses enclose our explanations of *what is going on.*

EXAMPLE 1

Situation

The wife, Ellen, has accepted an invitation from another couple, Sarah and Josh, to come for cocktails next Saturday. Ellen's husband Morris has just gotten home from the office, and she is telling him about their social commitment.

Ellen: Morris—(Smiles brightly but a little hesitantly.) Sarah called today and asked us for cocktails on Saturday. At five.

Morris (Absentmindedly and only half-listening; he is looking at the paper): Um. (Pause—as the message gets through.) You turned them down, of course.

Ellen (Frowns; looks nervous. Starts rearranging the magazines on the coffee table.) ["Oh, Lord—he's angry. What have I done *now*?"]: Why, no. I accepted. I thought you'd enjoy it.

Morris (Gives her a dirty look. Throws down the newspaper.) ["Can't you keep *anything* straight in your head? You always manage to louse up my weekends with stupid social engagements."]: You thought I'd *enjoy* it! You know perfectly well I can't stand Sarah. She's such an idiot. All she can do is blather on about nothing or else cut everybody to pieces. Besides, I'm going fishing on Saturday and I'm damn well not going to put myself out for them so I can be there at five.

Ellen (Cringes. Is close to tears.) ["I've done it again. But why can't we ever do what *I* want to do? Why does it always have to be *his* weekend—not mine?"]: You never told me you didn't like Sarah. And I didn't know you were going to go fishing. Why don't you ever tell me anything? (Now she is facing him with her fists clenched and her jaw set.)

Analysis and explanation

This argument could go on and on, getting more heated and angry as it progressed. The argument (at least its shape if not its specific content) is one which probably is familiar to both of them. But when Ellen and Morris simmer down or cool off all together, neither is likely to know exactly what went wrong or why it went wrong. If that is so, then sadly enough, this same kind of argument is almost bound to repeat itself again and again, since neither of them is aware of the dynamics of their communication and interaction. They just argue when the occasion arises.

What are the dynamics? What did happen and why? How could Ellen and Morris have handled the situation more constructively?

1. Ellen makes an assumption, does not check it out with Morris, and acts on her assumption that Morris would want to and would be willing to go. She also makes a decision without consulting him, which leaves him no really workable alternatives.

2. Morris makes the assumption that Ellen refused the invitation. When he learns that his assumption was incorrect, he is furious.

3. He reports another assumption to Ellen—that she *knows* he cannot stand Sarah and that she knows why he cannot. However, Morris does not report all of his feelings, and the ones he fails to report are the feelings that lie at the heart of all their arguments of this type. He feels Ellen is stupid ["Can't you keep anything straight in your head?"], and he feels that she deliberately thwarts him by lousing up his weekends.

4. Ellen gets defensive and claims Morris never told her about his feelings toward Sarah or about his fishing trip. Then she drops the whole matter back into a long-standing pattern of disagreement between Morris and her ["You never tell me anything . . ."]. But Ellen also is not reporting all of her true feelings.

5. Three basic flaws become clear from this interchange:

   a. Each person makes assumptions without checking them out or getting any feedback.

   b. Each person reports only *selected* feelings; thus neither Ellen nor Morris has enough to work with to communicate clearly. Neither has much knowledge of what is going on inside the other. Therefore they cannot possibly deal with the real feelings running beneath the immediate argument, and they cannot negotiate any kind of workable settlement because neither is sharing his insides with the other.

   c. Ellen and Morris assume they are arguing about a situation and the immediate feelings aroused by that situation. In actuality, they are really fighting on the basis of long-standing, deep-seated, and unresolved feelings that do not have much to do with the immediate situation. They are *patterned* to fight this way.

Suggestions

Although Ellen's and Morris' relationship and feelings are complex, tangled, and not simple to deal with, there are certain constructive measures each of them could take that might help them communicate better and come to understand each other better. What we suggest here are not cure-alls. One or both of them may not be able to implement the following suggestions; they may not want to. These are, however, more effective ways for each of them to act, and if they try to use these other ways, their relationship may improve.

1. Both should try to avoid assuming that they know what the other person feels. Instead they should check out and listen to the feedback.

2. Each should try to report as honestly and as fully as he can what he really feels.

3. Each should try to look beyond the immediate situation to the feelings and attitudes that have been aroused by the present situation.

EXAMPLE 2

Situation

Maria and Ricardo have been married for about two years. He consistently works late at the plant at least three nights a week. Frequently, he calls around dinner time and says he cannot make it home and that she should go ahead and eat without him. This is the fourth night in a row that he has called this week. He arrives home around 10:30, tired and irritable. Incidentally there is no "other woman" involved; there is just Ricardo's work.

Ricardo: Hi, honey. Boy, I'm really bushed. (Sinks into the nearest armchair.) How was your day?

Maria (Glares at him but says nothing. Walks out of the room.)

Ricardo (Looks startled and annoyed. Gets up and follows her into the other room.): What's the matter? Aren't you going to speak to me? [Now he is getting angry.]

Maria (Turns on him and curls her lip. Is shaking.): What's the matter? How can you stand there and ask me that?

Ricardo (Stares at her, frowns, and then paces around the room.) ["What the devil is wrong with her? All I did was ask her what the matter was."]: I don't understand.

Maria: I'll tell you what's the matter! (Bursts into tears.) You don't love me—that's what's the matter. All you ever do is work, work, work. You don't care about me; all you care about is your precious work!

Ricardo (Totally puzzled now.) ["Oh, my God—what do I do now?"]: But—but—honey. I *do* love you. The reason I work so hard is that I want to be a good provider. I want to buy you the things you want. I want to make you happy. (Begins to get angry; speaks coldly.) But obviously you don't care what I do or how hard I work; nothing seems to satisfy you. I'm only trying to take care of you the best way I can, and you don't even care. How do you think *I* feel, working my tail off at a job I hate?

Analysis and explanation

It would not take much to escalate this situation into full-scale battle. Although Maria's and Ricardo's relationship (as is true of the relationship in example 1) is a complex and long-term one built up over a period of time, it is possible to sort out the key features of this particular exchange. Although these features have been building up a long time, *now* rather than five years hence is the time for them to deal with their problems of communication and interaction.

Whatever other factors are contributing to the problem between Maria and Ricardo, the crux of this fight is that apparently neither Maria nor Ricardo ever had any clear idea of what the other's expectations for the marital relationship were. Apparently they also never have discussed their individual expectations and desires about the relationship—at least not insofar as they relate to the connection between his work and his and her emotional needs.

To the objective, impartial observer it is fairly easy to see the gap between what each of them wants and needs. Maria wants and needs to have Ricardo with her more, and she wants reassurance that she is more important to him than his work. Ricardo, on the other hand, needs and wants Maria to view him as all-important and satisfactory in his role as her provider and protector. His feeling is probably strongly tied to what he views as the man's role in this society. So he has sacrificed what he wants to do (in his choice of work) to fulfill the role he views as essential to his good relationship with Maria. What is happening instead is that neither partner is getting what he or she wants or needs.

Suggestions

Although many other factors are operating in this relationship and even in this particular aspect of the relationship, it is obvious what has gone wrong here. Although Maria and Ricardo have to discuss many other matters, where they can constructively start is clear. At this point, the most practical measure they could take would be to stop dead for a moment and then start communicating with each other about their inside feelings. For example, if this argument continues along the same lines, Maria might next say sarcastically, "Well, you never could have proved it by me that you hated your job. Looked to me like you'd married it instead of me." However, suppose instead she stops in her tracks, takes a deep breath, and replies in another way—a different and unexpected way (unexpected by both her and Ricardo).

Maria (Looks anxious but determined.): Ricardo, wait. I-I-I don't exactly know how to say this. I don't even exactly know what I want to say. Will you stay with me while I try something different? ((She checks him out.))

Ricardo [Has been taken off guard. Is puzzled, still annoyed, but interested.]: Yeah. Why not? Yeah—go ahead. ((Some feedback.))

Maria: Well, I think it would be a good thing if we could both try to hold our tempers and maybe try to talk about—about what we've just been fighting about. Are you willing to try it?

Ricardo [Is now intrigued but not fully convinced.]: Yeah. Okay. But I don't know as I really understand what you're up to. But go ahead. I mean, what have we got to lose?

Maria: Ricardo, I honestly didn't know you hated your job. (He looks angry and disbelieving. He starts to protest.) Ricardo, please wait. Just let me say a couple of things and then you can have the floor. Okay? (He nods agreement; looks resigned.) Look—I'm sorry I burst out at you like that, but everything just suddenly got to me. And what I'm saying is *not* to blame you. Now I begin to see what's been happening. When we got married, I had visions of your coming home every night at the same time, like my father always did, and I'd have dinner all ready and flowers on the table, and I'd be dressed up and kiss you at the door. Oh, you know—a kind of romantic picture of married life. But as the weeks and months went on and you kept calling and saying you'd be late or you'd grab a bite on the way home, my dream began to crumble. For a while I thought there might be another woman, but I didn't really much believe that. And slowly I just got to thinking that all you cared about was getting ahead and making money. And that I came second.

Ricardo (In wonderment): And all that time I kept thinking you were dissatisfied because I wasn't getting ahead fast enough, and so I worked all the harder. Oh, my God, Maria—how crazy can two people be?

But they are not crazy, and they are not stupid. Maria and Ricardo are just two human beings who did not communicate well with each other. What happened to them is inevitable if you recognize that here are two people with different expectations, life-styles, and roles who enter into a relationship but do not communicate with each other to any significant or effective degree about those expectations or much of anything else. We are not saying that all of life's (or of a relationship's) problems and misunderstandings can be cleared up so quickly or so easily. What we are saying is that people can learn to communicate with each other, that people can learn to deal much more effectively with themselves and others, that people can grow toward emotional maturity, and that people can learn how to grow. Finally and most importantly we are saying that honest, open, clear communication is the key to that growth.

EXAMPLE 3

Situation

Carol and Geraldine are college juniors. They live in the same dormitory, two doors down from each other. They have known each other for about three months. They have occasionally discussed such matters as trust, freedom, responsibility, honesty, patriotism, and other similar ideals. During one of these conversations, they agreed that each of them believes in honesty in human relationships. At the moment, Carol has just come back to the dorm from a shopping trip downtown, and she is modeling her new dress for Geraldine.

Carol (Flushed; excited.): Well, How do I look? How do you like it?

Geraldine (Looks uncomfortable. Stares at the floor, shifts her feet, and nibbles at a fingernail.): Well. Um—to be absolutely honest about it—um—I think it makes you look kind of chunky. I mean, it kind of makes your hips look bigger than they are.

Carol (Gets red in the face; her lips tighten into a thin line.) ["Well, you so-and-so. And I thought you were my friend!"]: Well, that's a crummy thing to say. What kind of thing is that to say to a friend?

Geraldine (Looks confused and sort of frightened; frowns.): But—I thought—I mean—well, I thought you agreed. I mean, didn't we agree that honesty was really important in human relationships?

Carol (Huffily): Of course we did. But I should think you'd be able to tell the difference between honesty and cruelty! (Stalks out of the room.)

Analysis and explanation

Words like honesty, love, trust, freedom, responsibility, patriotism, communism, and democracy, are emotionally loaded terms and have many different meanings to different people at different times. Fundamentally Carol and Geraldine never really communicated clearly or thoroughly about the emotional possibilities represented by the simple word "honesty." Although it is probably never possible to cover all the potential shadings of meaning a word may have or take on and although it is not possible to foresee what a person's particular feelings may be at a given time, it is possible to do some checking out of the other person's feelings before sailing into the verbal arena and letting go with an emotional broadside. Perhaps the best rule of thumb here is as follows: thoroughly check out people's definitions, do not rely too heavily on prior definitions, and check out your own and the other person's feelings before you act on the definitions.

EXAMPLE 4

Situation

Dave and Karen have known each other for about a year and have dated each other occasionally during that time. He is a senior and she a junior in high school. He is asking her for a date.

Dave: Hey, Karen. There's a great horror movie playing downtown. You want to go Friday night? [He is excited about the movie and is looking forward to having a date with Karen.]

Karen (Her face expresses nothing.): Oh—okay. What time do you want to go?

Dave [Disappointed.]: Seven-thirty. But, gee, Karen—you don't sound very excited about it. Do you want to do something else instead?

Karen (Her voice is flat, except for a slight tinge of annoyance.): No—no. The movies are fine. Anything you want to do.

Dave [He feels vaguely uncomfortable but does not know why.]: Okay. I'll pick you up at seven.

Analysis and explanation

The probable reason Dave feels uncomfortable is that he has no way of knowing whether Karen really wants to go to the movies. She says the movies are fine with her (although without much conviction), but she also says that she will do whatever he wants to do. That puts the burden of decision on him. He must decide without any emotional help from her (i.e., he has little knowledge of how she really feels about the whole matter).

Suggestions

Dave has already tried to find out if there is something else Karen would rather do ((both an informational and emotional question)), and she has given him feedback that does not sound convincing. Also her feedback (if you can call it that) avoids revealing anything that she may be feeling about herself, about Dave, or about the situation. Dave can just let it all go by (as he does in the example), or he can get mad and tell her, "That's what you always say. Why do I have to make all the decisions?" Or he can try to find out what is behind Karen's avoidance. If he tries to do that, he might act in the following way:

Dave: You know, Karen, you often react to things I suggest by saying you'll do whatever I want to do. For a while I was kind of flattered by that. But then I got to feeling sort of edgy when you'd say it. I'm not exactly sure why—but I think it's because it kind of dumps all the decisions on me. And I'm never sure what you really want to do or what you really enjoy. ((He is reporting his "insides" here.))

Karen: But, Dave. I really don't care what we do. I mean—I enjoy doing whatever you decide we should do. ((She denies having much feeling about the matter; which fits her style.))

Dave: Well—okay. But could you try looking at it from my point of view? I mean, how I feel when you always agree? ((His "okay" indicates his acceptance of her denial, but he now swings the communication back to his feelings. If he can't get at *her* feelings, he may be able to get her to consider *his* feelings, which he already has access to.))

Karen: Yeah, we can do that, if you want to. ((True to her style, she throws the ball right back to him.))

Dave: Well—but—I feel uncomfortable, for one thing. It's like I always have to run the show and I never can tell if what I decide we should do is what you really want to do. ((Now he is identifying a feeling position.)) So sometimes I think you're just putting up with me and my suggestions because you can't think of anything better to do. Do you see what I mean? And I don't mean all this as an attack; I'm simply trying to tell you what I feel. ((He elaborates on his feelings and suggests that she may be feeling passive. Then he starts to check out but veers off for a moment to reassure her.))

Karen: I—I—think I sort of see what you mean. I never looked at it that way. I've just always felt that you're smarter than I am and that you should make the decisions.

Now hopefully they are on their way to communicating about what goes on between the two of them. Their communication may bring them closer together, or it may help both (or one of them) decide that the relationship is not what they want. Whatever happens, however, at least if they communicate with each other, they have a chance to get in touch with what each of them really feels, a much better chance than they would have if they just go along as they have gone along all year.

EXAMPLE 5

Situation

Ralph and Greg are college roommates. They have known each other for one and one half years and are fairly close friends. Greg has just come into the room. It is about 11:30 p.m. His girlfriend has just told him she wants to break off their relationship and that she is interested in another person.

Ralph: Hi. Where ya been?

Greg (Scowls.) ["None of your business."]: What? Oh, I've been at Tony's (one of the local gathering places—a pizza and beer place).

Ralph: Didya have a good time?

Greg: Yeah. It was okay. ["She can't treat me that way. How could she have been dating him all this time without my knowing it?"] Yeah—fine. (Sarcastically.)

Ralph (Hesitates for a moment, looks puzzled.): You don't look or sound like everything was fine. Is anything wrong?

Greg (Speaks sharply and angrily.): I just *said* everything's fine, didn't I? (Looks unhappy and angry but does not turn away from Ralph.)

Ralph: You look awful miserable for somebody who's just had a fine time. Are you sure you're okay?

Greg (Snarls at Ralph.): How many times do I have to tell you I'm fine? You stupid or something? Get off my back, will you? (Greg stomps out of the room; Ralph throws his book down on the bed.)

Analysis and explanation

It is possible to argue that Ralph is insensitive; it is also possible and more probable to argue that he is concerned but does not know how to handle the situation. It is a miserable one for both Ralph and Greg: Greg is saying one thing but is sending off contradictory signals and messages. He *says* everything is fine; nonverbally he conveys intense anger. Ralph, of course, has no way of knowing what the anger is about, and as long as they communicate in this manner, Ralph will not be able to find out. Instead he probably seems to Greg to be prying or needling him. What happened (as frequently happens in situations like this one) is the following: Greg's anger is *appropriately* directed toward the girl who has rejected him and who has dated another person behind his back. However, by the time they are halfway through their interchange, Greg has *inappropriately* turned his anger on Ralph.

The obvious reason for the breakdown in communication is that Greg simply does not want to talk about what has just happened or what he is feeling. That, of course, is his prerogative. Probably the major reason Ralph pursues his attempts to get through to Greg is his concern for his roommate. Besides, it is not all that easy to pretend that nothing has happened when a tornado enters the room. The ultimate problem is that Greg completely denies the existence of any problem at all.

Suggestions

The simplest and probably the most effective way to deal with the situation would be for Ralph to ask Greg if anything is wrong. If Greg denies that there is anything wrong (as he does in the example), then Ralph could proceed as follows:

Ralph: Look, Greg, I'm not trying to pry and I don't want to force a conversation on you. But even though you say everything's okay, you act like the world's fallen apart. I'm concerned about you, so just let me ask you this—do you want to talk about whatever it is? Do you want me just to say nothing? Do you want to talk about the weather? Or would you like me to go off and study somewhere else for a while so you can be alone?

Just what and how Greg answers is up to him. But Ralph has probably defused things enough so that Greg can give him some kind of answer without entering into major hostilities. Ralph has made that possible by doing the following:

1. He has clearly stated his own position—that he does not want to force the issue and that he is concerned.

2. He has distinctly identified the credibility gap between Greg's denials and his nonverbal signals and messages, but Ralph has done so without blaming Greg.

3. Ralph has offered Greg four different alternatives from which he can choose. In addition, by saying what he says and by

saying it without harshness or anger, Ralph has implemented his concern for Greg and has set a tone of friendliness rather than hostility.

Greg may choose to be alone and may decide never to talk to Ralph about what has happened; technically that could be adjudged noncommunication. But there are many times when *not* talking about certain subjects or when giving someone the option to be alone or not communicate are the most constructive ways of acting.

Good communication does not result from using force or deceit or from pushing too hard. Part of what enables good communication to exist and flourish between people is a sense of freedom and a feeling that one's inner privacy will not be violated. In this case, the suggested way for Ralph to act certainly shows more promise for a constructive resolution than does the fight of the original example.

EXAMPLE 6

Situation

Matt is a junior in high school. Although he is fairly bright, he tends to not study much and to slide by whenever he can. In this instance, he did not make it: he took and failed a history test. He has gone to his teacher, Mr. Gilman, to complain that he does not think he deserved to fail.

Matt (Shifts from one foot to the other, looks everywhere but directly at Mr. Gilman and chews at his lip.): Mr. Gilman, sir—ah—I'd like to talk to you about something. That is if you have time, sir.

Mr. Gilman: Sure, Matt. Is it about the test?

Matt (Looks startled.): Y-yes.

Mr. Gilman (His tone is friendly.): What can I do for you?

Matt: Well, sir. Ah—you—that is—I don't think I deserved to fail it.

Mr. Gilman: Was there a mistake in my adding up the points?

Matt: No, sir.

Mr. Gilman: Do you feel that I graded you unfairly?

Matt: Well—not exactly. What I mean is—I think I knew more than you gave me credit for.

Mr. Gilman: But, Matt, I gave you credit for every, what I call, "significant contribution." See—here in the margin. That's what those check marks are for.

Matt: Yeah, I know your system, Mr. Gilman. But I still don't think I should have failed.

Mr. Gilman (He looks directly at Matt who in turn looks directly at the floor.): Matt, how long did you study for this test?

Matt (His voice is somewhat muffled because his head is down.): Pretty long.

Mr. Gilman: Matt, how long is "pretty long"?

Matt: Well, long enough, I thought. I studied as long as Stan Gellerman did.

Mr. Gilman (Patiently): How long did Stanley study?

Matt: Well, I don't know—but a long time.

Analysis and explanation

This conversation is obviously beginning to go around in circles. Where it goes from here will depend almost totally on what Mr. Gilman says and does, since Matt is obviously not going to direct it into honest channels.

Mr. Gilman has asked straight questions to get both information and feelings from Matt. He has checked out (or has tried to check out) exactly what Matt is objecting to. But when Mr. Gilman approaches the heart of the matter—how long Matt studied for the test—Matt gives Mr. Gilman an informational runaround. In fancier terms, Mike's responses may be called "defensive avoidance." As long as Matt responds that way, he will of necessity be dishonest. With that, any real communication stops.

Suggestions

If we look at this exchange from Matt's point of view, our suggestion would have to be either try to be honest or do not bother. If we approach the exchange from Mr. Gilman's point of view, there are various possibilities. Mr. Gilman can simply end the conversation by saying he is sorry Matt is disappointed with the grade but that he (Mr. Gilman) still feels it is a fair grade. If he feels, however, that Matt used the test to come to him to talk about something else or that Matt's evasive pattern should be challenged or interrupted, then Mr. Gilman can at least try to develop some honest communication between them. Suppose that instead of just closing down the conversation, Mr. Gilman intervenes in Matt's defensive avoidance pattern.

Mr. Gilman: Look, Matt. We could keep going around and around like this. But we wouldn't get anywhere. (His tone is friendly and concerned.) At this point, I'm not really particularly concerned about how long you did or didn't study for the test. I assume from your rather evasive answers that you didn't study very long for it. Did you study more than two or three hours?

Matt (Shrugs his shoulders; speaks in a sullen voice.): Well, we had team practice the week of the test—and my little brother was sick—and—

Mr. Gilman: Matt! Wait a minute, will you? I'm not challenging you. And I'm sorry if that's the way my comments came across to you. (His tone is reassuring and noncensuring.) What I find is that you keep avoiding answering me. I don't care what the real answer is. What I do care about is that you're either so afraid of me or of the truth or of I don't know what that you can't seem to give me a straight answer. Are you aware of that?

Matt (Pauses. Looks at the floor.): Yes, sir. I am. (He now looks directly at Mr. Gilman; Matt seems slightly relieved.)

Mr. Gilman: Is there something else on your mind? Something other than the test that you want to talk about? Or do you want to let it go?

Where this communication goes from here is now up to *both* Matt and Mr. Gilman. Mr. Gilman has managed to clear the air enough for Matt and to convey enough reassurance to him that Matt is now freer to be honest. Matt may choose to drop the whole matter, or he may choose to open up and share whatever is bugging him with Mr. Gilman.

Notice the ways Mr. Gilman has set up the possibilities for fuller and freer communication:

1. He is honest.
2. He checks out.
3. He reports what he feels (what he does and does not care about).
4. He reassures ("I'm not challenging you.").
5. He gives Matt alternatives ("Do you want to talk or do you want to let it go?").

You can argue (and you may feel) that since Mr. Gilman is a teacher and an adult he *ought* to know how to do what he has just done. But, sadly enough, being an adult (or anything else—teacher, wizard, or shaman) does not guarantee that a person will have the kind of communicational skill Mr. Gilman has just exhibited. Happily enough, however, such skill can be learned and can be practiced until it becomes almost second nature. It does not really matter who you are, how old you are, or what your ethnic, religious, racial, or economic background is, you *can* come to understand and use to one degree or another the dynamics and skills of communicating effectively.

EXAMPLE 7

Situation

Alex and Sam are good friends; both are medical students. They bump into each other in the student union.

Alec: Hi, Sam! How ya doing?

Sam (Looks miserable and angry.): Lousy. I just got my anatomy midterm back. (Makes the thumbs down sign). Got a *D*.

Alec: Uh-oh. (Sympathetically.) That's rough. How do you feel about it?

Sam: That prof has it in for me. Do you know how the curve went?

Alec: No. How?

Sam: 65 was the lowest *C*. And I got a 64.

Alec: How do you feel about it?

Sam: Yeah—and get this! That idiot, Jack Barnes, got a 65!

Alec: But how do *you* feel about it?

Sam: What am I going to tell my parents when grades come out?

Alec: Sam—listen to me! I'm asking you how you feel about the grade.

Sam: Well, at least I've got a *C* in lab so far.

Analysis and explanation

It could be argued that Sam is telling Alec in his own way how he feels about the *D* on the midterm. However, that is not exactly the point. This is hardly an example of good, clear communication. Rather it is an example of what is aptly called "sliding off." Every time Alec directly asks Sam what he feels, Sam slides right off the subject and thereby avoids answering Alec's questions. The way Sam slides off is to project (blame the professor) and to drag in various "red herring" worries and annoyances (Jack Barnes and his parents). There can be no doubt that plenty of strong feelings are sitting beneath the surface of these various topics; the problem is that as long as Sam operates as he does, he does not feel or deal with his emotions in any direct or constructive way.

All of this raises certain vital questions. If Sam wants to "slide off," does he not have the right to do so? Yes. Sam and *only* Sam is ultimately responsible for what he does or does not do. He and he alone has the right to choose how he will act. But what if Sam does not realize that he slides off; what if it is an automatic pattern? Where does the responsibility lie then? To say the least, that is a tricky, if not impossible, question to answer. (We are not trying to slide off the answer ourselves at this point, but we do want to make it clear that we believe there is no pat answer to this question.) If we go back to the situation and the dialogue between Alec and Sam, the question of responsibility in this particular case would seem to rest with Alec. That is, Alec is aware of Sam's sliding off; thus Alec is the only person at the moment who is in a position to point out this automatic pattern to Sam. However, Alec is not responsible for Sam or the way he lives his life. Alec may feel that as a friend it is his responsibility to point out the pattern, but how sharply or insistently he points it out or how strongly he pushes Sam to deal with the pattern is a choice Alec must make. One reminder, however: even if Alec were to really "lean on" Sam, it would be difficult if not impossible for Alec to break down Sam's defenses if Sam does not want to let Alec in.

A greater risk occurs if Sam does let Alec in, and they find that Sam's feelings are so supercharged or so complex that neither of them feels (or is) qualified to handle those feelings. This may be the time for Sam to seek a professional, since Alec is not a psychotherapist.

Suggestions

If we pick the dialogue up at the point at which we left off, Alec is the only person who can make a significant decision. What decision he makes depends on many different factors. For example, is Sam's set of responses a pattern Alec has seen again and again? Does he see Sam as a fairly stable person? Does he see Sam as a person who might want to learn about an automatic pattern? Does Alec want to get involved in this way? Does Alec have the courage to take the initiative and point out what may be unpleasant to Sam? These are just some considerations that are related to Alec's decision-making.

All these considerations perhaps made Alec's decision and implementation sound impossibly risky, but there are ways to minimize those risks. These ways are the techniques of good communication. If Alec decides to go ahead and try to help Sam become aware of his feelings and help him to start feeling and working with them, then Alec needs to proceed slowly and carefully. He needs to report his own hesitations and feelings (his insides) to Sam, and he needs to check out and get feedback at every step of the way. He needs to share with Sam his own evaluation of what is occurring in the communication as it is occurring. That way Alec minimizes the risks and maximizes the possibilities of communicating meaningfully and helping Sam to begin to grow. Another choice Alec has is merely to point out to Sam that he is sliding off and to explain what sliding off consists of. Then they may just drop the whole matter. But at least Alec will have pointed out the automatic pattern to Sam; Sam is free to do whatever he chooses from then on.

EXAMPLE 8

Situation

The mother, Myra, comes stomping down the stairs and into the kitchen where her 12-year-old son, Kelly, is sitting, staring out the window. She has just come from his room upstairs.

Mother (Stops when she sees Kelly sitting at the table. Her facial muscles are tense; she looks harassed and disgusted.): Oh. There you are! I want you to go upstairs this very minute and clean up your room. It looks like a pigpen. Do you hear me? (Her voice rises.)

Kelly (Sullenly.): Yes, Mother. I hear you. (Does not move.)

Mother: Well, then, get going. (Her voice is like a whiplash. Kelly slowly begins to get up from the chair. Myra watches him, glaring all the while.) Why don't you ever hang up your clothes or put your dirty clothes in the hamper?

Kelly: But I do. I just forgot to these last couple of days.

Mother: That's what you always say. You don't seem to care how I feel or appreciate how much I do for you.

Kelly (A despairing note in his voice.): I *do* care, Mother. But why do you always have to pick on me?

Mother (Glares at him.): Don't be so disrespectful toward your mother! (Pauses, takes a deep breath, and then sighs.) There you go again—you don't have the slightest idea of how much I do for you.

Analysis and explanation

And so on—and on and on. To say the least, Kelly and his mother are not communicating in any meaningful or constructive way. However, they are communicating or sending messages of despair, pain, anger, weariness, and futility. The blockage of clear and constructive communication results from their making assumptions about each other, from not checking out anything, from making accusations, and from not talking about the feelings boiling underneath the surface. What these two people are doing is communicating their age-old, patterned feelings—feelings that are so automatic, so repetitive, and so stereotyped that neither of them really is able to feel the feelings. But the feelings are there, corroding the relationship so that eventually all that is left is a bitter taste.

Suggestions

If Kelly were older, we would suggest that he is the one who might break into this automatic patterning of the relationship. If Myra, the mother, were more aware of Kelly's and her own feelings, she would be the logical one to break in. However, assuming that neither one of these two people is likely to break into their patterns, we suggest that some outside force—an event or another person—would be necessary to interrupt this relationship's destructive patterning. It is possible that a crisis, such as Kelly's suddenly falling seriously ill, might shake matters up enough so that Myra could get a different perspective. Perhaps her husband, another sibling, a neighbor, or a clergyman might intervene. We are suggesting that probably the situation between Kelly and his mother will not change unless something outside of each of them influences at least one of them in some significant way.

EXAMPLE 9

Situation

Mr. Engle is sitting in the living room after supper. His 14-year-old daughter, Pam, comes in to talk to him.

Pam (Pouting slightly, but her tone of voice is fairly even, not unpleasant or whiny.): Dad. (He looks up at her and appears to be interested and willing to listen.) Can I talk to you about something?

Mr. Engle: Sure, honey. Have a chair and let's talk.

Pam (Slightly hesitant but looks determined.): Dad, why can't I stay out later than midnight on Friday nights? All the other kids' parents let them stay out as late as they want.

Mr. Engle [Surprised at the subject—which they have discussed before. He thought the issue had long ago been settled.] (Slightly annoyed.): Because I say so—that's why. I just don't think it's good for you to stay out later than that. [I'm afraid for you. You're so young and vulnerable.]

Pam [Angry and frustrated.]: That's all you ever say. You don't seem to care anything about what *I* want or what *I* feel. All you care about is how things look!

Mr. Engle (Frustrated and annoyed): That's not true. But I know what's best for you. [You don't know how much I *do* care. But I don't know how to tell you.]

Analysis and explanation

These two people are following rather set patterns of talking with each other. Pam asks a question and then applies social pressure. Her father answers first from a totally authoritarian point of view, then adds a reason that is so vague as to be almost meaningless—"I don't think it's good for you." Pam then accuses him of not caring; she is assuming that he does not. He denies this and then reverts to his vague but authoritarian position. They both make assumptions; they fail to negotiate.

Suggestions

From what is going on in Mr. Engle's "insides," we may gather that he is capable of stepping out from behind his authoritarian mask of defense. All he seems to need is a slight push and a little knowledge about effective ways to communicate. Or he may just decide that now is the time for him to say what he really feels to his daughter. Maybe he is tired of playing and being cast in the role of the local tyrant, or maybe he suddenly looks at the situation from Pam's viewpoint for a moment and gets a fleeting notion of the discomfort and annoyance of her position. Whatever the impetus, suppose he decides to try to communicate.

Mr. Engle (Consciously speaks in a calmer tone of voice.): Pam, I'm sorry. I guess I really haven't listened very carefully to what you're trying to say to me. A lot of my own feelings and worries get tangled up in all this and they tend to make it hard for me to really listen. Can we try it again—but differently?

Pam [Puzzled but interested.]: Sure, Dad. But I don't exactly know what you mean.

Mr. Engle: Well, let's go back a little. You said I don't care about what you want or what you feel. I do care, but let's leave that for the moment. Could you—and will you—try to tell me what you do want and what you do feel?

Pam [Overwhelmed. Doesn't seem to know where to even begin answering—or how.]: I-I. I don't know what to say.

Mr. Engle: Let me see if I can help. What do you want? Do you want to be completely free of any time limits? Do you want later time limits? Do you want the exact same freedom that all the other kids get?

Pam (Sullenly.): Would it make any difference? I mean—what if I said I wanted complete freedom? Would you give it to me?

Mr. Engle: I honestly don't know at this point. But what I feel is that neither of us can possibly negotiate about all this till we each know what the other wants and feels. Is that fair enough?

Pam: Yes, it is. Well, let me think for a moment . . . .

That is one way the communication could get rolling. Another would be if Pam were to interrupt their usual ways of talking.

Pam (Softens her voice.): Dad, you say you

know what's best for me. I don't want to argue about that. I really don't. But could I ask you to conduct an experiment with me?

Mr. Engle [Intrigued by this sudden change in the usual ways of their arguments.]: Sure. Go ahead.

Pam: Suppose you pretend you don't know me. We've never met before. We're total strangers, and we meet during the local festival. I tell you about my wicked father who lives in a castle on top of the mountain. My wicked father won't let me do what I want to do, which is simply what everyone else in the kingdom is doing these days. Now suppose I ask you to play the role of my wicked father—your job is to tell me (the daughter) I can't do what I want, but you also have to say what you really feel. That is, why you wont' let me do those things.

A little far out? Maybe. But humor in the right places can do wonders. If we get technical, Pam is asking her father to role play himself but to interact and communicate with her in two ways—giving both his outsides and insides. This can be a productive way of getting at what each of them feels. If they do this, they have a real chance to negotiate in a constructive manner. And they might have some fun along the way.

EXAMPLE 10

Situation

Ginnie (23 years old) and Walt (25 years old) meet at a discotheque in San Francisco. Both of them are of average attractiveness.

Walt: Hi! My name's Walt. What's yours?

Ginnie: Ginnie. How are you?

Walt: Fine. Where're you from?

Ginnie: Wisconsin. How about you?

Walt: The City. How do you like living here?

Ginnie: Not much. How about you?

Walt: Oh, fine. Say—what do you do?

Ginnie: I'm a research assistant with ____________ Magazine.

Walt: That sounds interesting. Do you like it?

Ginnie: It's okay. What do you do?

Walt: I work for an advertising firm.

They have gotten through all the preliminaries and are starting to discuss a movie.

Walt: Have you seen "________________"?

Ginnie: Yes. I just saw it last week. (She laughs.) I finally caught up with it after all this time.

Walt: Did you like it?

Ginnie: Yes. Very much. Did You?

Walt: Yes. I thought the photography was great.

Ginnie: I thought it was an awfully good character study.

Analysis and explanation

This conversation is dull. Yet it is typical of the conversations that people so frequently engage in, especially when they first meet but also at any time during relationships that stay on a basically superficial level. What these two people are doing is mostly trading information. Even the tone of the trading is flat and lifeless. Information is fine, and some information may be necessary, especially on first meeting someone. But too often people tend to stay on this level because it is safe. It may be safe, but it sure is dull. The basic reason it is so dull and flat is that there is little feeling tone; neither of these people has conveyed or talked or asked about feelings.

Suggestions

Life would be much more interesting if these two people traded some feelings along with the information. They have had various opportunities to branch off into feeling questions—opportunities they did not take advantage of in the conversation. For example, what does Ginnie dislike about living in San Francisco? Is she lonely? Does she feel closed in? Does she miss the smells, sights, and sounds of Wisconsin? Has she found it easy to meet people? How does she react to the accents she hears around her?

As for Walt, what kind of work does he do? Does he enjoy doing it? What part of his work interests him the most? What about it interests him? Does he feel frustrated, satisfied, happy, or disappointed in his job? Has he ever lived outside of San Francisco? Would he ever want to live outside it? If he did, where would he choose to go? What would make him choose that particular place?

Although some of these questions may seem personal, it is possible to preface what you say to another person with the statement that you have no desire to pry but that you *are* interested in who he is and what he is like. It is also possible and desirable to check out with the other person whether he feels you are being too personal. But certainly it would seem worth the risk of appearing a bit personal in your approach as opposed to appearing as though you could not care less about who and what the other person is and what his feelings are.

These ten examples present a wide range of communicational and interactional experiences. Hopefully they will sensitize you to the more common forms of distortion and help you to make your own communication (and therefore your interaction) clearer, more effective, and more open. These goals are worth working toward; distorted communication helps solidify closedness, whereas effective communication is the necessary instrument for using The System so that you can change and grow.

GLOSSARY

acquiring insight Achieving personal understanding, which results from putting together in conceptual form one's thoughts, feelings, and actions; gaining a grasp of what is going on and what certain experiences mean —an "a-ha!" experience.

acting (behavior) A person's acting function, which is always in operation acting on his information, his feelings, and his own and others' responses.

Adult The part of a person that negotiates between his Child and Parent parts so that neither of them automatically dominates; the guiding force that helps a person think, feel, and act as a whole, mature, autonomous individual.

alternating relationship An essentially complementary relationship between two people in which they alternate between the two dominant life-styles of the relationship.

ambivalence Emotional state that occurs when two contrasting feelings exert comparatively equal power.

anxiety Generalized, unfocused feelings of uneasiness, apprehension, and discomfort.

audible body language Any signals a person sends by making (or by refraining from making) nonverbal sounds.

autonomy Health, maturity, and responsible functioning resulting from an appropriately balanced blend of thinking, feeling, and acting.

backing off The conscious and deliberate process of pulling back from that which is new and unknown and temporarily returning to that which is familiar.

backsliding The unconscious process of pulling back from that which is new and unknown and temporarily returning to that which is familiar.

building in Through repetition and practice, incorporating what one learns into one's self-system and/or life-style.

checking out A basic communicational method of making sure information and perceptions are clear and undistorted, carried out by asking and answering questions and giving and receiving feedback.

Child The part of a person that thinks, feels, and acts in ways similar to the ways he did as a child.

Child/Parent/Adult balance The proportional relationship among the three parts of a person; the balance among these parts.

closed family style Disharmonious jamming together of family members' personal life-styles that conflict or a harmonious but nonconstructive blend of neurotic styles, which results in an unhealthy or dysfunctional dynamic equilibrium.

closed marital relationship A marital relationship based on demands for conformity, little freedom, a lack of awareness and in-touchedness, and ineffective, often destructive communication and interaction.

closed marital style A marital style characterized either by a disharmonious jamming together of two individual life-styles that conflict or by a harmonious but nonconstructive blending of neurotic styles. Either kind results in an unhealthy or dysfunctional dynamic equilibrium.

closed person A person who has little self-awareness and awareness of others and who is governed largely by unconscious, automatic, and repetitious inside and outside forces.

closed society A society based on a structured, authoritarian, patriarchal system; one that maintains its stability and the stability of its members by means of a restrictive system of accepted beliefs, expectations, rules, and values.

cohesive relationship A functional or dysfunctional relationship of the kind and quality that tends to draw two or more people together, i.e., to attract them to one another.

communication A specific and specialized form of interaction involving the conscious and unconscious process of giving and receiving verbal and nonverbal signals, messages, and responses. This process encompasses both objective and subjective content drawn from the three aspects of human functioning—the intellectual, emotional, and behavioral.

complementary relationship A relationship between two people in which each person's life-style fills in or supplies much of what is lacking or seems to be lacking in the other's life-style.

composite PFL A dominant PFL that synthesizes the directions given by all the interrelated individual PFLs in a packet into a powerful basic prescription about how the person should think, feel, and act.

compromise A form of decision-making in which one of the parts of a person (e.g., Child) or one of the people in a relationship yields and agrees even though he may not be satisfied with the decision.

conflicting PFLs PFLs that belong to the same packet because they deal with the same subject matter but that clash with one another.

dating Any nonmarital, two-person relationship (dating, going steady, being engaged or living together).

dating games People's predetermined, automatic, repetitious sets of actions and reactions in a dating situation that help the partners achieve certain psychological ends: the establishment of intrapersonal and interpersonal dynamic equilibrium.

decision-making Making a choice from at least two alternatives after prior negotiations (whether conscious or unconscious).

developing alternatives Making a conscious, deliberate attempt to discover, identify, and evaluate all the possible alternatives in a given situation.

difference A way of thinking, feeling, or acting that is not exactly the same as a person's usual way of thinking, feeling, or acting.

differences Those qualities of each person that make him unlike another person.

directive A precept that sets up restrictions which try to cover every occurrence of a situation and which implies that those restrictions should always apply.

divisive relationship A dysfunctional relationship of the kind and quality that tends to drive people apart.

double-bind A situation in which there seem to be only two diametrically opposed alternatives, each of which has great emotional force.

dynamics The relationship between activity and the forces that cause and influence that activity.

dynamics of family interaction The forces (e.g., each member's self-system) that create and constitute the activity (interaction) between or among two or more family members and the interplay among these forces.

dynamics of human interaction The forces that create and constitute the activity (interaction) between or among two or more entities and the interplay among these forces. These forces consist of communications, thoughts, feelings, actions, and reactions, which are determined by each person's self-system and life-style.

dynamics of marital interaction The forces (e.g., each partner's self-system) that create and constitute the activity (interaction) between marital partners and the interplay among these forces.

dynamics of relationships The forces that create and constitute the activity (interaction) between or among people in a relationship and the interplay among these forces.

dysfunctional life-style The style of a person whose functioning is limited, impaired, or both, thus making his life-style less qualitative, less healthy, and less constructive than it might be.

dysfunctional relationship A relationship in which the dynamic equilibrium is based on minimal effective communication and on little information about or awareness of the other's thoughts and feelings. The results of this limited and/or impaired functioning are often a tenuous, conflictual, neurotic, or destructive dynamic equilibrium.

expectation PFLs PFLs commonly communicated through the word "expect." They are also frequently expressed as "should" or "ought to."

extended family Any grouping related by descent, marriage, or adoption (i.e., grandparents, aunts, uncles, cousins) that is broader than the nuclear family.

family Any group that operates in ways designed to foster group unity (e.g., members live together or near one another and have some commitment to one another) and that fulfills some or all of the functions designed to promote and protect the well-being of the group and its members (e.g., care, nurturing, socializing).

family Child/Parent/Adult balance The overall balance created by the interlock among family members' individual Child/Parent/Adult balances.

family concept The way each person in a family perceives and feels about the family relationship based on each member's self-concept and on the way he perceives and interprets the other members' thoughts, feelings, and actions.

family core characteristics Characteristics that are intrinsic to the nature of family relationships: intellectual heritage, biophysiological heritage, religion, race, ethnic background, number of parents' marriages, age of present marriage, family members' ages, number of children, and children's sex and sibling rank. These are always present and exert continuing and significant influences on each other, on the ways members interact with one another, and on the development of members' relationships.

family dynamic equilibrium The interpersonal balance that the family members establish between or among them, which is based on how each one's self-system and life-style fit with the others'.

family games Series of preprogrammed reactions and interactions between or among family members that help them achieve intrapersonal and interpersonal dynamic equilibrium in and in relation to the family. These games result from the harmonious or disharmonious interlock between or among members' self-systems and life-styles.

family identity What the family relationship is at present, how it became the way it is now, and what it may become in the future.

family identity crisis Occurs when family members' usual ways of maintaining their dysfunctional dynamic equilibrium are challenged or shaken up. The results are a forced partial awareness of the dysfunction and a tendency to reevaluate the family relationship.

family insides The private, inner thoughts and feelings each member has about himself, the other members, and the family relationship and each member's intrapersonal patterns.

family interaction The verbal and nonverbal activity (action) that transpires between or among two or more family members.

family intrapersonal patterns A person's consistent, private, inner ways he thinks, feels, and acts within the family.

family life cycle The various stages that family members experience during the development and life of the family unit, including infancy, youth, adolescence, young adulthood, maturity, and old age.

family outsides Each member's conscious and unconscious external expressions and manifestations of his insides; each member's interpersonal patterns and the interlock between or among them.

family PFLs Internalized expectations, rules, and values that each member has about himself as a family member, about other family members, and about the family relationship.

family roles The roles most basic to the family relationship and interaction, which are parent (mother, father) and child (daughter, son).

family style The basic interlock among the members' life-styles. This interlock forms a larger observable network of interpersonal patterns, which determine how each member will function in regard to the others and to their relationship. It is the dynamic equilibrium established by the meshing of the members' life-styles.

family system The internal functioning of each member plus the ways each one's insides affect each other member's and the whole family's internal functioning.

fingertip material An individual's ideas, feelings, and actions that are just beneath the surface of consciousness or that he knows about but cannot quite get at or has not yet implemented.

functional Marked by functioning (thinking, feeling, and acting) based on in-touchedness with insides and outsides; functioning that is essentially qualitative, healthy, and constructive.

functional life-style The style of a person whose functioning (thinking, feeling, and acting) is basically qualitative, healthy, and constructive.

functional relationship A relationship in which the dynamic equilibrium is based on clear, undistorted communication and on patterns of interaction that are not automatic or repetitious but are under each person's conscious control. The results of this functioning are a qualitative, healthy, and constructive dynamic equilibrium.

gathering information Collecting data that is relevant to whatever is being considered.

getting in touch with Becoming aware of, identifying, evaluating, understanding, and appreciating one's inner thoughts, feelings, experiences, and self-system.

giving and receiving responses The reciprocal communication and responses between a person and his inner and outer environment.

guideline Proposal about living that suggests various possibilities and alternatives, allows for exceptions, and leaves the choices and decisions about appropriateness of the alternatives up to the person who subscribes to the guideline.

holistic orientation A perspective in which the focus is on both the individual and his interrelatedness with others, especially in marriage and family life, and with his society.

human interaction Activity (or action) between or among two or more entities (entities may be parts of one person or two or more people). This activity includes everything that transpires between or among two or more entities, i.e., all verbal and nonverbal communication as well as all conscious and unconscious thoughts, feelings, actions, and reactions.

humanistic approach An approach that focuses primarily on the individual: how he functions, how he affects relationships and groups he belongs to, and how these relationships and groups affect him.

identifying feelings The process by which a person is able to identify and get in touch with both strong and subtle emotions and with multiple feeling positions on an ongoing, moment-to-moment basis.

identity Who a person is in the here and now, how he got to be who he is now, and who he may become in the future.

ideology The ideas, attitudes, views, theories, expectations, rules, values, and feelings or sets of these that shape, direct, energize, or govern the ways a society, a group, or an individual conceives of self, feels about self, and acts.

implementation Acting on a decision (no matter how large or how small), i.e., putting the decision into effect.

individual core characteristics An individual's natural endowments that comprise his essential makeup: sex, race, intellectual heritage, biophysiological heritage, and age.

inductive method The process of acquiring pieces of information and details, categorizing them, and eventually drawing certain general conclusions from and about them.

insides Intrapersonal phenomena, i.e., a person's inner world of both conscious and unconscious thoughts, feelings, and experiences (his self-system).

insight The personal understanding resulting from being able to put thoughts and feelings and the meaning of actions together in conceptual form.

intellect (thinking) A person's thinking function, which is continually used to analyze, synthesize, imagine, project, and evaluate anything and everything.

interactional therapeutic system (ITS) A conceptualized, systematized, practical approach to teaching and learning how to change and grow, how to become more open and autonomous, and how to develop and maintain qualitative relationships with self, others, and society; often referred to as *The System* in the text.

interpersonal communication A process in which two or more people are simultaneously engaged in intrapersonal communication, the fruits of which they share with one another; that is, each person is giving and receiving verbal and nonverbal signals, messages, and responses to and from the other person.

interpersonal dynamic equilibrium The balance in a relationship that results from each person's maintaining his own intrapersonal dynamic equilibrium while at the same time taking into account, making allowances for, and adjusting and accommodating to the other person.

interpersonal negotiation When two (or more) people work together to discover what each of them thinks and feels and what they might do in relation to whatever they are considering at the moment.

interpersonal patterns Consistent, public (outside) ways a person thinks, feels, and acts with and toward others.

intrapersonal communication The conscious and/or unconscious process of giving and receiving verbal and nonverbal signals, messages, and responses within self.

intrapersonal dynamic equilibrium A vital balance by which a person keeps his sense of self and stability intact while at the same time allowing for and adjusting to newness, to difference, to change, and to the unfamiliar.

intrapersonal marital patterns A marital partner's consistent, private, inner ways he thinks, feels, and acts within the marriage and toward the marriage.

intrapersonal negotiation A process within oneself to figure out what one thinks and feels and what one might do in relation to whatever is under consideration at the moment.

intrapersonal patterns Consistent, private (inside) ways a person thinks, feels, and acts within and toward himself.

life-style The observable network of consistent interpersonal patterns that determine the ways a person functions (thinks, feels, and acts) in the interpersonal sphere.

living the process (The System) Building in such familiarity and expertise in using The System that using it becomes second nature.

long-term growth toward openness and autonomy The cumulative effects of the small growth gains that occur from moment-to-moment experiences with difference, newness, and change.

marital Child/Parent/Adult balance The balance created by the interlock between the two partners' individual Child/Parent/Adult balances.

major components of human interaction Motivation for growth, expectations, roles, patterns of communication, patterns of interaction, and decision-making processes; useful categories for evaluating self and others.

major mini-matters All the little details of everyday living that are repeated day in and day out.

marital concept The way each partner sees (perceives) and feels about the marital relationship.

marital core characteristics Characteristics that are intrinsic to the nature of the marital relationship: intellectual balance, religion, race, ethnic background, socioeconomic class, partner's ages, the number of marriages, and the number of children. These characteristics are always present, exert continuing and significant influences on each other, on the partners' interaction, and on the development of their relationship.

marital dynamic equilibrium The interpersonal balance that marital partners establish between them, based on how each one's self-system and life-style fit with the other's.

marital games Series of preprogrammed reactions and interactions between marital partners that help them achieve intrapersonal and interpersonal dynamic equilibrium in and in relation to their marriage. These games result from the harmonious or disharmonious interlock between the partners' self-systems and life-styles.

marital identity Who the partners are (as a marital couple) and what their relationship is like now, how their relationship became the way it is now, and what their relationship may become in the future.

marital identity crisis Occurs when a marital couple's usual ways of maintaining their dysfunctional dynamic equilibrium are challenged or shaken up. The results are a forced partial awareness of the dysfunction and a tendency to reevaluate the marital relationship.

marital insides The inner thoughts and feelings each partner has about himself, the other partner, and the marital relationship and the intrapersonal patterns of each partner.

marital interaction The verbal and nonverbal activity (action) that transpires between marital partners.

marital outsides Each marital partner's conscious and unconscious external expressions and manifestations of his insides; his interpersonal patterns and the interlock between them.

marital PFLs Internalized expectations, rules, and values about marriage that each partner has and brings with him that direct how he should think, feel, and act in and in relation to the marriage.

marital style The balanced interlock between the partners' life-styles. This interlock forms a larger observable network of interpersonal patterns that determine how each partner will function in regard to the other partner and to their relationship.

marital system The internal functioning of each partner plus the ways each one's insides affect the other's and the marriage's internal functioning.

marriage The one long-term or permanent heterosexual couple relationship sanctioned by religion and society. In this book it is also used to refer to all relatively long-term, two-person relationships.

metamessages Meanings resulting from the combination of signals (nonverbal messages) and verbal messages; they either reinforce, expand on, or undermine the meaning of the verbal message.

mixed relationship A relationship that is a combination of complementarity and supplementarity: each person's style has some aspects that complement and some that supplement aspects of the other person's style.

moment-to-moment influencing factors (MIFs) Phenomena that are potentially present in all moments of living and that influence a person's thoughts, feelings, and actions at a given moment. They include motivation, psychological desires, goals, intent, mood, social situation, opportunity, time available, societal pressures, and significant others.

negotiation A process whereby an individual or individuals try to assemble, identify, and examine all the thoughts, feelings and actions that are relevant to whatever is under consideration. It has four purposes: (1) to better understand the options; (2) to evaluate appropriateness and workability of thoughts, feelings, and actions; (3) to develop and evaluate alternatives; and (4) to jointly decide what decisions to make.

newness A big or noticeable difference.

nonverbal communication The process of sending and receiving signals and messages by means of the body but not the voice.

nuclear family Commonly consists of two married adults who are parents to one or more children (whether created by the spouses or adopted), all of whom ordinarily live together as an interrelated group. A one-parent family may also be a nuclear family.

open family style An essentially harmonious meshing of personal life-styles, which results in a healthy and functional dynamic equilibrium.

open marital relationship A marital relationship based on respect for individuality, responsible use of freedom, intrapersonal and interpersonal awareness and in-touchedness, and effective, constructive communication and interaction.

open marital style A marital style characterized by the harmonious meshing of the partners' personal life-styles, which results in a healthy and functional dynamic equilibrium.

open person A person who is available to new experiences, willing to take appropriate risks, accepting of individuality, flexible, freedom granting, and free from the restrictions of a rigid, automatic and repetitious life-style.

open society A society that is based on a non-authoritarian system and that is flexible and tolerant enough to allow for the existence and encouragement of alternative ways of thinking, feeling, and acting. An open society maintains its stability and the stability of its members by means of guidelines rather than strict rules and by means of negotiation rather than authoritarian pressure.

openness Being aware of and honest with self and others; being willing to experience difference and newness and to try to use these experiences to change and grow.

outsides Interpersonal phenomena, i.e., a person's conscious and unconscious external expressions and manifestations of his insides.

packets of PFLs A number of individual PFLs that naturally group themselves together because they are closely related to one another according to one or more of the following: specific subject matter, attitudes, emotions, or behavior.

Parent The part of a person that thinks, feels, and acts in ways he has learned from one or both of his parents and from other significant persons; the part of a person that responds as he believes his parent figure(s) would respond in similar or similar-seeming circumstances.

parental dynamic equilibrium The interpersonal balance between parents, which is based on both the match between the marital partners' individual self-systems and life-styles and on their marital system and style.

parental identity Who the parents are *now* and what the relationship is like *now,* how the relationship got to be the way it is now, and what the relationship might *become.*

parental insides Each parent's private, inner thoughts and feelings about self, the other parent, and the parental relationship and his intrapersonal patterns.

parental outsides Each parent's interpersonal patterns of thinking, feeling, and acting in regard to the parental relationship.

parental style The observable network of consistent interpersonal patterns that are underpinned by the parental system and that determine how each parent will function in regard to the other parent, to their relationship, and to the children.

parental system Each person's parental insides plus the interlock between those insides; the internal functioning of each parent plus the ways each one's insides affect the other parent's and the relationship's functioning.

parenting The process of a parent's (or other adult's) caring for, protecting, socializing, and giving physical and emotional nurturance to a child.

pattern discovering Identifying a pattern.

pattern watching Searching for and attempting to discover consistent ways of thinking, feeling, and acting.

patterns The consistent ways a person thinks, feels, and acts.

personal and interpersonal competence Having the ability, the psychological equipment, and the know-how to get in touch with and work constructively with your insides and outsides so that you can modify or alter rigid and limiting influences on you.

personality The dynamic interaction between and among a person's biophysical and psychological components, the results of which inform and control both his characteristic and his unique thoughts, feelings, and actions.

personality traits Static descriptions of a person's interpersonal patterns.

physical appearance A specialized category of body language referring to what a person looks like and what he does (or does not do) to his body to make it look a certain way.

power play A form of decision-making in which the stronger part of a person wins (e.g., Parent) or a stronger person wins and the decision is made according to the preferences of that stronger part or person.

prescriptions for living (PFLs) Both conscious and unconscious internalized expectations, rules, and values that provide the content, the shape, the impetus for, and the direction of the ways a person operates and manages himself.

psychological defenses Particular ways of thinking, feeling, and acting that a person (consciously, unconsciously, or both) employs to protect himself against anxiety. Every part of the self-system and life-style has the potential for being used defensively.

psychological games A person's specific but distorted application of intrapersonal and/or interpersonal patterns of communication and/or interaction that set up a series of preprogrammed (automatic, repetitious) reactions and interactions to achieve certain psychological ends.

psychological work Any and all efforts directed at becoming more aware, bringing thoughts and feelings to the conscious level, using one's skills and talents of communication and interaction, and using The System.

relationship The outcome of moment-to-moment ongoing interaction between at least two people (their self-systems and life-styles). This interaction involves achieving and maintaining some kind of intrapersonal and interpersonal dynamic equilibrium.

respectful settlement The most mature and healthy form of decision-making in which an outcome is reached by means of negotiation.

rule PFLs PFLs commonly communicated through "do" and "don't." They are also frequently expressed as "must/must not," "can/can't," and "have to."

selective processes Processes by which a person consciously or unconsciously chooses what stimuli he will and will not respond to.

self-concept The ways a person sees and thinks about himself (self-image) and the ways he feels about himself (self-esteem).

self-esteem The way a person feels about himself.

self-fulfilling prophecies Beliefs a person holds that he makes come true because he believes and feels them to be true.

self-image The way a person sees and thinks about himself.

self-system A person's insides, his internal functioning (thoughts, feelings, actions, and responses), and his intrapersonal dynamics. The self-system is comprised of PFLs, intrapersonal patterns, self-concept, and Child/Parent/Adult balance.

signal A brief, nonverbal communication message (conscious or unconscious) that is limited to a few comparatively simple and specific meanings, which are determined by their context.

significant person Any person in an individual's life who exerts a substantial influence on him.

silent body language Any signals a person sends by means of his body without using words or sounds.

similarities The common things that all human beings have thought about, felt, and done (or thought about doing).

situational triggers Those factors in a situation (e.g., another person's reaction, a comment) that set a person's pattern in motion.

social being A person who has at least some knowledge of and feeling for who he is as a person and for who he is in relation to other people and to society; a person who knows the PFLs and roles that his family and society prescribe and who is capable of trying to fulfill them.

societal PFLs Expectations, rules, and values formulated and enforced by society.

supplementary relationship A relationship in which two people have significantly similar life-styles, and therefore each person's life-style or parts of it adds to, completes, and enhances the other's life-style (or parts thereof).

teaching one's competence Either intentionally or unintentionally teaching others how to communicate and interact more effectively; includes teaching The System to others.

transference A strong feeling response to a person that is based on similar feeling responses to another already familar person.

uniqueness The particular manner in which a person combines and manages the ways he is similar to and different from other human beings.

value PFLs PFLs commonly communicated in the form of "good" and "bad," "worth something/worthless," "important/unimportant," and "right/wrong."

verbal messages Communications that employ spoken words to convey meanings. (In intrapersonal communication, the words may not be spoken aloud, but the person does conceptualize the meaning of the verbal message.)

whole family The combination of two, interlocking, mutually influencing parts: the family's insides and outsides.

whole marriage The combination of marital insides and outsides.

whole parental relationship The combination of parental insides and outsides.

whole self The two interlocking and mutually influencing parts that comprise the human being: his insides and outsides.

INDEX